WHAT PEOPLE ARE

Tours and Cures o.

There is much to be applauded in this book, from the courage it takes to follow your dream, to the bravery of standing up to those who seek to destroy it and to then speak about untruths that still exist in this world masquerading as fact. Take encouragement and guidance from this book and live your truth today!

Barbara Meiklejohn-Free, author of bestselling book *The Shaman Within* (Moon Books)

I have been very lucky to meet and work with Alexander who is a true healer. I highly recommend his book as it will inspire many people and help those in search of the loving truth of the deep spiritual wisdom that is always available to us when we work with our hearts wide open.

Gaetano Vivo, author of *Messages from the Angels of Transparency* (Axis Mundi Books)

I had many negative periods in my life: suffering in family life, difficulties at work, problems with friends too. But thanks to Sascha's (Alexander's) revelations and healing I have discovered how our views of life can change and with it suffering and conflict can be removed and even prevented.

Francesco Giovine, Assistant Professor at the Politecnico di Milano, Faculty of Architecture

Working in the mainstream healthcare sector and as a spiritual counselor I sensed a striking authenticity in the author's experiences and applaud his open stance. The world of alternative healing can offer miracles, but delivered by regular people, so human failings, insecurities and egos can get in the way. People will make mistakes, and this book helps to identify and expose the most common so that the reader

i

may focus more easily on the real gems.
Mathew Tyler, RDNS Australia, Spiritual Confidant and channel

It's all laid out for the reader to decide; nothing held back and nothing hidden, a unique perspective that just may set alight a few internal flames.
Susie Anthony, author of award-winning book *A Map to God* (O-Books)

Tours and Cures of a LightSoldier

Surviving the Path to Enlightenment

Tours and Cures
of a LightSoldier

Surviving the Path to Enlightenment

Alexander King

BOOKS

Winchester, UK
Washington, USA

First published by O-Books, 2015
O-Books is an imprint of John Hunt Publishing Ltd., Laurel House, Station Approach,
Alresford, Hants, SO24 9JH, UK
office1@jhpbooks.net
www.johnhuntpublishing.com

For distributor details and how to order please visit the 'Ordering' section on our website.

Text copyright: Alexander King 2014

ISBN: 978 1 78279 982 5
Library of Congress Control Number: 2014958366

A CIP catalogue record for this book is available from the British Library.

Design: Stuart Davies

Cover image: *Aegishjalmur Gold on Green Stone* by Brent Berry
Cover design: by Kate Osborne

Printed and bound in the USA by Edwards Brothers Malloy

We operate a distinctive and ethical publishing philosophy in all
areas of our business, from our global network of authors to
production and worldwide distribution.

CONTENTS

Dedications

To my wonderful Ultimate Good Healers, Helpers and Guides I offer many thanks for all the support, inspiration and wisdom. I ask and thank Ultimate Good for perfect protections for all readers of this book: perfect protections for them, their bodies and their lives. Ultimate Good, please help them to connect to the ultimate good wisdom both within and without. Give them the strength to discover potentially new truths and avoid getting confused/sucked in by any confusions I might have (unintentionally) included in this work. Amen.

Introduction

Why I Had To Tell This Story…

It has taken me years to begin to write this book, because I had to test and retest my beliefs/conclusions and their effects on my life, before committing them to paper. I am sincerely hoping that this book shall bring more clarity, and not add to the tangled mass of confusions out in the Mind-Body-Spirit (MBS) market, which often lacks open, critical thinking. People seem afraid to question esoteric or spiritual teachings, especially if they are claimed to have been channeled by Angel X, Spirit Guide Y or enlightened Alien Z; forgetting that these teachings have been channeled through human beings, and we are not infallible.

I don't doubt the ultimate goodness of the Divine, but I am cautious about people's perception, understanding and teachings of all things divine. That is why I have my mind to filter out the true, good and wise intuitions, from all the other input I receive when opening up. I urge you too to keep your head screwed on, feet planted firmly on solid ground, while perusing my thoughts, explanations and beliefs. Feel free to question and test them as often as you like. I have seen and felt too much suffering coming out of what first seemed liberating esoteric or religious ideas to be offended by any caution on your part.

I write about my experiences, my thoughts and ideas, which have shaped my beliefs and understandings. I am aware it's not a 'movie star's' life, still I believe it has interesting and entertaining elements, that might just help you to understand how I have come to see the world and what life on this planet is about. The examples I use in this book are just that, examples. In the past, maybe because of my German heritage, I would take many things very literally, which sometimes led to unnecessary fears or feelings of guilt. So please read my examples with a pinch of salt and consider that 'exceptions make the rule' i.e. examples that may be suitable for some might not be all applicable for another. The same applies when trying to find a balance between connecting to you the reader and not sucking you in, but leaving you room to make up your own mind, whether you choose to agree with my conclusions or have your own – if I do say 'we' and you do not feel comfortable seeing yourself as a part of that 'we', please feel free to assert your own belief.

Whereas many prominent esoteric authors, healers and lecturers lay claim on having been born with the gift, having had some life-changing spiritual experience, such as a visitation by an angel or perhaps having 'hooked up' with some spiritual being during an automatic writing session, I am one of the many more who just happened to start reading about 'Lightwork', 'Spiritual Healing' etc. and decided to learn and understand more about it.

On my path I have encountered countless, seemingly bottomless abysses of guilt and doubt. Were it not for my innate stubbornness and a good deal of help from 'Above', I might have given up on Spirit or Life altogether, long ago. The main reason for this book is to hopefully spare you a few of those mind traps and feelings of paranoia that can be so debilitating. And if you have come to the same conclusions as I already, then perhaps you will get comfort from discovering you are not alone.

I am aware that, from say a psychiatrist's view, some of my experiences could possibly be diagnosed as bipolar, paranoid and/or schizophrenic – but then one just ends up with the same old debate of whether there are divine powers/spirit(s) (which one can communicate with) or if we live in a purely materialistic world. I am not a radical creationist. I do see the merit and worthiness of science. However, if we look at scientific history, we will often find many a scientific accomplishment would never have been possible without scientific visionaries, who pursued their ideas against all odds. If something cannot be measured yet, that does not disprove its existence; it just points out that the proper measuring tools are yet to be discovered.

I hope that this book will help you get some fresh perspectives or give you healing tools you might not have considered yet. For me the spoils of wandering the spiritual path are diminished fears, serenity, having fewer questions and knowing who, what and why I am. I'm much less likely to be shaken up, by what seem unfortunate events now, because there is a certainty, rooted deep inside me, that all is going to be good. My spiritual path has also taught me greater patience and to manage my expectations. 'Ultimate Good' is working full speed on the fulfillment of my harmonious dreams, and they are allowed to be 'big', but for all sorts of reasons they can still take time to manifest. It's not that miracles don't happen, just that they can take a lot longer to manifest than one is often led to believe when reading other esoteric books.

The spiritual tour can be stressful and sometimes perilous. My own journey definitely got worse before things started to come together and improve. Initially I ended up in a cult and afterwards for almost ten years I suffered from ME, so my experiences with spiritual tools and techniques could be said to have gone through some good stress tests, which have helped me to sort the wheat from the chaff. I often feel that I am in the midst of a battle between 'Lighter' and 'Darker' energies. I feel though that with Ultimate Good support I am as safe as can be during these battles, but that does not mean that they are always pain free. This book may well shake up your belief systems and rattle your peace of mind. If you bear with me, I hope you will find peace in my conclusions. To those who might get upset about my writings and criticisms – I am sorry. I pray you'll come to forgive me, as I have forgiven all those who have caused me upset and pain with some of their spiritual wisdoms, beliefs and ideas, which I found to be wrong or incomplete.

I am a great optimist and think all suffering can be overcome with the right approach, help and patience. Spirituality, spiritual healing tools are complementary forms of healing though. So if you are ill in any shape or form, this book does not suggest you flush away all your medicines and shout, "I'm healed!" never to set foot in a doctor's practice again. If you believe you have been healed, get it verified by a doctor. I studied medicine and saw the compassion in my fellow students and our teachers. Furthermore I spent a year in a medical research facility and saw the love and unpaid overtime that went into research by doctors and scientists there too. There are ongoing developments for medical treatments to become less invasive, more effective and with diminished potential side effects etc. I do not think that generally doctors are out there to poison their patients.

Where medical treatment of one's physical body should be one's own decision (where possible), I would never recommend ditching your doctor. Sure, educate yourself about your ailments, different treatment options, do not just trust blindly, get a second opinion etc. In my opinion it's likely though that medical treatment, if one is sick, will often buy time, give more strength or diminish some pain and hence enable you to resolve other issues causing the dis-ease, which might have to be approached with complementary means.

I see that the true purpose of our being is simpler and far more positive than many religions/belief systems purport. It is perfectly alright to strive for happiness in life. That includes striving for, affirming and living creational essences, such as intelligence, creativity, beauty, abundance and sex. Our bodies were primarily created for us to enjoy and to experience the world around us on physical, emotional and sensory levels. On this planet we can choose to take our bodies on a roller coaster of suffering, but once we decide that we have had enough, we are allowed to fully utilize their potential for joy. My moral compass points to the notion that what I do not want others to do to me, I do not do to them. And this book is my tour of discovery, which I hope in some way will make your journey less fearful and ultimately more joyful as well…

Book One

Battlefields & Tours

Chapter 1

Conscription

My early years weren't extraordinary, but I mention them simply because some believe they are critical in forming the emerging adult. However, I believe that any part of our life is just 'a part' of the whole experience. If a part is testing, it is best to learn potential lessons, forgive and move on.

I was made in Rome and born prematurely into a middle class family in Germany in 1971, slotting between two sisters: one three years older, the other nine years younger. My German father worked as a psychologist while my Croatian mother kept the home front in order. Though my father didn't say he loved us every day, or play with us every chance he'd get – I love him for always providing well for us. His love is demonstrated in actions rather than words. He has always been very reliable and helped me immensely by exercising my scientific brain, always trying to explain with reason and scientific thinking when any of us would come home with some idealistic, harebrained idea. He'd keep us grounded. Mum is more emotional. She would be responsible for cuddles, mending scraped knees and always having an open ear and heart for any problems we might face. She had her hands full with me being born with severe strabismus and knock-knees. During the first years of my life she ran me patiently and lovingly to doctors and therapists.

Other than that I was low maintenance. My mum just had to give me a toy car and I'd happily play by myself for hours. At school I was self-motivated, loved learning, and even if not at the top of the class always did well with very little parental super-vision. My strabismus was mended, but never to the point of me gaining three-dimensional vision. I didn't miss it (never having known any different), but it did impair my abilities in any kind of ball games or activities that require quick hand-eye coordination. By the time my eyes and brain told my hands the ball is coming, it had already flown past. These days this does not pose a problem, not too many flying objects in everyday life. Back then all the boys were spending most of their free time playing football or hockey. Since I was a useless addition to any team, I did not have many 'mates'. Girls were playing with Barbie dolls and did not want any boys around either. When I was eight years old I started playing the piano though, which kept me fairly busy and happy. Finally, around the 8th grade, girls became interested in socializing with boys and I acquired many great (girl) friends. I guess me being gay made me an attractive, sensitive male person to talk to. (Even though I did not really know then that I was. That dawned on me when I was 17, several years later.)

Even though I was a pretty well-behaved child, a little more introverted perhaps and often praised by elderly relations for my maturity, I was not the perfect little angel. I had my share of quarrels with my older sister. I exploited my favored status as the only son and could be certain that, if annoyed by or in a fight with my sister, loud crying would get my mother's attention and mostly she'd side with me. And at times I vented pubescent frustrations on my baby sister too. Despite that she still admired me. Looking back I could have been more understanding towards my parents and shown more gratitude. I did not really understand and see the effort it takes to raise and support a family.

As for my spiritual upbringing – my mother is Catholic and my father an ex-Protestant. They had the foresight not to christen us kids though. They wanted us to have a say in the matter when more capable of making an educated decision. I loved singing and spent years in church choirs. If we ever sang during a full service, I'd usually nod off during the sermon though.

After doing my 'Abitur' (the German equivalent of A-levels) I spent countless hours worrying about which direction to go with my life. Initially I spent 15 months doing civil service as a 'conscientious objector', which gave me a bit more time to ponder the decision. During those 15 months I worked on a repertoire of piano pieces to get into the Music Conservatory, but I was unsure if I was good enough, or patient enough, to practice sufficiently. If anything I wanted to be a concert pianist though I didn't believe 'just' being a piano teacher would be fulfilling enough. An arrogant attitude I admit. Studying music meant I needed a second instrument, so I took voice lessons, but again my somewhat restricted range was an issue too.

My other idea was to study medicine. This promised to feed my hunger for scientific knowledge and would enable me to work with people – something I enjoyed. I was a bit of an intellectual snob. An academic education was taken as a must. I generally wanted to live a meaningful life – helping people as a doctor seemed to me more meaningful and worthy than, say, being a sales representative flogging nails. The fact that we'd be hard-pressed to build houses without nails and that our economy needs more than just the medical profession to prosper – eluded me back then. Or perhaps I felt that people less intelligent than me could do those things?

The battle inside me between music and medicine was decided by the government or better the ZVS (Zentralstelle für die Vergabe von Studienplätzen – the Department for the Allocation of University places). When finishing my civil service I thought I'd have another year to prepare for an audition with the Music Conservatory, however, I received a letter informing me that I had moved forward on the waiting list and had to enroll within the week with the University of Hamburg or lose my chance of studying medicine. Hamburg had been number one on my wish list of cities to study in too, so I packed my bags and moved up north.

Spiritually I could best be classed as a skeptic in my early years. I was an adherent to common scientific explanations of the world. That said, at times some esoteric books would land in my lap. I remember a book about the power of the subconscious when in my mid-teens: Joseph Murphy – *The Power of Your Subconscious Mind*. The idea of manifesting wishes through affirmation and visualizations seemed appealing. It did not seem to work for me though. I focused on being more muscular, but nothing much happened. I did start to do some occasional push-ups and chin-ups in my room which helped some, but I expected more. I figured that if I became more muscular through exercising hours a day, I would not need the affirmations, that it would be pure biology. I did not understand that the affirmations might help me to find the motivation and strength for regular exercise. The book promised visible, palpable results if one just affirmed. Furthermore I fought the budding 'gayness' inside and tried to affirm that I get aroused by the opposite sex, but that did not really succeed either. So I put the idea of 'affirmations' on hold.

A year or so later I came across a book about Rosemary Brown, who supposedly auto wrote dead composers' compositions from their afterlife – *Unfinished Symphonies: Voices from the Beyond*. I found it fascinating. I especially enjoyed the bit where the composers apparently told her that there is no hell! Everyone goes to heaven. Everyone is psychic in heaven, so a person, who had lived a life of lies and deceit, going to heaven, where everyone can see through them, might initially experience heaven as hell. The Divine does not put any pressure on us to find our belief in it during our physical lifetime, being confident that with an eternal afterlife we will come to understand the truth again. Today when I Google her, I find mixed reviews. I have also listened to some of her compositions and find that an original Chopin does sound more inspired and genial than her version. She might have been a spoof…

I read another book about Ouija boards. This was interesting at first too; people who apparently had gotten in contact with enlightened spiritual beings who dictated whole books, fascinating. The last three chapters ended with dire warnings though; players having become possessed by evil spirits and the recommendation to deeply bury any Ouija board (supposedly the damn things just won't burn). I did have to sleep with the lights on for a week or so and decided that the spiritual worlds seemed far too dangerous. I went back to 'normal' living, having enough hopes and dreams that seemed accomplishable by ordinary means.

My initial years of medical study were filled with excitement; discovering the joy of helping patients, studying for exams, embracing the new life away from the parents' hearth, making new friends and sometimes having more than one part-time job trying to keep a comfortable lifestyle. My life seemed all mapped out – I'd finish my studies, specialize and either open a private practice or become the head of a hospital. I always saw myself in a blue pinstripe suit driving a Jaguar. I also relished the status that came with my field of study; being respected and sometimes even adored when saying I was studying to become a doctor. University was tougher than my school years. Medicine required a faster pace. In school we were taught critical, analytical thinking to understand concepts and ideas – easy for my analytical brain. University demanded a lot of memorizing, not my greatest strength. Yet, I managed to pass all the exams.

During my first year at university my grandmother died. I had moved into her flat in Hamburg, as she was in a nursing home being too frail to live on her own. It was a rather posh place in one of Hamburg's affluent suburbs. I visited her regularly, but the fancy façade of the home soon turned out to be just that. She was in a little loft room which got incredibly hot during that summer. My dear 94 year old grandma was sitting in just her underwear when I arrived one afternoon. Always having enjoyed her food she complained that they were very stingy with the rations. The service was pretty lousy too and considering that she missed her friends and relations, plus the fact that this home was costing her an arm and a leg, we decided she should move back home again. She had a few more happy months, looking after me as much as I looked after her.

I had not 'come out' to her and did feel guilty lying to her when she enquired about girlfriends. I am not good at living any kind of lie and soon developed quite severe juvenile cardiac arrhythmia for a few months, perhaps because of this? By then I had settled in Hamburg and had started working as geriatric homecare nursing help. At the end of the semester I had also found a room of my own, nearer to university and then went back to my parents' during the summer. A week after I had left, my grandma died. Her warm heart and zest for life had been an inspiration.

I considered myself a romantic back then; guess I had watched too many chick-flicks. I desired the perfect romance, to find the perfect man and planned to be faithful to him till the end of my days. But every couple of months I'd be heartbroken. Usually the object of my affections would fall out of infatuation after a week or so, or vice versa, or the guys I fancied were not interested or 'taken'. Between the ages of 18–25, I only managed two noteworthy relationships, of no longer than six months each. It was all very frustrating, if not depressing, especially because subconsciously I was convinced I would never be completely happy without being in a great relationship. I was attractive, intelligent, sensitive and studying to become a doctor. Not a bad catch I thought. On top of that the sheer endless amounts of knowledge I'd have to retain, to become a responsible doctor, became ever more daunting. Before my first big clinical examinations I got mononucleosis – and ended up having to postpone my exams by a semester.

Then I met my perfect man – attractive, intelligent, dressed well, a great lover and he seemed to genuinely like me too. After a week he confessed to me that he was financing his studies as an ecstasy wholesaler. The moment he told me, my feelings for him just vanished. He went back home to Berlin and stopped dealing – for my sake! Allegedly he dumped hundreds of pills down the toilet, but I could not resurrect my feelings for him, however hard I tried. Was there something wrong with me? You see my father had always told us that according to twin research studies, about 80% of our character/being is genetic and 20% environmental, i.e. there is not much we can do to change ourselves. I was led to believe that if there was anything I did not like about myself and my character, I better get used to it. I would likely have to live with them for the rest of my life. Perhaps, these theories/scientific teachings were another reason why I felt so stuck with myself and in life at that point. It all made for fertile ground – for new, potentially more liberating ideas and concepts.

In the autumn of 1995 I met Carl. A very handsome guy who raved about some esoteric books he had read. He said he could sense that I was a 'good' person (always nice to have that confirmed from the outside, especially in times of self-doubt) and recommended these books to me. Carl also told me that our thoughts have creative potential! In other words as children of God/the Divine, through our thinking, we have the same creational powers. This struck a chord with me.

Two of the recommended books were written by a woman who claimed to have connected to wise and loving entities from the Pleiades constellation, who had channeled the books' contents through her. These Pleiadians have supposedly come to Earth (in spirit) to help humanity evolve and transition. Carl advised me to read these books one chapter at a time and let the 'knowledge' sink in. I devoured these books though. They talked about humans discovering their true, long forgotten potential. Our DNA morphing from 2 to 12 strands and that humans (or at least those following the Pleiadians' advice) would also discover great gifts: psychic abilities, even flight or levitation. Another claim centered on the 'reptilian conspiracy', that the top tier of the richest and most powerful people on Earth were hiding their true, dark, destructive reptilian roots. I just gobbled it all up, without question.

I was naïve. I trusted that if someone claims that they channel extraterrestrials, then they would (I would be far too embarrassed to claim something like that without being certain of my claims). I did not consider that such authors might only be talking to their subconscious, could be deluded or simply be telling porkies. These days I feel that the books were (mostly) channeled, but I am less certain about the motives of the entities dictating them. I have come to be very wary of manipulative techniques used in spiritual contexts. These books ask the readers to keep a completely open mind – as a lot of information would be conveyed to the reader from 'between the lines' (however that is supposed to work – but it did have a somewhat hypnotic effect on me). There was no recommendation asking the readers to request 'good protection' before embarking on this spiritual quest. I believe that you should ask for divine protections before any spiritual adventure, be that meditation, mind-altering exercise, attending an esoteric lecture or just reading some spiritual text. Call me paranoid but you'll soon see why I have become so cautious…

I tried to tell my friends about the newly discovered ideas. The great potential we, as humans, are now able to rediscover. Instead of being grateful though, they started to shun me. Today I can see that I was annoying with my continuous proselytizing attempts, just repeating what I had read, without giving it any thought. I read other more 'sensible' books too. I still remember one about ancient Hawaiian Huna philosophy, *Urban Shaman* by Serge Kahili King. Explaining how we can all be shamans for the benefit of our lives, that we have the power to change our lives with our thoughts, through visualizations and by communicating with (all) beings. Communication that is possible because everything has consciousness and can communicate spirit-to-spirit: plants, animals, rocks, computers, the wind or the waves in the sea. At least this book was backed by millennia of indigenous tradition and experience – whereas the extraterrestrial channeled book had far less of a proven track record.

What hooked me though was the Barbara Brennan book *Hands of Light*, an inspiring 'textbook' about spiritual healing. I did not really have any psychic abilities back then i.e. I did not see any auras, feel energies, have visions or hear voices, but the author claimed that with proper, supervised training everyone could (re)discover innate psychic abilities. That sounded very appealing, especially as with my medical studies I had learned that most medical diagnoses, and with them treatments, are based on statistic probabilities. If a patient comes to a doctor and describes their symptoms the doctor might decide for the 'most probable' diagnosis or order some more diagnostic tests. But even with further investigation, plenty of diagnoses are not 100% guaranteed. Psychic diagnosis could be 100% accurate – which sounded awesome to me!

Furthermore many illnesses, especially cancer or chronic diseases, are hard to manage, available help potentially has grave side effects and some cannot be helped at all. Now supposedly spiritual healing could tackle any problem, side effect free! Combining Western Medicine with Spiritual healing therefore seemed to be 'The Answer'. Plus, I learned that all illnesses have spiritual, mental and/or emotional roots and that without discovering and healing these causes one could never really get better. What might feel like a healing effect through most Western medical therapies would potentially just mask the symptoms.

Barbara Brennan did repeatedly stress that you needed proper training and supervision to become a good healer. If improperly used, spiritual healing could be just as dangerous as a surgeon operating without the proper skill set. I had no reason to doubt that she was right. I concluded that if I wanted to become a Spiritual Healer, and I really did, I had to learn Spiritual healing.

That meant I had to acquire knowledge and find someone to offer supervised training. Plus I would have to rediscover my psychic abilities. 'Luckily' Barbara Brennan was running a four-year healer development program – there was a place where I could learn!

Her courses were rather expensive though. Furthermore her school was in the United States. This meant I'd have to find the funds to pay for the courses, as well as for the flights and accommodation. I was only a penniless student, but I was visualizing and praying for the funds so surely creation would get me the money? I did not win the lottery in the next few days, but I did have the intuition that I could maybe find a spiritual healer in Germany, even Hamburg, who could teach me instead… I did find a spiritual healer in Hamburg (around the corner from my house, in fact). I just did not know yet that I was not skipping merrily into a harmless healing circle, but marching blindly into a cult.

Chapter 2

Boot Camp

Now I was on the lookout to find a good healer in Germany. According to the 'Heilpraktikergesetz' (a German law about healing practices) only Doctors or Naturopaths, approved by the German authorities, are allowed to diagnose, treat and 'heal' the public. Just being a spiritual healer and treating the public could lead to incarceration. It was hard to find someone in the phone book in 1995. Nowadays this law still exists, but the German courts have declared that spiritual healing should not be included in it. I therefore asked about healers in a New Age bookstore in Hamburg. The nice lady at the counter gave me Peter V's telephone number, remarking that Peter had been highly recommended to her just that day! It all felt like divine providence to me, so I set out to contact Peter and ask for an appointment straight away. I could hardly wait and was glad when he called me to arrange a session.

I was impressed by our first meeting. Peter seemed to hit the nail on the head. He commented that I was impatient (true, but then again how many 25 year olds aren't). He also said that I might get frustrated in the medical field... How could he know I studied medicine? In retrospect I cannot recall what I might have said on his answer machine, when calling for my appointment. Perhaps I mentioned getting his number from the bookstore? He did have time to go there and speak to the lady who knew what I was studying. When I exclaimed, "Funny you say that, because I do study medicine!" He replied, "I know, I can see everything!" He also said that my right side seemed weaker than the left and that if having accidents I would tend to hurt my right side. I do have a scar close to my right hand so even with long sleeves he might have spotted this?

16

I really wanted to learn healing though and being naïve I decided in my head and heart that Peter had just shown genuine signs of psychic ability. I decided that I had found my 'teacher'. I cannot remember any alarm bells ringing, like getting bad vibes or a funny feeling in my stomach. I assumed that to develop (or keep) your psychic abilities you needed to be of good character (Barbara Brennan had insinuated such in her book), so Peter's psychic feat had me conclude that he must be a good person. A few months later Peter affirmed this belief by claiming that if a person is given psychic or other spiritual abilities and misuses them, the Divine will strip that being of them.

I told Peter that I wanted to learn healing and Peter was happy to take on the role of teacher. He claimed all our healing and psychic abilities are already inside us. They cannot be taught, but only rediscovered. I would not find them in books, but inside myself. He recommended that I sit in on his biweekly healing circle and learn by observation, received healing etc. I told him that I wanted to meditate regularly, believing that this was essential to discover my healing and psychic abilities, but that I had problems actually doing it! He encouraged my desire and supposedly did something during my first healing session to unblock my ability to meditate. After that session I had no more problems and meditated twice a day. I did not really 'feel' anything during my first session with him, but was told that that was quite normal.

Peter seemed a genuinely caring person. Wise, very intuitive and he often wore a knowing, amused smile. Sometimes there seemed to be a warm, kind, palpable glow emanating from him. He must have been in his 40s. His appearance was always well turned out. He had longish curly, fluffy grey hair and a bit of a beard. He did appear very well adjusted, without getting stifled by social norms or fashion rules. His practice was very well presented too; it reminded me of my last piano teacher's house. She was a bit of an environmentalist and her house was furnished with bespoke solid wood furniture. No flat pack chipboard anywhere. At Peter's practice I recognized the same. Most of the furniture was made of pale woods, like pine. It was all rather eco-conscious and practical. Plus I knew from my piano teacher how expensive such furniture was, even if not the prettiest. Everything was kept in light colors, and there were usually plenty of flowers around. It was warm, unpretentious and welcoming. The healing circles were usually held in the large healing room. This was just a big comfortably carpeted, open space with two large crystals and a treatment couch for one-on-one sessions. For larger gatherings we'd carry in foldable wooden chairs and meditation cushions. What really gave the room great atmosphere though was a large mural on the ceiling – a mural of a pond with water lilies, which was pretty, serene and calming.

About 10–30 people attended each healing circle. Some regularly like me, some sporadically and others only showed up once. I was eager to experience and witness healings and spiritual diagnosis, and I was not disappointed. Peter would often ask two of his other students/clients to help with the psychic diagnosis, in order to help them hone their abilities. These were mostly two ladies, both of whom I befriended and do not suspect to have been 'fakes'. They would read something he'd call the 'somatic strip', and supposedly they were able to see the patients' auras, see inside the body, communicate with their organs etc. I was impressed. The regulars, attending the healing circle, seemed nice, gentle and intelligent and came from all walks of life. Everybody appeared welcoming, friendly and genuinely desiring to do 'good'. I could not wait to learn and discover more about spiritual healing.

Just going to the healing circle, twice weekly, soon felt like it wasn't 'enough' anymore. I heard though that Peter ran other circles. One was called 'Intensive Circle' (a seminar held on the third Saturday of each month) and the other the 'Shamanic Circle' (held on the first Saturday afternoon of each month). I asked Peter if it was okay for me to come to these and Peter had no objections. I started attending regularly. After a while the 'Easter Circle' was established, where attendance was by invitation from Peter only.

The Intensive Circle would start off with a meditation followed by Peter lecturing. He would often 'prove' his teachings, with someone from the group performing a past life regression. Sometimes he'd tell us stories. There was no prescribed structure or program; everything supposedly happened as divine intuition told him. The Shamanic Circle would start with a meditation too, followed by a little lecture, smudging with herbs and then the group going on a shamanic journey. While we travelled in our minds and spiritual bodies, he'd drum. Travel experiences, things we had seen, felt or been told during our shamanic journeys would then be shared. We'd finish with an 'animal dance'. Peter would drum again and we'd channel, handing over our bodies to be used by our animal spirits and guides. After that there would be a nice buffet of vegetarian dishes brought in by all the members. The Easter Circle was the inner sanctum of the group. Only regulars (true devotees) would be allowed to attend. The main topic was Jesus' life (Peter as an incarnation of Jesus) and how his disciples (the rest of us) had failed him 2000 years ago.

During a circle meeting I told Peter that I was thinking of quitting my medical studies. He discouraged this, saying that he had been told (by Upstairs) that it was my divine mission to stay in the medical field. I should become a doctor and then help heal the profession, turn the whole Western medical apparatus around. Medicine needed to become more alternative – more herbs, spiritual healing, acupuncture, more intuitive, less expensive diagnostic machinery, healing from the heart, less healing with machines, no more chemicals and so forth. I felt honored; I had been given a mission from the highest echelons of Spirit. They must really trust in my abilities. At the same time it was quite a daunting task and none that promised to be much fun. I thought that if with Ultimate Good help I could do whatever 'I' enjoyed, I would much rather 'just' be a spiritual healer. Plus I had visions of opening a little café, revive my musical interests. Still who was I to argue with the Divine? So I did my best to fulfill my destiny. If I had to convert the medical profession, I felt I needed good proof that spiritual healing worked. I thought I knew in my heart that it did, but I acknowledged that to reach most doctors, I needed more than a feeling!

I figured it would be a good start to look for proof where I was, with Peter. If diagnoses he made spiritually turned out correct, if regressions performed could be proved, that would be a good starting point. I decided I would start by just observing. It felt as if I did not really develop any (reliable) psychic abilities yet, so I could not test Peter's diagnosis from a spiritual perspective. No 'patients' ever got up, walked out and/or openly disagreed with what was said about them though. I remember one occasion where I complained about bleeding gums in a healing circle. Peter 'had a look' and said my toothpaste had too much fluoride. I changed to a fluoride free version and the bleeding stopped. Had he accurately diagnosed actual fluoride hypersensitivity, or was it just a common sense lucky guess? Whenever I ask a dentist about this they say that fluoride allergy is extremely rare. Yet when I forget and use fluoride toothpaste again, my gums bleed.

On reflection no 'miracle' healings ever seemed to take place in the circles either. Comparing Peter's 'healing results' with other renown healers, from (scientific) literature I have read, his results seem rather lame. However, there was a lady with cancer (colon, I believe). She had been given about three months to live, but two years later she was still with us. She did have to go back into hospital for numerous operations for metastasis, and finally passed on about 18 months after I joined. In contrast, a 23 year old woman who had kidney failure, and was on regular dialysis, died about a year after joining Peter's circle. She collapsed on the street after one healing session and could not be saved.

Peter's clients were not directly discouraged from seeing or consulting doctors, but the medical profession was frequently criticized as disharmonious, e.g. chemotherapy was described as highly toxic and damaging. It was propagated that if your beliefs were pure and strong enough, everything could be healed. As Peter did not say that some healings might take years, even if one's faith is strong and pure, I (and probably most attendees) interpreted delays in healings as simply a lack of faith and/or the presence of too many lingering doubts. Peter preached reincarnation and that supposedly all illness has spiritual roots. You get sick because you act or have acted disharmoniously. Everything is karmic and there are no coincidences!

I stopped wearing my glasses for about a year. I figured that by wearing my glasses I just kept reaffirming my poor sight. I had to believe that I did not need them. I told Peter and he encouraged me, but did not ask me whether I ever had to drive a car for example. Fortunately I was farsighted and still had about 85% vision without my glasses, but my eyes were more tired and strained than usual. I looked more cross-eyed most of the time too. At one point on a trip, to Maui, Hawaii, some of us took an excursion to the top of the volcano. On the way up I was driving (without my glasses) with three passengers. Nothing bad happened, but I was very relieved when someone else offered to drive back down.

In the Intensive Circle Peter's main doctrine was that we are all 'slaves' of our 'subconscious', that we are usually only 5–15% conscious. We walk through our lives in a daze. Apparently the degree to which we are controlled by the subconscious can be read, in real time, in one's somatic strip. Peter demonstrated his theory by insulting one of the members (while another 'capable' person read the somatic strip). Her subconscious supposedly made her react (to the insult) and took over. Every time we 'react', i.e. are not calm and consciously choosing an action, we are supposedly ruled by subconscious energies.

Not only are there 'negative reactions', but also pleasant, positive ones, when listening to a piece of (cheesy) music for example. These reactions were said to come from our past. So both pleasant and negative reactions make us live in the past. This universe (and several others), Peter claimed, have been created and are ruled by Subconscious Forces. Our aim is to overcome these and be allowed back into a Central Universe. Supposedly we have been 'kicked out' of this Central (Holy) Universe, for having misbehaved – become greedy, selfish, vain or whatever. Anything we experience was said to be a repeat from the past, there is not really anything new... ever.

There are many worlds stuck in different stages of ever-returning cycles. Right now there are worlds with dinosaurs as well as futuristic ones, and we have supposedly experienced them all before, again and again. Our future, Peter taught, is predetermined by our actions, and if our actions are led by subconscious decisions we'd live the same experiences, make the same mistakes, over and over again. Even if, in this life, we were to move to another city say, our e.g. subconscious programs of loneliness, trouble with the boss, wrong partnerships, and so on, would follow us, catch up with us, just acted out by different people. According to Peter there is no escaping our subconscious programs, which rule and determine our life experiences. Peter also said that when going on the spiritual path the first lesson is to realize that we don't know anything.

Supposedly there are great benefits to ridding yourself of subconscious rule. Besides being happier and an enlightened being (we all thought Peter was), you would become 100% 'conscious', and could stop a war by just sitting in the middle of a battlefield. I did wonder why Peter did not just travel to war zones, become all conscious and stop wars... According to him, he did not want to take the learning process away from us. Still I was not sure if all the suffering created by wars could be justified for the satisfaction of a 'complete' learning process? On top of all the above, we might actually be allowed 'home' again into the Central Universe.

I soon ran into real problems with Peter's teachings. I became unable to criticize anything or anyone (including myself), fearing I would just be projecting my own subconsciousness. Furthermore I had learned to 'not resist evil', but look straight through it into the Divine behind it. Doing so was said to stop feeding the confusion with energy and strengthen the truth behind it. Was I strengthening subconscious programs simply by identifying them and giving them my attention that way? But don't you usually have to identify and potentially name something that is wrong at first, so you can start with the relevant healing or improvement processes?

I hit many walls. If I had problems with an individual, for example, I would practice forgiveness and pray for healing etc. If the disharmonious actions of the individual, towards me, did not change though, did I have the right to say anything? Ask the individual to change their disharmonious behavior? Was I not just being impatient and simply needing to work more on myself, to resolve the problem? I felt supremely guilty just thinking critically about anything! If I thought *gosh he is in a real bad mood today*, did not that potentially create (or definitely strengthen) the bad mood in the other person? After a while I had the epiphany – thinking is coupled with intent.

There is contemplative and projective thinking. If I ponder something this should be okay. Actively thinking ill of someone coupled with the conscious or subconscious desire to harm that someone is to be avoided! Confusion is temporary. Never deny someone's or something's divine core. However evil a person might act, one should never forget that they are still an individualized divine being and that all evil is temporary, even if it takes that being eons to 'overcome' that evil. Admittedly it takes more energy to remind yourself of the divine core of an evil dictator or gruesome murderer than an alcoholic, homeless person that has lost their way.

According to Peter our goal was to 'defuse' all emotional triggers from this and past lives, so that we would not 'react' anymore and be released off the shackles of our subconscious. This could be achieved through forgiveness, of ourselves and others. Peter claimed that past life regression was one such forgiveness tool. By viewing past lives (excerpts) and particularly important events in such past lives, the emotions (stuck since these past lives) were said to be released. Peter called it an act of 'active forgiveness'. Plus one might supposedly 'learn' why you felt and acted in certain (unfavorable?) ways in this life, by seeing the roots of these feelings and behavior patterns in previous lives. Not to mention the potential healing effects when strengthening your faith in your eternal spirit/existence. If we are eternal, then chances are greater that we are indeed individualized, divine spirit. One might take more responsibility for one's actions too. Peter liked to say that someone destroying the environment in this life might think twice if he/she could be certain that they might have to come back to a ruined planet...

Past life regressions were frequently performed in front of the group. One of the followers would lie down and Peter would lead them very quickly to a previous life. He'd ask them to tell the rest of us what they saw and experienced. Peter did mention that these regressions usually had been done prior in one-on-one sessions, and that they were re-done for our benefit in front of the group. These regressions were usually very vivid and emotional. One could hear, from the voice of the person being regressed, how involved they were in the plot. Regressions spanned centuries, continents, some animal reincarnations and even different planets.

Frequently the lesson for all to be learned was that we needed to believe strongly, have unshakable faith, and that if we were advised by a spiritual leader, especially one like Peter, we should not question! We saw several regressions where terrible things befell the person being regressed, or their loved ones, because they did not believe enough, or follow their guru's instructions to the letter! For example in one regression two people from the circle were supposedly killed in Auschwitz's gas chambers. They then reported what else happened after they left their bodies. They were at peace despite the trauma and met their guides/angels. Their angels supposedly told them that had they believed stronger/truer, they would have survived the gas chamber.

Peter claimed that all of us had met in different constellations in prior lives. In some 'critical' lives all of us had been together. Supposedly he had been our spiritual teacher several times already, but due to our inability to follow his instructions, develop spiritually and truly believe, he would have to return to help us, over and over again. Peter would 'prove' his point by showing us past lives, where the person being regressed was listening to famous spiritual teachers. At the end of each of these regressions Peter would ask the participant if they could recognize their past life master from this life. Peter told the regressee, "Just look into his eyes," and they always exclaimed, "It is you (Peter)!"

Peter was identified as having been Jesus, Buddha, Mohammed, Lao Tzu, Socrates, Moses, a few Native American medicine men and many others. But Peter stressed that he was not claiming he was Jesus himself, as so many other confused, deluded gurus out there supposedly do, but that he had been identified as such by the participants. Peter also claimed (himself) at one point to have been Sir Francis Drake. He boasted how generous he had been in that incarnation – having built orphanages and other charitable institutions. Years later I saw a BBC documentary about Devon, which mentioned Sir Francis Drake as one of the local, historic celebrities from there. The moderator told his viewers a little less known darker fact about Sir Francis Drake: he was one of the original initiators of the slave trade with the Americas. Perhaps Peter should have listened to himself a bit more, during his Jesus incarnation…

We were told that allegedly we are one of a handful of major groups/players responsible for the spiritual development of all mankind. (I guess we had to be important, having the true reincarnated Jesus there with us!) According to him we were catalysts. If we were to evolve fast enough, we could save about one billion people (our core group had about 40–60 permanent members, so that is at least 16.6 million each member of the group was responsible for). Should we fail in our efforts, mankind would not survive past 2012.

We were urged to meditate regularly (each meditation missed would be like a missing stone in a bridge, i.e. years of meditation could be undone by missing just a few) and practice forgiveness by saying, *I forgive myself, I forgive xyz, I let go in love and thank creation that everything is wonderful, Amen.* To hand over a current fear one would say, *I hand my (current) fear to creation and thank that this fear and all related subconscious programs be processed and deleted. Amen.* One would then start to breathe deeply and exhale these disharmonious thoughts or feelings. These were claimed to be secret and very powerful tools, which antique Egyptian High Priests had used already.

Peter soon not only read minds, but implied he would always be consciously connected to all of us. We only had to think of him. If in trouble he'd hear our plea and would interfere. Just as Jesus is said to hear and answer all prayers directed to him. It was also implied that besides looking after all of us, he was able to still carry out all his other Jesus obligations too, i.e. helping each and every prayer that billions of Christians may send Jesus' way. That sounded virtually impossible, I still had problems doing two things at once; but who was I to say he could not? There are plenty of Christians who believe that their Jesus can accomplish such feats; I never heard that they think Jesus will have those abilities taken away, should he ever reincarnate.

Apparently humanity had already destroyed Mars and Venus mainly because our group failed there too. Furthermore our group was responsible for the 'dark' Middle Ages and all the current unrests, wars, poverty and other injustices worldwide. Peter showed us an 'alternate' regression – what would have happened over the course of the last two millennia had we not all allegedly denounced Jesus, or had just worked that little bit harder on our spiritual developments, while under his tutelage 2000 years ago. The result would have been lasting peace and interracial, inter-cultural and interfaith understanding every-where. We saw Columbus discovering the Americas and, instead of killing the indigenous peoples, they embraced them and they shared each other's cultures.

I was soon very busy praying and practicing forgiveness in every spare second I found. Whatever I was doing in the outside while awake, whenever possible inside my head I'd use Peter's spiritual tools. I must have done this hundreds of times each day. There seemed to be plenty that required forgiveness. Considering, as we had been told, that the outside world is a mirror of our inner thoughts, emotions and beliefs, I dreaded watching the news, hearing about wars, famines or just seeing homeless or unhappy people on the street. I felt I was respon-sible for their suffering. Something still had to be inside me that caused these suffering. If I could dissolve enough aggression, poverty and sadness inside me, the outside would heal too! Since there was hardly ever any praise for work done, only reiterations of our past and present failings, I kept on fearing that we were all underperforming.

I had (as strongly recommended by Peter) become vegetarian and only bought organically grown foods. The cost for attending Peter's healing groups and circles, and buying from the organic shop, was quite high on a student budget. I saved by not going out partying anymore and buying fewer to no new clothes, but still soon maxed out my overdraft. Worldly pleasures, like going out with friends, soon seemed too frivolous. There was no time for parties until humanity and the world had been saved.

Peter mentioned that there might be those who call our circle a cult. As I had not the slightest suspicion that we were a cult (not that I knew much about cult mechanisms and psychology back then), I thought he was kidding. He was quick to add though that the greatest cult of all is Humanity. Should outsiders criticize us, this would obviously just stem from their subconscious programs, resisting our more enlightened ways. If someone would say anything critical or bad about us (or anyone else for the matter), we were told they'd actually just be projecting and talking about themselves.

In the main Peter's teachings followed Christian lines, with emphasis on reincarnation and the frequent mention of Karma. Our Universe was claimed to be ruled by subconscious powers – but due to Karma, it was supposed to still be just. Between lives there seemed to be a reprieve. Between lives we were said to be in a pretty much enlightened, all-knowing state again and would meet our Guides and Angels – discuss our last incarnation and prepare for the next. We would not really have a say about what we were to experience in the next life. They would be our lessons! In a poor man's incarnation the lesson to learn would most likely be humility and sharing, for example.

Peter did affirm that humans had 'free will' – well free will using the average 10% of consciousness free and available. He also said that all humans have an innate inner sense for right and wrong, i.e. there is always a voice inside ourselves telling us if something is right or wrong. It apparently is up to us to either listen to this voice or ignore it. That sounded great to me; the only slight problem for me personally was that with increasing amounts of guilt pressure, time pressures and the associated fears and paranoia, I really was not all that sure what I was feeling and hearing anymore. Also with all these new concepts, teachings and philosophies, I was still busy sorting, reevaluating and rearranging just about everything I knew (and had taken for granted) so far.

Peter claimed that every time we thought we had overcome a subconscious behavior, we would be tested (by the Divine) to see if we have actually, truly overcome or were just wishfully thinking. According to him doubts (that devilish opposite of beliefs) are built into the spiritual development process, to be overcome again and again. Oh, and there obviously was frequent mention of that old devil – the mind – our rational thinking. As mentioned, during healing circles Peter often used a couple of female helpers, who would read the attendees' somatic strips for him. He would apparently monitor them and berate them saying, "Yeah that is it, you just had it there. Ah, but now you have let your rational mind interfere again!" It seemed that our mind was okay to do math, but other than that it was just a bloated, subconsciously ruled organ, whose purpose was to cut us off from 'truth' and divine intuition.

Peter recommended the book *The Sermon on the Mount* by Emmet Fox. It is a Christian Science analysis of Jesus' Sermon on the Mount. Not a bad book. Most of it is basically a list of metaphysical rules like 'Don't resist evil, but look through it into the divine behind it.' As mentioned earlier, by taking away one's attention from the 'evil' and only giving energy to the ubiquitous divine essence behind it, you help dissolve, heal or send away the confused energies. 'Energy follows thought' and we supposedly create and attract those things into our life that we think about or which we believe. The book did talk about how, if you do not dissolve negative thoughts, emotions or beliefs straight away, they can dig in and are then harder to remove, but it failed to mention that embedded evils might take a fair amount of time to dig out. Rather it too made you believe that if a healing does not happen there and then, your beliefs are not strong enough. Reading the book also had me assume that if you forgave yourself completely for an erroneous behavior, then all other prior behaviors should be automatically dug up and dissolved too. An experience I did not seem to create myself though. However, the book exclaimed, *Ask, and it will be given to you; seek, and you will find; knock, and it will be opened*, which I found to be a very empowering concept.

This *Sermon on the Mount* challenged quite a few of my beliefs. If everything in life is self-generated by beliefs and emotions, but can bow to the power of the mind ('Beliefs can move mountains!'), what could that mean for me and my life? Call me shallow, but one of the first things that came to my mind was (and still is) ageing. I had lived with my grandma, worked in old people's homecare for some years and had seen what age could do to the body, health and mind! Does ageing only exist because everybody believes in it? Considering I believed in human reincarnation now, I asked myself, "Why do we need ageing?" If we have been humans before, why go through childhood and old age again and again. I suppose childhood can be great, if you have loving parents, a whole load of toys and friends. On the downside one forgets so much stuff and has to relearn it. I might have been a professor, a philosopher, a holy man or a king in my previous incarnations, but one will likely forget most of those experiences and have to start all over again, savants excluded.

Creation does seem incredible; humanity has not even managed to completely understand all the different processes and workings of a single cell organism, not to mention why and how multiple cells come together to form organs, organisms etc. If creation can do all that, would it not just be one small step further to turn us into beings that don't age? Surely creation is capable of such a feat. I had read about some aborigines and Buddhist monks whose bodies aged, okay, but who know/knew when it is/was their time to go and to leave their bodies. Once they have decided it is time to go, they consciously leave their bodies – they just shut down all bodily functions and die. That just sounded so right, natural and desirable to me. I decided to work on that, plus to stop believing in ageing there and then.

Seventeen years on, I think I am doing alright. I believe I look younger than most people my age. My mum did keep her young looks well into her forties too though, so potentially I just have good genes? And before you think me irresponsible, which world could support 7+ billion humans that live forever? That is not what I strive for. I pray either to find the skill to know when to leave my body consciously and will do so then, or that creation just takes me in my sleep when my time has come!

I was happy to have found spiritual anti-ageing principals and revelations for other reasons as well. It seemed that so many people are stuck doing the same job all their lives, because of restrictions they impose on themselves, by believing that learning new things and skills becomes harder with age, and that one has to work for years to build a successful career in something. But do they not build their own cages of mono-professionalism? There are many things I still wanted to do and achieve besides healing. Learn a few more languages, become a professional musician, an architect and or perhaps a designer – all things that interest me. If I can stay young and energetic, and attract all the funds and support I need, I can possibly still fulfill all of them. Especially after the Divine and Peter had apparently dumped the 'Heal the medical profession' task on me, there was still hope that I might get a few decades of my life, where I could do things I enjoyed more!

The *Sermon on the Mount* book triggered a thorough investigation into my whole life and my beliefs. I understood that if we were created in God's image, what we should strive for was perfection! Theoretically we could all do at least as much as Jesus is said to have done and potentially more. Since everything starts in the mind, I started to monitor every thought and emotion. Well, that is whenever I did not sleep or was too occupied with the outside world. So besides practicing forgiveness, everything that was not harmonious, loving, fearless etc. was 'handed over' to creation with Peter's handing-over-to-creation tool. Any single belief that was restrictive to my abilities or freedoms was weeded out. I got quite creative, sometimes perhaps handing over thoughts or emotions which today I would not consider abject anymore, but I thought it better to be safe than sorry. Plus if I mistakenly handed over something that was actually a part of my divine essence, I trusted that creation would not take it from me as my divine self would be indestructible!

Using the 'handing-over-to-Creation' tool taught me two things. One, when using the tool a few times in a row, I got a feeling as if a pipe inside me, in my core, was blasted free. As if I was pulling energy through this pillar of light inside me. I could feel uncomfortable energies in my body shifting and being taken out. And two, there was a feeling of 'linking in' – connecting with the Divine or cosmic energy. Not only did it feel like being linked into a divine flow, but I felt more connected to everything. I just had to intend to connect to the purest divine good core (soul star) in another being and I'd usually feel a connection from it to my divine core. My breath would slow and there'd be a sense of more peace and comfort. It is a very 'true' or authentic feeling. I strived to always feel it. It felt, and still feels, utterly right! Today I also call this state being in healing mode or meditation mode.

This feeling and Peter's teachings made me see all beings – in spirit – like little suns. But most of these little suns are surrounded by clouds. Clouds which are our subconscious programs, beliefs, emotions and other confusions. We should, I felt, strive to sit inside the sun bit, the divine bit of our being, rather than the cloudy bit. And the brighter we make our light shine, the more we blast away the clouds around us, and the harder it becomes for the clouds to make us believe they are what we are.

I should mention though that when sitting down and

spending an hour or two on just handing-over stuff, I could get into a bit of a manic rush. My mind would come up with an ever-increasing number of thoughts, emotions, traits which needed handing over. Sometimes it all sped up and I pretty much tumbled over myself. I would also end up with what felt like clogged up energies. As if I was 'releasing' too much energy at once and they would all pile up at some energetic bottleneck, like a chakra. Then nothing much seemed to flow at all anymore. Was there a spiritual-physical limit to how much one could shift at any one time?

All this mindfulness also taught me to better control my emotions and thoughts. Disharmonious thoughts and emotions should be cut off as soon as one realizes them, so that they cannot dig themselves in. I did my best to do so. I learned that I can either 'give in' to an emotion or cut it off before it can get a hold of me. Naturally it's a skill that one improves at with the years. Strong emotions cannot always be prevented or stopped in their tracks; they started to pass quicker though then they used to. Writing this I get the image of a rodeo, some strong emotions will ride you (again and again), but with practice one gets more skilled in staying on the beastly emotions and not being thrown off – eventually even taming or subduing them. One might start with riding a bull and end up with a puppy dog.

'Handing over' meant that potentially I would have fewer emotions like a fear. As opposed to cutting off a fear and suppressing it, pushing it deeper down in my being, I 'released' them. (Even though for years it felt as if there was an inexhaustible well of negative emotions inside myself.) I also came to agree with Emmet Fox's understanding that on the path to becoming one's true divine self again – guilt (over things done incorrectly in the past) is an affront to one's divine self. Guilt usually includes a degree of hopelessness and resignation – whereas one should instead remember (and strengthen) one's awesome divine nature! One's incredible capacity to self-love, self-forgiveness and self-improvement – one should not wallow in guilt, but rather feel remorse and change one's behaviors now and in the future.

I became pretty much celibate for about a year. Apparently male ejaculation depletes you of your Life force, so being celibate might speed up your path to enlightenment. Considering that I (according to Peter) was responsible for the spiritual well-being and development of so many humans, I figured I would have to do everything possible to grow spiritually and fulfill my obligations as a 'catalyst'. So I stopped going out or meeting guys, and if masturbating (at all) I worked hard on achieving 'dry' orgasms and channeling the orgasmic energy up my spine. Doing so, I had read, would fuse them with cosmic energy above my crown chakra resulting in a 'cosmic' orgasm. But all I ever got was the feeling of a frustrated orgasm. I tried for a few months, and then finally gave up, for I had bigger things to worry about...

Chapter 3

The Frontline

After several months of intensive spiritual work I noticed my thoughts becoming more separate from me – they felt more like separate entities now. Some might call it 'voices in your head', but they were still within context. However, I could communicate with them. Before my thoughts were pretty predictable, but when communicating with these voices I sometimes got surprising answers. I took this as a budding psychic ability. I realized too that the thoughts in my head weren't necessarily just coming from inside me. I understood that when talking to the Divine, it would talk to us through our 'inner voice'; at least that is the way I had always heard devout believers describe it.

From what I had read and heard by then, to communicate with the Divine one just has to ask to be connected, evoke divine protection and all such communication is then safe and secure. To me it did not seem to be that easy. Sometimes I'd get enlightened and loving answers to questions, at other times they were rather strict and condemning. I believed the Divine was all-knowing; but when testing the communication e.g. during my studies (trying to get medical answers/facts) or during healing circles, I mostly got incorrect answers, compared to the medical books or what Peter would report.

Guilt, which was more or less an unknown feeling to me before joining Peter's circle, became a major player in my emotional body. Guilt about not knowing if I could ever be forgiven for prescribing potentially 'harmful' pharmaceuticals to patients, while still in training, to feeling guilty when flies met their death on a car's windscreen (I was travelling in – or even on the trucks that delivered the food I ate). It might all sound a bit loony, but I had just discovered my relation to everything, even the flies, one of which might be my dead grandmother... The guilt made me fear that any human, plant or animal I might harm (directly or indirectly) could constitute GBH or murder from a divine perspective. I even worried that a patient peeing out medication might damage the environment somehow. Most of my guilty pangs were very uncomfortable emotionally, mentally and physically, and they took up a lot of my time, which I could have spent more effectively studying or simply being content and happy. Obviously I did not want to wallow in guilt; as discussed I aimed to just feel remorse, change necessary behaviors and move on. It just seemed that in a lot of circumstances I had little choice about what to do. Just to get my medical degree e.g. I would have to learn, reiterate and practice loads of healing methods, which I considered wrong!

I acknowledged everything Peter said and scrutinized my life accordingly. If he mentioned people were not praying enough, I took it personally and prayed even more. Or when he spoke of greed I took that as a sign to reduce the only thing I still did plenty of, and that was to eat. I did have a high metabolism and was pretty much always hungry, still I prayed to be guided to eating the right amounts of food. As a result, for a week or so, I became super-aware about anything I ate. With this came the feeling as if Spirit was physically choking me (to teach me modesty) every time I ate without sufficiently strong bouts of hunger. It felt like some spiritual hand grabbed my windpipe and squeezed. Not enough to totally cut off the airflow, but definitely palpable, uncomfortable and scary. For a few days I went with it. As a result I went from about four large meals a day to one or two small ones. I was very hungry in the end and ended up eating a big portion of semolina, which in turn gave me acute gastritis. Peter did appear to manage to heal it the next day during a healing circle though. I ate normally again after that, was quite confused about the whole thing though and over the next two or three years there were more eating related crises.

At one point, when communicating with Spirit, I asked the big question, *What is the meaning of life?* The answer I got was *Happiness!* It seemed we should enjoy our lives and be happy without harming anyone/anything else in the process. What constituted harm to other beings though? That was a question that seemed far less easy to answer and seemed to require a great deal of evaluation. For example, I hoped that it was okay to eat plants at least. On the other hand I had heard about Buddhist teachings that humans should actually overcome any desires of the flesh, else they might not be able to stay in spirit (perhaps angels do not eat?), but will have to reincarnate again and again. Was I supposed to eat and enjoy it or overcome it?

Overall 'happiness' seemed quite the revolutionary concept to me though. Obviously I was looking for some happiness in my life already, but especially after listening to Peter I had started to assume that 'duty' was the big 'must', with an added big dose of 'redemption' on top of that. To have happiness as my main guiding light was new to me! But then again, as this had been an intuition in my head only, I was not sure for a good while longer if Peter's duty and redemption should be my guide, or happiness?

According to Peter we were the catalysts and should lead by example, and he sometimes did talk about the greed of modern industry and pollution. In my mind modern living became more and more disharmonious. It seemed totally fixated on human well-being and did not appear to consider the well-being of animals, plants, the planet etc. Should our group therefore not lead by example, return to an Amish way of living – self-suffi-cient and independent of electricity and fossil fuels? (I guess these kinds of thoughts are why some cults actually do end up giving up 'modern' living, move to the countryside and attempt to be self sufficient. Perhaps even try to totally overcome their bodies and commit mass-suicide?)

At one point I felt so guilty for leading a 'modern' life and supporting the exploitation of the planet, that I thought I'd have to walk to the woods somewhere and meditate for six years (like Buddha). I asked Spirit (or the voices in my head) if my thinking was correct. I prayed thoroughly to be connected to the highest source (or Heavenly Father, as I called it back then) and asked for heaps of perfect protections. A very stern, strict voice bellowed in my head, saying I should leave everything behind and go to the woods – NOW! I went to Peter for advice. I was obviously feeling extremely guilty already for doubting the divine (well, I assumed it had been) voice I had heard. Was I a coward, ruled by my subconscious for not going through with it? Peter did not say much, just performed some healing on me. I was a bit calmer after that. It seemed okay to stay and keep on living a 'normal' life – well that is to use some electricity, the telephone and such. It was yet another issue though that left me confused, and would come back to haunt me over the next few years.

One of the worst side effects of all this guilt was my doubt about whether I was still lovable or forgivable by the Divine. Were my divine helpers nauseated by the mere thought of me? I felt like the biggest loser and a thorough disappointment to God when failing to go through with some 'intuitions', like retreating to the woods. Perhaps we, Peter's circle, were staying to help the rest of humanity by staying in their midst? But if everything is spiritual and we were the catalyst, would the biggest shift not happen automatically, once we as a group would leave 'modern' life behind? Then there was my family, the flat I rented and friends, should/could I just break those bonds and contractual agreements? On the other hand I felt guilty for doubting Peter (who was leading an apparently normal life). If he was Jesus, would he not know best?

Every year, around Easter, the group would take a trip to Maui, Hawaii. The first time they went, after me joining, I did not go. The year after that, I felt it my duty. I prayed for the money, around £2500.00 (DEM 6000.00), a lot for me! As a student I received DEM 1000.00 per month from my father, which paid my rent and I earned about another DEM 1000.00 per month nursing. The majority of which went to paying for healing circles and other Peter seminars. Peter claimed that if we were ready, the money would come to us. Creation would provide! Well, no money came to me. Contrary to my beliefs, visualizations and prayers, I ended up having to go to the bank and take out a loan. It did not really feel right to take out such a loan, but I was stuck between a rock and a hard place. By not taking out the loan, would I not be affirming lack instead of abundance? Abundance was just being held up somehow. Peter claimed that going to Maui was imperative for our spiritual development, and had he not told us enough times that not listening to him could only lead to disaster!

The plane trip to Maui seemed such a waste of fuel and so polluting, why could we not just find a sacred place in Germany? Could one not connect to the Divine anywhere? Peter claimed that the energies on Maui were better and cleaner, but was it worth the 'sin' of air travel? When questioning Peter why we had to go so far, he just said that Mother Earth had given her blessing and that we'd do more good by being there. My old circle of friends had pretty much all run away, after my repeated attempts of trying to convert and proselytize them, and soon the 'group' was the only real social network left to me. In the shamanic circle one member saw us rowing in a boat, and every time someone dropped out of the boat, everybody else had to row even harder. That seemed clear enough instruction to not leave the group, even though to do so had not crossed my mind yet anyway.

Maui was quite the horrific experience. I could see it was a beautiful island, but spending 24/7 with Peter and the group made things very uncomfortably intense. Peter obviously claimed that that was a good thing. I had quite a few rebellious thoughts there. I was getting tired of watching one regression after another – telling us that we were eternal losers and utterly incompetent. I was also doing a lot of shamanic journeys; I figured it could only help to get as many heavenly beings and helpers onside as possible. For good measure and because of increasing mistrust in Peter, I had started to travel before going to sleep. I intended to travel into and sleep inside the energy of Heavenly Father (the purest I could think of). I am pretty certain I asked to be taken back into my body before waking up again (or when God saw fit).

Considering that when awake you simply imagine travelling back into your body (after journeying in spirit), I did not think it would be troublesome for God or my angels to send me back into my body when sleeping. Peter reprimand me in front of everyone though, saying that I shamanically journeyed too much (not sure how he knew, maybe I had told someone in the circle who had passed it on?). If one did travel outside his supervision (like in the Shamanic circle) one was supposedly in danger of losing bits of the soul. Really? I asked for divine protection; was Peter more capable than my angels or God? I was not feeling well, the fears, guilt and constant criticisms left me feeling more and more detached from my very being. I felt chock-a-block with negative energies. I literally felt detached, as if my consciousness was hovering somewhere outside my physical body rather than in its midst. Still I refused to attribute these feelings to 'incorrect' spiritual travel.

I kept on working on communicating with Spirit, but it continued to be problematical. Asking the same question I might get one answer one day and a different one the next. Wouldn't it be great to be able to give up studying and get all necessary medical knowledge from all-knowing divine Spirit? But asking any question, which required answers that were outside the scope of my (accumulated) knowledge, would usually just result in gibberish, affirming my concerns that I was still mostly just talking to myself. I believed it must be all that old, bad karma I must still be carrying and having to forgive myself and everybody else for, which screwed up my connection to the Divine. Any incongruities were obviously down to me and never Peter… Peter never offered me any one-to-one sessions. I was as blind as a bat regarding my third sight.

I spent my free time trying to heal the world, by meditating, praying, practicing forgiveness, doing shamanic journeys or trying regressions by myself. Once during such a regression, at home, I was 'told' I had been a doctor in Berlin. I asked for a name, address and birth date and was given some. (Peter had once asked a follower during a regression to look at her passport and read her name. She did, but it was never followed up.) Since it was my mission to convince Western medicine of spiritual concepts, as it seemed to play such an important role in most illnesses, I sent the given data to the German National Archives, enquiring if the person had actually existed. The enquiry came back as 'not known'. When asking Peter about this, he just shrugged his shoulders.

I had often started feeling quite 'stupid' in the group now, any critical question I would ask (usually this was not to question Peter, but to understand better) would be answered with a look and comment along the lines of, *Are you still not believing and trusting enough? Would your mind not constantly blabber and interfere, you'd find the answers in spirit yourself. You are too impatient.* Anything that went wrong, anything that I did not understand or seemingly did not make any sense, any inconsistency would be personalized and put down to me still being imperfect.

During one healing circle Peter commented that some of us are just here to overcome our bodies, another comment that threw me into turmoil. Certainly suicide would not be Christian. But would it not be the perfect way to prove that we were ready to leave the body – leave food, drink and sex behind? Had my suspicions not to eat and/or leave modern life behind been right all along? I was not certain. I prayed to the Divine to take me out of my body, if that was the most enlightened thing to do. Surely they had ways to arrange that, even at my age and general health, perhaps grow a brain aneurism and have it burst? Quick, efficient, pain free!

One thing Peter had said was that to protect ourselves against negative energies we just had to pray: *My energies are perfectly protected. I send all foreign energies back.* But what were foreign energies and how did I send them back? In case we were not sure whether something we prayed for was harmonious or not, we should just add – *if it is best for me and Creation* – to our prayers. I did put out a repeat request to always harmonize all my prayers and all my spiritual work as required.

At one stage I started to include Peter in my forgiveness prayers. I thought it might improve our relationship, help him cope at having to bring his energies 'down' to our level. I was instantly hit by feelings of terror, panic and guilt though. It was like being zapped with a punishing spiritual electric shock telling me, "How dare you include Peter in your forgiveness prayers. He is perfect!" Back then I thought there was something wrong with me. Now I think it is more likely Peter is a sociopathic guru. It took me years to overcome fears of him and the energies he seemed to associate with if I just thought about him critically.

One night I woke with a buzzing noise and menacing presence in my bedroom. Then something flew into my ear, there was a physical popping sensation and I felt paralyzed. I started praying, mainly to Peter. Soon a 'pop' followed and the energy left my ear again. Another weird occurrence was triggered on a day out with Peter. The whole group was out walking in the woods. I asked Peter about the book that I had read before joining, that was supposedly channeled by the Pleiadians. He claimed there was much danger in working with these entities, and that he had recently been attacked by some of them. He supposedly still had burn marks on his ankle. I asked to see the scar and he just gave me one of those punishing looks. The following night I had the most severe panic attacks, thinking these aliens would be coming for me as well. I spent the night in my neighbor's flat; unsurprisingly, the next morning there were no signs of an alien invasion in my flat though.

There was not much joy in my life back then. I did try to keep as happy as possible and not let my frustrations out on anybody else. One positive lesson I had learned on my spiritual path so far was that if I am grumpy it's not usually anybody else's fault. I don't need to be bitchy towards the world because I am having a bad day (or two, or three). But some of my prayers seemed to bear fruit. My main mode of transport was my bicycle. Before Peter, I would ride along the local streets any direction I wanted, be that with or against the one-way signs (they were wide enough!). It saved a lot of time. Now I felt guilty for going against the Highway Code. So I had prayed a few times for the laws to be changed and hey presto, a few months later, the one-way street sign had this new sign underneath stating 'Bicycles Free'.

I had also visited a Gospel workshop. Good fun. The choir-master was this nice, large lady. Supposedly her knee always played up when she had to stand for a few hours in a row, like when conducting during our workshop. When we went for a coffee she complained about her paining knee; she had already discussed and planned surgery for it with her GP, but I told her I'd be happy to try some laying-on-of-hands, to help it heal. She accepted, but admitted she did not really hold out much hope. I prayed to the angels and asked them for healing, to look through the 'evil' and confirm divine health behind it, to look at and confirm her divine, perfect, healthy knees. I am not sure if my hands got hot or anything. No immediate comments came from my friend.

I left early, before she or any of the other choir members got up. When I got home, I had an excited message from her on my voicemail. She said that after I left, she got up to go to the toilet and her knee pain had vanished. I met her again two years later. She was still pain free. When I did some laying-on-of-hands in the homecare with my elderly clients though, it did not usually get any immediate palpable results. I felt somewhat ashamed, even though I had not made any promises to them or created high expectations. It also left me with many questions as to why it would not have worked…

I tried my best to do as much spiritual work as I could at medical school. But it was difficult to concentrate and stay attuned to divine energies there. I felt it was more important to meditate, pray and do other spiritual work rather than study. Besides working in homecare nursing, all my spiritual work efforts and Peter's courses, there was not much time and much less energy left to study anyway. In most medical courses I felt even more stupid than at Peter's; rightly so. I felt under a lot of pressure, after all 2012 was not all that far off and I felt guilty enough even just still being in my body.

I was never a great fan of expending energy on undertakings that had no real long-term value to me either. Now why should I spend a lot of time and energy studying medical information and skills which, after all, according to Peter, were disharmonious anyway? I would have to learn it all, to then forget about it all as quickly as possible again, and to learn a whole new skill set of healing, naturopathy and so on. Furthermore I did not really improve my situation by gathering all my courage and attempting to talk about spiritual healing with some of my lecturers. It might have been more impressive had I been a medical prodigy, but to start criticizing as some rather mediocre student, who did not really know enough yet about either medicine or spiritual healing, was causing me to become an irritant.

Looking back I forgive myself; I was under a lot of pressure. I should have just done my studies and kept a low profile until I might have been in a position where I could convincingly effect change. I could have just done taciturn spiritual work. As it was, I tried to do so some spiritual work, but it was hard to while in a hospital environment. Just thinking about healing seemed to trigger all sorts of nasty stuff and I would feel like an utter fool and charlatan. I had not experienced many incredible spiritual healing results yet, but I felt in my heart that spiritual healing is real and can be incredible! It was strange too that in a hospital my doubts felt near insurmountable, but at home I did not have them.

In two years with Peter's circle, there was only one indirect compliment, for all my efforts, from Peter. At one healing circle Peter asked different members how often they used the forgiveness tool each day. Peter's future wife and favorite said she used the tool about five times a week. He then asked me, with a knowing look, how often I used the forgiveness prayer, and I was allowed to tell that I did 'practice forgiveness + hand over' several hundred times a day. My memory could be warped on this, but if I remember correctly most of Peter's attentions (and eventual praise) were usually spent on female and the more affluent members!

As Peter supposedly read everyone's mind, communication with him was often cryptic. I often felt as if fully verbalizing an issue or question would be to doubt his 'mind reading' abilities. It is hard to remember exactly when and how he ever showed signs or proof that he could read people's minds, or how much I just interpreted into his comments and behaviors. As an example, when my bicycle got stolen I went to his practice for advice. He 'had a look' and told me that it had been taken to the gypsy travelers' camp. I gathered all my courage and went to retrieve it. I got there as quick as I could but did not find it. When I told Peter that I was not successful he simply said that I got there "too late".

Then during my summer holiday away, while meditating, I was told that I had been Moses. I was elated at first, a celebrity pre-incarnation! When I got back I asked Peter, "Is it true?" He confirmed it! Two months later though, he was identified as Moses during a past life regression in front of the group and I was confused (again!). Skeptics say that the reason why so many regressed people see themselves as some historic celebrity is they probably feel so ordinary in this life that they try to make themselves feel important by imagining themselves as Napoleon, Cleopatra, Alexander the Great and so on. There might be some truth in this, but I have to say that, back then, compared to constant extreme guilt pressures in the circle, the possible claim to fame for having been one of Jesus' disciples really was immaterial. It did tickle my ego a bit, admittedly, but I was also very much aware that no one would believe me anyway. I'd just alienate myself more from the outside world. Had I gone around claiming to have been Moses I would possibly have ended up in a psychiatric ward.

Peter made us very aware that often every little detail had a meaning and would be 'telling' about a person's state of mind, e.g. the colors they would chose when they dressed could tell you if they were confident, happy or confused. He claimed that wearing the color combination of red and black showed highest degrees of confusion – is that why the Devil and Dracula are often depicted with such colored costumes? This extended to the things one attracted, seemingly coincidentally. Well, when we were on Maui, when picking up our rental cars at the airport, everybody's cars were white, except for his. His was more menacing, larger than anyone else's and black. That same trip he kept on telling us that we had to stick together. If people wanted to split into smaller groups and see different sights that was very much discouraged. The same rule did not seem to apply to him though. He would speed ahead and also stay in a separate compound.

There was also the issue of all his wives. From what I learned he had been divorced twice already. One of his ex-wives was a member of the group. Another lover of his was one of my best friends in the group. She had very developed psychic abilities and according to regressions was formerly Mary Magdalene. She had been his lover for a year or two. She had left her husband and two kids for him! Yet he had cheated on her with another woman in the group, who ended up being his third wife. I.e. on the previous Maui trip he had shared his bedroom with my friend, but she caught him sneaking to the other woman's room in the middle of the night. These somewhat shady morals were once explained by him as having been dictated by subconscious forces. In other words he just behaved badly, so that his energy would be lowered and we could bear being around him or some such.

Were we supposed to do what the subconscious forces wanted us to do or behave harmoniously? I thought we were supposed to be catalysts and paragons of excellence in our behaviors. It seemed though that whenever Peter acted suspiciously, he would make it look as if it was to our benefit. He would imply that it was simply his intention to trigger a subconscious reaction in us, and that it would then be easier for him to remove these energies from us. I believed him back then, but in retrospect that argument was pathetic. My healing work now seems to function just fine without aggravating my clients.

Peter told us that one could tell if someone was in subconscious or conscious mode by looking into their eyes. The more lifeless and dull the eyes, the more one is stuck in some subconscious program, and the brighter and shinier the eyes, the more conscious one is. When I looked into the mirror, most times, my eyes looked very dull! There seemed to be something else occupying (at least parts of) my body. When I relaxed the control over my facial muscles, they would somehow slip into somewhat of a devilish grimace; it took me years to get rid of it. I was not levitating or spinning my head like scenes from *The Exorcist* though, plus I could control my actions and (verbal) communications.

I continued with my frequent shamanic journeying – I trusted Heavenly Father more than Peter now. I had grown increasingly unsure of Peter. The initial blaming of any incongruities (in observations and his teachings and behavior) on myself and my karma was giving way to a more critical view. I now allowed my mind to consider that he might make mistakes.

Another concept I was pondering was 'unconditional love'. What was divine unconditional love? Does unconditional love imply total forgiveness? I was still at a loss trying to imagine that I should emotionally love a mass-murderer for example. That I should go and embrace such a being or tell them I love him/her. I believed that love is not necessarily all cuddly and guaranteed to be pain free. If one does an intervention and tells the addict what harm they have done – it is probably going to hurt. Were 'tough love' and forgiveness one and the same thing? Considering the time restraints (just 16 more years until the end of the world) and the major sins that humanity apparently conducted, a bit of tough love seemed almost unavoidable. But how tough does tough love get? There was another problem. How do unconditional love and Karma work together? Are we supposed to love and forgive or 'teach' perpetrators a lesson and make them taste their own medicine? I figured that sounded like revenge. Or was it not revenge, if it was free from anger? I figured I better leave Karma to the Divine to dish out. Could one even 'dish out' Karma to anyone without creating more Karma for oneself?

I believed our group was more knowledgeable and doing a great deal more good than the average person. Regardless, some members of the group were being picked on constantly. Shortcomings were put on display and they featured in a lot of regressions as the incurable losers. It seemed sadistic. Others were apparent favorites – and thinking back, again, most of them seemed to be amongst the more affluent members of the group.

Having performed the forgiveness prayer tens-of-thousands

of times by now, something clicked inside me. Since joining the circle, I had started to see myself as a major, almost despicable sinner – but was I really that bad? I had had fights with my sister when I was small, was not always the nicest son to my mum during puberty, occasionally had grumpy days, but overall I always had been a 'nice' human being. If I really had been such a bad human in prior incarnations and accumulated that much bad karma – would I not have been an utter bastard up to the time I joined the group? Tortured little animals while a child? (I have to admit I did stomp a few ants and once locked a wasp in a half-full Fanta can to drown. I am not proud of it, but I hardly think it shows dictator or mass murderer potential.) When Peter claimed that every shortcoming we saw in a regression was to be taken personally, by each member of the group – maybe he was going a little too far?

I was fed up with all the guilt and suffering, but I kept on going. The whole reincarnation teachings became more and more questionable. I could not really put my finger on it yet, but it made less sense to me and just seemed sadistic. Why would an all-loving God/Creator devise such a system? Supposedly we were much more enlightened and knew about all the spiritual laws in between lives – but then we would enter another embryo and forget all about these spiritual laws again. We always had to pretty much start from zero, which usually resulted in years of making all the same mistakes again, rather an ineffective and stupid system.

On one hand I was supposed to realize/understand/believe that I was a son of God/Creation – made from his/her flesh and hence had all his/her potential and abilities – on the other hand I was supposed to believe that, regardless of this, we apparently were all abject failures? How an utter unconditionally loving, perfect divine individualized spirit could be so incompetent that he/she/it could not, according to Peter, heal, learn and improve for millennia, across endless lives, on different planets; it all felt less and less probable to me. Still, I had not cracked that nut yet – and was a slave to reincarnation and Karma fears for another year or so.

The last big incident that occurred, during my time with Peter, was because of another regression I performed myself at home. During said regression I was told, by a very stern and loud voice, that I had been Josef Mengele: the most infamous doctor in Auschwitz, responsible for selecting Jews for the gas chambers or as forced laborers. He had also conducted many (often gruesome) experiments on e.g. identical twins. As soon as I was told this, I felt a hundred tons of 'guilt bricks' rain down on me. I prayed for forgiveness, still the crushing sensation remained. I tried to telepathically communicate with Peter to verify this revelation. It was near impossible to stay calm and objective, so I got both yes and no answers. I decided to consult him in person. When I got to his practice, he was with a client, appeared annoyed and queried why I was there. I just asked, "Is it true what I have just been told?" He replied, "Yes, but why do you worry, this is another life?" How could I ever make up for all these deaths? Would I have to save millions of lives as a doctor?

I contemplated suicide. Maybe by showing that I could overcome my body I could strike Karma off the record. I grabbed Peter alone after the next healing circle and asked him specifically, "Are you sure it is true, Peter?" "What?" was his reply. "That I was Mengele?" Peter laughed, "Nonsense, who ever told you that?" To say I was confused would be an understatement. Either he had not 'read my mind' properly or he had knowingly left me with the false belief that I was Mengele. If the latter was true, it had gone beyond 'teaching me a lesson' and was an act of pure cruelty.

I went to the library and learned that researchers had exhumed Mengele's remains. He died in 1979 somewhere in South America. Genetic testing identified Mengele, with more than 99% accuracy. As I was born in 1971 it seemed highly unlikely I could ever have been Mengele. But without the genetic tests being 100% accurate, Mengele could have died before 1971, and I was frequently attacked by the fear that I might have been him. In those moments my mind came up with the most paranoid parallels. I was studying to become a doctor and my father was greatly interested in twin studies (in conjunction with his work as a psychologist). Through my father I had had a fleeting interest in the topic. Had I not, at least for a few ignorant years, not objected to animal testing, could I not have taken the next step to human testing, such as Mengele did? Today I'd resolutely say, "No!" Back then, having been worn down by Peter's continuous accusations, I was not all that sure. It almost appeared a relief to just admit to all the guilt that was heaved upon us; perhaps that was the quickest way to get rid of it and make the emotional, mental and spiritual pains stop?

I mustered the last scraps of resolve left in me and decided not to let this matter rest. At the next Easter Circle, Peter reiterated that he had a clear channel to the highest divine ranks. We were asked to listen to him and follow his instructions without a shred of doubt or a second's hesitation. We allegedly were in crucial times. All these orders prompted me to ask him a simple question, *What if our teacher makes a mistake?* In return he screamed at me (in front of everyone) that this question was not permissible! I got up and left. I did not go back. I went from entertaining thoughts of *Peter might make mistakes*, to *Peter might be evil!*

Chapter 4

Going AWOL

After my time in the cult I read a few books about cults, cult mechanisms and their leaders. Looking at the common personality traits of cult leaders, anger when questioned is very typical. Peter told us we were one of the few 'true' healing and spiritual development groups on this planet. My ego had been flattered by this elitist notion – there was not much else to feel good about. Peter claimed that much of the esoteric scene just triggered positive subconscious reactions. People participate and walk out of them feeling good, but they do not actually change themselves for the better or for the greater good. He would usually refer to such seminars as 'fluff'. People failed to confront their sordid pasts. Only suffering through these again seemed to promise forgiveness.

With this logic Peter generally justified the sadistic methods he used. From what I read, most people ending up in cults get abused spiritually, mentally, emotionally and/or physically. And some of the examples I read were worse than mine; at least I had not been physically raped and put to slave labor. I am sure that the majority of those cult members bear such abuses in the distorted faith that all their suffering is necessary.

Peter also frequently discredited other esoteric personalities. For example he claimed that Barbara Brennan's drawings weren't all correct and Louise Hay cannot heal and has ghostwriters writing her books. He made himself out as the only true, trustworthy source. In my cult research this appears to be another of the very common techniques to create dependency. I am aware that I too criticize plenty of things I have encountered in the esoteric scene. I do not think that critique is per se 'bad'; it is often required for things to get moving and improve. Peter's way of doing so was rather different though. He claimed he was the Son of God. He made his followers believe that he was infallible and that they did not have to read any other literature. Free thought was mostly stifled by burying his disciples under tons of guilt.

A potential sign that one has been buried under a ton of guilt or responsibility, or else radicalized, is that you lose your sense of humor. I definitely had lost most of mine during my 'Peter' years. Sure, Peter gave us the prospect of eternal life too. You would think that with an eternity at hand, to dissolve all your problems, you could relax, but then we supposedly had to do it all in this life – or else! Furthermore plenty of other cults predict the end of the world or that following the leader is the only hope of salvation. Commonly, major tools of control are fear, guilt and shame – looks as if Peter's group has no monopoly here.

I spoke to advisors about cult affairs, both from the Church, psychotherapists and state institutions. There are hundreds of Jesuses out there and I am sure they all have a very good explanation as to why they are the only and true reincarnation. Scientology founder Ron Hubbard supposedly claimed to have been Buddha too. Note to self, very entertaining TV viewing might be 'mud wrestling between cult leaders', after a heated debate of: *"I was Jesus!" "No, I was Jesus." "You lying son of a ****, I was Jesus and I have been clearly identified as such in regression." "Ha, I have been identified too, plus my organization is worldwide, you are only in one single city. Clearly I have the backing of the highest heavenly echelons…"*

Looking back, identifying Peter as Jesus by looking into his eyes was not a very scientific or careful method of recognizing someone across lifetimes. In comparison, confirming a child as the reincarnation of the Dalai Lama, it has to be born under predicted star constellations and then has to go through rigorous testing before being accepted as such. I doubt Peter's victims of regression applied anything but wishful thinking (and mental coercion) when identifying him.

If someone I know well died today, had a transplant card and their eyeballs were transplanted into another human being, I doubt I'd recognize their eyes on anybody else. In Peter's group those undergoing regression always identified Peter with such vehemence though – I never doubted them. Peter always accepted these identifications too – no hesitation whatsoever.

To anyone involved with Peter's group (or thinking of joining), I recommend reading up on Mind Control and Cults. Alternatively you can contact specialists for advice, such as government or cult advisors. A simple Internet search can reveal a lot. The same applies if you suspect that you might have been brainwashed, suspect that a group you are interested in might be a cult or if you suspect that a loved one might be involved with a cult. I am pretty confident that, had I done my research into cult dynamics and psychology earlier, I could have spared myself emotional and psychological problems. Sure, I have learned from my experiences and problems, but I am certain that there are plenty of other, less masochistic ways to learn the same lessons.

Peter's circle can be classed as a destructive cult: a cult where Peter is the self-proclaimed Master, he exercises mind-control and manipulates his followers and is provided with a very good income. Back in 1995/96 Peter's hourly rate was DEM 100.00. He tended to see up to 3–4 people at the same time, in different rooms (i.e. one might pay for a one-on-one session with him, but end up lying on a couch, alone in a room, receiving distant healing). Peter claimed it was easy for him to treat more than one person at a time, as he was (like God) omnipotent. Healing Circle attendance was charged at DEM 100.00 per person too, and there were up to 30 people there per two-hour session. I am not aware that he ever did any 'free' work, as a lot of healers in the UK do, or like Harry Edwards, who worked on a donation basis. To be fair, after a while I enquired about a potential student discount and was granted one. I had to ask myself though!

Peter justified his prices by saying that people expect to pay for a service and that the healing would not be accepted and valued enough if no fee were levied. I agree that healers should have the option to charge – they are, if nothing else, giving their time! Especially if healers work full-time! Considering that there are plenty of anecdotes about distant healing working on people, who weren't even aware of it, Peter's argument that healing would not really work, unless paid for, could be seen as an oversimplification though. He once explained how a client had paid him double his fee for a particularly well-received session – Peter could then see that the healing effect doubled instantly. Whereas I cannot say that that is impossible, it makes little sense. If actual healings worked on such mechanisms, they would be nothing more than a placebo. I am confident though that healing is not just a placebo, but an actual energetic process, regardless if someone believes in it or not.

I never saw Peter's actual home. Supposedly he lived in one of Hamburg's most affluent, riparian suburbs. Any kind of charitable work was paid for by the group. Members were urged to pack Christmas care packets for the poor in Hamburg, for example. There was a once-weekly soup kitchen too, which as far as I am aware was funded through donations. After about six months in the circle two 'charities' were founded (Peter being their director) and the entrance fees for the weekend seminars (DEM 50.00pp) were donated to them. This source of income must have made up the smallest bit of his general income though. He may have even charged a fee to those charities for his lecturing services.

No real mention was ever made about Peter's past either. He practiced healing without any qualifications; he wasn't a Doctor or Naturopath, as was actually required by German law back then. After some time members and patients had to sign a declaration of indemnity against any possible physical, mental or emotional damages sustained during treatment or membership. His lack of qualifications did not seem to bother anyone;

obviously his work was far too important and time-consuming to fret about formalities. Considering that he claimed to be connected to 'all knowledge' though, qualifying as a Naturopath should have been a walk in the park for him, right?

The healings I witnessed weren't impressive, certainly nothing that would match the miracles performed by Jesus, as described in the Bible. Any lack of healing was simply explained away as a very complex subconscious problem which had the backing of so many 'past lives' problems that it would need a long time to heal. In one meeting Peter explained that he was here to help us, and that he could just as well make an excellent living by getting rid of people's warts in one session (a common feat, said to be accomplished by herbal women and still quite normal in the German countryside), but that he would be sticking to his divine strenuous duty of leading us. I told him about my warts and asked for his healing. Despite two years of 'treatment' they still remained.

Retrospectively not all my problems back then necessarily came through Peter though. I can e.g. still experience some negative emotions when visiting my family in Germany. For years I got eating related problems just before travelling, like feeling guilty about consuming meat. It used to be a 'joy' for my mum when every Christmas I would come home with new dietary requirements. Now that I understand these patterns, I ignore these feelings and eat as normal. The funny eating ideas simply vanish a few days later. I doubt that Peter could still affect me today, so there must be other forces at work...

We were catering to Peter's expectations. I refer to the often publicized phenomenon from America, where suddenly a large number of patients start to believe they have been abducted by aliens or molested by relatives as children. This may be a self-induced phenomenon where patients subconsciously try to fulfill what they think the therapist expects. I do strongly feel that the setup with Peter would have worked in exactly the same way –

the pressure to comply with his expectations would possibly have been even higher, considering that we believed that poor Jesus had to come back down from paradise to help us because we were just too stupid and renitent to get it.

I do not have any proof that the regressions performed weren't true, but no proof was delivered by Peter that they were either! Just as with everything else initiated by him – they were unquestionable. I believe there was a good chance that those regressed started seeing things they believed they were expected to see, not factual events. There are other theories as to where regressive information might originate from too. One theory says that all historic experiences, even each individual's, is stored in the 'Zero Point Field', like a life movie, including thoughts, emotions and all sensations. So even if actual events were viewed, there is no telling if they were indeed experiences from the regressees' past lives or information picked up from the Zero Point Field, and in fact someone else's experiences. Furthermore most people will have seen countless movies and/or read plenty of stories to feed their subconscious and imagination.

I am no quantum physicist and trustingly just reiterate what I have read, especially in *The Field* by Lynne McTaggart. Supposedly the Zero Point Field is an energy field connecting everything, animate or inanimate, and which (potentially) stores information about all events. The Zero Point Field is so-called because even at the absolute zero point (at 0° C in a vacuum) some energy can still be measured. This energy is ubiquitous, and all permeating. It can be depicted in waves, and waves supposedly have near infinite ability to store information. Lynne's book could just be pseudoscientific; I did have an experimental physics professor as a client though, who was generally interested in spiritual matters too. When chatting with him I mentioned her book. It turned out that he had read it and endorsed it.

Two regressions stick in my mind, both performed by my

'Mariy Magdalene' friend, who I do not think would have consciously 'faked' a regression. One was about an archangel coming into a church and warning the priests and their congregation that, if they did not look after the poor, hungry and helpless, sell their greedily acquired possessions, he would be back to destroy the church and its sinners. Supposedly the priests chose to hide the churches' treasures instead of feeding the poor. Most of the congregation kept their riches too. There is no fooling an archangel though, so when he returned, he made the church roof collapse on all present, just as he had warned. Only those who had followed his instructions were miraculously saved.

Now my friend had studied religion as a primary school teacher. Years after, I skimmed through the Bible, a rare thing for me, and found that exact story. It could easily have been that my friend had read the story, forgotten about it and relived it as a regression with Peter. The question would just be if and how Peter could know that she had read the story? Peter tended to (very quickly) guide the individuals into regression by giving them a few facts to get them where, he thought, they should be. In this case something like, *Now go back into the life and time when you sit at mass and an Archangel appears in front of the altar.*

In another regression on Maui, Peter regressed my friend to a life where she was part of a Hawaiian tribe and Peter was their shaman. She was given a task by him, during which she died because she did not perform it to the letter. She had been given the task to bring offerings up to the edge of the volcanic crater. The volcano had rumbled and seemed on the edge of erupting – it needed to be appeased with these offerings. The shaman (Peter) had warned her not to go all the way to the edge of the crater, but put the offerings down a few yards away. My friend wanted to show extra devotion though, walked all the way to the edge, the earth shook and she fell into the crater, perishing.

The next day we travelled to the other side of the island, which had an indigenous history museum with a model historic village. My friend was amazed. She told me afterwards that the huts at the museum looked exactly like she had seen her village in the regression the day before. She did not believe to ever have seen a native village like it before. They were wooden huts with I believe palm leaf roofs. I did not think they were too special and unique – one could easily have learned a mind template from an old Pacific WWII movie.

The memory, it seems, can be mystical and powerful. I once tried to access cosmic all-knowing at an elderly patient's house. The patient was bedridden, clinically depressed and at times aggressive. I asked 'Spirit' if there was an herb she could take. The voice in my head replied, "St. John's Wort." I looked it up at home and it turned out to be an herbal antidepressant, result! I suggested it to the patient's family. Their physician did not think that adding St. John's Wort to her regular medications could do any harm, so it was. It did not really make any apparent difference to her behavior though. Still, it was one of the rare occasions where the 'voices' seemed to give me usable information. Years later I reread a favorite children's book of mine. It mentioned St. John's Wort as an antidepressant. Did that mean that I had just remembered something I read 20 years prior?

Peter did not forbid us from praying to the Divine directly, but mentioned several times that he was there for us 24/7 for any kind of spiritual difficulties and needs. And since I did not want to question his abilities, he was my first point of call in any spiritual emergency for a good while. Since I very much doubt his spiritual purity or that he worked with Ultimate Good powers, I doubt that going via him linked me to Ultimate Good powers. As to Peter sometimes having a strong warm and apparently loving energy emanating from him – my explanation for this is that it was an illusion. According to the Bible the devil is but a fallen angel   perhaps Peter could fake 'Good'? Or was it projected onto him by his disciples' erroneous (holy) beliefs about him?

Another typical cult setup was a double standard of practices exercised by the leader and the followers. Peter was able to carry on with a handful of women and go along with the 'subconscious flow' – a taboo to be avoided by his followers. It was generally agreed that if Peter had come down to Earth without these 'failings', we as mere humans would not have been able to stay in his presence. But would this not also mean that his teachings might still be 'infiltrated' by the 'evil' subconscious programs as well? Yet neither he nor his teachings were allowed to be critically examined! And whereas it was perfectly alright for him, for us to give into 'subconscious temptation' was seen as detrimental to the salvation of humanity, leading to the end of this world…

Isolating members from the rest of the world to create a 'them and us' mentality is another common cult practice. It is desired for members to think that the outside world is the enemy. Cult members actually feel strengthened in their beliefs if criticized by non-group members. This was certainly the case for me. Any critique was interpreted as the other person's truth-resisting-subconscious. Peter told us that if a lesser-developed spiritual being encountered a higher-developed one, it would not be able to stand its presence and run away. If a group of lesser-developed beings encountered a more enlightened person, they would turn into a mob and try to kill the more enlightened human. According to him persecution against religious groups was based on this programming. So every person who had turned away annoyed, when I tried to 'convert' them, was just put in the 'running away' category.

Nowadays I see plenty of people that live or work happily together regardless of faith. The key is tolerance. If one does try to enlighten others, sharing information that adds to their current worldview or uncover illogical ideas in their beliefs, one has to be sensitive. Twisting people's arms, when it comes to questions of faith, can easily just backfire. I do personally feel that, being a strong believer, I frequently trigger people's resistances. There might still be places on this planet where religious fervor and disagreements of faith (or lack thereof) can become violent, but we, as Peter's group, were sat in Hamburg, Germany. The chances of a stoning mob of atheists, storming his practice or chasing any of us down some dark alley were relatively slim.

Regarding the power of the subconscious, I was never more a slave of negative emotions, guilt and fear than during my time in the group. Scared about being greedy, I had sorted out six bin bags of clothing for charity. Who needed the joy of fashion and variation when the end of humanity was near and the divide between the classes was increasing! I did regret this later, as I loved my clothes; and considering that Peter had a wonderful collection of expensive cashmere sweaters, my sacrifice seemed a bit pointless. Any positive development was accredited to Peter and his divine influence, but any negative development was blamed on the non-dedication of the group. When the 'cancer-lady's' health got worse, we were all responsible, due to our lack of sufficient spiritual work.

I can easily identify other cult traits such as Peter's tendencies to preach in a way that created double binds. Conflicting teachings applied to the same situation and which made me freeze up in indecision. Not knowing what to do, the only solution was Peter. It was made very clear that without Peter we would be lost. According to him, if we failed in this life, we would have to go through millennia of tending sheep on a lonely mountaintop somewhere, before we would be allowed to reunite with him and his guidance. Not only would we forsake him and ourselves, but we would also jeopardize the other group's members' chances of salvation. Not to mention that we would condemn the rest of humanity.

In my opinion Peter's group shows multiple signs of being a destructive cult. For me personally, my membership did not just cost me two years of my life, but was at least partly responsible for a lot of suffering in the following years too. At least another ten years, where I had to fight depression, extreme fatigue and exhaustion and self-esteem issues. For years I'd wake up totally distraught and shattered every morning and frequently feared that I might be forsaken by the Divine. If Peter's teachings were true, would the Divine not be cross with me for ignoring its true son?

On the other hand my cult experience has made me stronger, and definitely less naïve and gullible. It has taught me the potential ill effects of just teaching esoteric, spiritual knowledge that has not been double-checked or which one consciously uses to control and manipulate people for one's own benefit. I have learned that even if something has a pretty, apparently holy façade, it does not necessarily mean that the holiness extends beyond its façade. I know now that psychic abilities are not necessarily proof of good character, as I had initially assumed. It has taught me to ask for 24/7 spiritual protections, and I ask Ultimate Good to be the only judge of what energies are allowed to pass these barriers.

Perhaps the pressure exerted on us through Peter got me to practice my mental and spiritual skills? Control my emotions and thoughts? I cannot say for sure that without Peter's pressures I would have developed as quickly and efficiently as I believe I have. Generally I feel that guilt and fear are poor teachers though! I choose to believe that I am pretty dedicated to being a good human and healer in all I do, and would be too not having gone through Peter's school of guilt. Not to forget that I had developed a passion for becoming a healer before I even met Peter.

I would not wish my experiences on anyone, and feel for those that remain or have joined Peter's circle since my departure. I am aware that a current member of Peter's group might just interpret the above as the subconscious ranting of some ex-member who just did not have the strength to walk Peter's path of the righteous. However, they might one day discover similar feelings and discrepancy as I have experienced, which got me out in the end. My heart and love is with them. I am not saying that all Peter is preaching is wrong – it is specifically this mixture of truths with exaggerated or incorrect teachings which seem so dangerous, and certain techniques he uses are textbook brainwashing.

One such technique involved meditating before he started to lecture. Meditation supposedly lowers your rational thinking; it can make you more open to manipulation. Peter mixed commonplace spiritual truth with questionable facts, such as him having been Jesus, and spiced them up with humongous amounts of guilt. By claiming he was Jesus and that our group was one of just a handful – with no mention of where to find the others – an increasing dependency was created.

Furthermore Peter propagated mantra meditation. Some say that when we pray we talk to the Divine, but when we meditate we listen to the Divine! Using a mantra could be seen as an attempt to drum out any 'true' divine intuition. The guru's teachings should remain the only input. We were being 'scared' into meditating twice daily. Any meditation missed would be like a missing stone when building a bridge. Just a handful of stones missing and collapse was a real threat, which would result in having to start all over again.

Today I believe that this is grossly exaggerated. Meditation is a spiritual shower, getting rid of energetic muck, but it also helps to be more receptive to healings and potential receipt of other Divine input. If one does not shower (physically) every day one might start to smell, even start to look dirty – one might need a good bath and soak to get rid of the dirt, plenty of soap and a few shower rinses to smell nice again – but missing a shower there and then won't usually end in irreparable body odor or discolored skin for the rest of your life!

Stereotypically most people look down on cult members. Having been brainwashed often comes with the label of having been somewhat stupid (to have believed in such nonsense teachings), feebleminded or needy. Most people will likely believe that it could not happen to them. Just about all cults target intelligent middle and upper class individuals though. They are seen as more useful to the group. They'll have better connections and usually greater disposable income than working-class individuals. There are not just spiritual cults but also political, psychotherapeutic or family cults to name a few. Unless one has actually met and experienced a charismatic sociopath, it's hard to imagine that someone can quite effortlessly circumvent a healthy individual's protective mind barriers without triggering any warning bells.

Unless one has had psychological, psychotherapeutic training, is a cult specialist or brainwashing techniques expert, or been on the receiving end of a charismatic sociopath, it is hard to spot them. You might think that you are immune because you are content and happy. But there are not many humans who are free of all desires which a guru could exploit. Moreover, is it not a basic quality of the human spirit to continuously be curious, seek, search and discover? Most people have some unanswered questions about life and its meaning. Peter's group was a good representation of the above. The members were mostly profes-sional, middle or upper middle class. Pretty much all were there because they wanted to do good. It was that openhearted attitude and belief in 'good' that made them fall for Peter – not because they were stupid.

I was never told to cut all ties to my family, but in time it was indirectly becoming more difficult to see them. For one I was scared to take the train home – fossil fuel – expenditure and all those crushed flies on the locomotive's windscreen. Once I got there, I insisted on organic food. My mum tried to accommodate me and claimed that all the vegetarian fare she prepared for me was organic. She did not take me too seriously though. The crisis I went through, when I found the Christmas meal's carrot packaging in the bin – and they weren't organic… Plus watching my family eating meat was pretty gruesome. Considering reincarnation, they might as well be eating some dead relative. I also believed that if they did not overcome their carnivore habits, they would probably end up as farm animals. I worried about them ending up like that! I was worried about my family, and they were worried about me – as our views were far apart though, we got into some pretty nasty arguments.

From what I last heard, in 2011, Peter's group continues. Some people have left; others have joined. I feel sorry for them. Initially I beat myself up for actually having stayed as long as I did; today I pat myself on the back for having gotten out that quickly. I credit my stubbornness, never resting mind and mostly a lot of help from my true guides and helpers. Peter has since established a publishing house and has brought out children's books, "to teach them to read". I did not have any problems learning how to read and write, back in my days, with government issued books.

I have fully forgiven myself and Peter for all the harm that has come to me. I believe we pre-choose our earthly experiences, and having pre-chosen those cult experiences I have no one else to blame but myself. I have learned to love and forgive myself for all pre-chosen suffering! But even having forgiven myself and Peter – had I the feeling that he would be attacking me again somehow – I would have no qualms to pray for his banishment or a strong rap over his spiritual knuckles. If to heal such an attack some pain would be irrefutable, I would rather he gets it than me!

Chapter 5

Army of One

Leaving the cult did not mean leaving all illogical teachings behind, at least not from one day to the next. It just meant the long and arduous process of sorting out which of Peter's teachings were true and which were to be discarded, altered or appended. I was still sold on the idea that the best way to achieve happiness was to seek enlightenment by striving for perfection. I believed enlightenment would be a very distinct event, like some Divine Power switching on a light. Suddenly all would be 'one' and I'd effortlessly and simultaneously know everything and be everywhere at once.

Today I think it is a process. If we truly seek to improve and rediscover our divine selves, we can also realize this bit by bit, have a little epiphany every day, week or month. Today I am just content to be healthy, safe and happy, any 'special effects' like psychic abilities etc. are nice if and when they happen, but I am not desperate for them anymore.

I was trying to shake off the shackles of Peter's guilt and responsibility constructs, but went the opposite direction for a while longer. I figured that Peter telling us we are the catalysts of this day and age was hokum. If Divinity, and with it 'truth', is in everybody and everything, it would be everybody's responsibility to (re)discover this for themselves. One could help and support, but why should I be responsible for what others did? I still believed in Karma, but I stopped short to take on the responsibility for all aggression, poverty, ignorance etc. I saw in the world.

I realized that by following Peter's teachings to the letter and believing the outside to be the mirror image of my inside I had practically made myself the middle of the Universe. A bit presumptuous perhaps? The blinkers fell off my eyes. Everybody and everything was conscious and thinking, feeling and believing, hence the state of the outside world was everybody's responsibility! Perhaps the accumulated anger of thousands of individuals can trigger a war? I had withdrawn my bit in this game though, as I had forgiven myself for the anger inside and asked for it to be removed. The same applied to poverty, injustice, illnesses, ageing, and so on.

I could only change so much by changing my thinking. In my heart I was now only affirming the true Divine and 'good' nature of everything and everybody. Sometimes some 'bad' illusions still sucked me in, but whenever I could, I reminded myself that the disharmonious illusions in the outside were only ever temporary. And when I had even more time and energy, I would meditate for as long as it took to 'feel' more of the goodness in everything.

Peter had not been the only one guilty of warping the 'mirror' teachings. I had previously succumbed to Barbara Brennan's image of our world being a hologram as well. She had written that our world is like a hologram; hence everything is contained in everything. If we become lighter and more colorful, supposedly the whole world becomes lighter and more colorful. Or, in turn, if we become more confused and dark, the whole picture becomes darker. There might be some truth to all of this, but it is a question of proportions. In my guilt-twisted mind I believed myself a major player. Now I started to see myself as one of over six billion influencing parts. Not only that, but I realized that if Earth is a hologram, then the whole of Creation – all of the universes, galaxies would be one hologram.

Cause and effect of my actions on things outside my immediate range were infinitesimal, so even if I shone with 10,000 watts, the overall brightening effect on the Milky Way would be virtually nil; just as if I became the blackest black, people around me might suffer, but I would not trigger a galactic implosion. However, we should let ourselves 'go'; it is still good to strive to discover and live one's true, divine, loving self. I still strived to be as responsible for my thoughts, emotions, and actions – but little mishaps in my (and others') behavior, on the way, were much easier to forgive now.

I figured that as long as one had all one's limbs, senses and a reasonable grip on one's faculties, one could be the master of one's own destiny. Everyone also had the option to ask for divine help themselves. Free of Peter's shackles telling me it was my divine mission to stay in the medical profession, I quit my studies. Being there just did not fit with anything I believed in at that time.

I shifted my attention from humans to animals. Being vegetarian, moving in spiritual circles and organic food shops seemed to naturally attract all the horrendous information about the inhumane rearing of livestock and 20 million animals supposedly tortured, in one way or another, through experimentation every year. There was also still the nagging fear that if animal husbandry and experiments were not abolished from this planet, I would not be karmically safe from potentially having to come back as an industrially reared chicken, pig, cow etc. Now most animals don't have hands or can't let their tormentors know they are suffering by telling them to their face. It seemed more sensible to dedicate my energy and time to help free all the animals from captivity... but how?

I made sure I dedicated my spiritual shamanic travels to helping the animals. I also tried to strip the use of any chemicals out of my life. Chemicals, in my mind, incontrovertibly meant animal testing. I did not use many cosmetics, but what I did (like toothpaste) was organic. Just like the cleaning products I bought. I even repainted my flat with organic paint. At one point I bought a pair of new organic cotton trousers (they only came in off-white) and dyed them myself, with organic dye. But I had not lost my fashion sense; after wearing them for ten minutes, they'd turn into a sack and any outlining of my nice (bicycle trained) behind vanished. To me 'beauty' is one of creation's essentials. I believe every being should do its best to portray its beauty to the world – for humans it means looking after their bodies and dressing nicely. It is not vanity, but a divine right and urge!

Well the good intentions (saving the animals, the planet etc.) became harder to maintain. Avoiding chemicals is costly. I quit my homecare job having annoyed all my nursing colleagues and clients by incessantly preaching recycling and organics at them. The advances had been very slow though – a few recycling bins had been set up, but most clients were not willing to swap their Nivea body lotion for organic alternatives. Each time I did their shopping, at a 'regular' chemist, or got them their conventional medications, I felt like I was committing a crime against the animals. Most people seemed so selfish and arrogant; knowing that animals were tortured, tested upon, but they felt they were above them and that animal testing was justified, if it might save human lives or keep you from coming out in a rash with your face cream.

I would rather have died then, than take medication tested on animals. I could not take it anymore; I felt so guilty every time I just did a client's shopping in a supermarket – I had to hand in my notice. I was not totally forsaken though and found a part-time job helping an organic farmer selling his produce on street-markets. I still wasn't at peace though. I would find some flaw with everything, and my guilt demons made sure of that too. Now said farmer was still using a regular petrol engine in his truck and there seemed better cleaner alternatives like rapeseed oil motors. At least he was aware, contemplating refitting his truck with such a motor. But first he bought new 'scales-and-cash-registers' in one. They looked and functioned like computers (God knew what environmental sins had been committed in their production) and the receipt paper coming out of them positively reeked of chemicals.

I felt at a total impasse. It seemed virtually impossible to escape modern life and its environmental sins. I was in debt, buying organic and still paying for two years of Peter's courses, seminars and the Maui trip! I could not just up sticks, buy some land and become an organic farmer. It might require a bit of training too. Even if I won the lottery, did everything totally without chemicals as an organic farmer, my guilt demons reminded me that most of the people who would buy my produce would still be committing chemical misdeeds. And I would have fed and strengthened them to do so. I could try to not sell them anything, but I would most likely always end up having to buy stuff from them, tools, seeds etc. anyway.

And I did not even want to think about what might happen if I kept money in banks; they might use it to fund arms deals, chemical companies etc. I had switched my bank account to the Öko Bank (an organic bank with strict ethical investments), but everyone else I dealt with might not be so careful. With all these modern-life problems, I started contemplating the 'walking into the next forest, sitting under a tree and meditating until life around me had changed enough' idea again. But was life not about being happy? I could not imagine sitting there would be very pleasurable; I'd be wet and hungry, and sooner or later picked up and transferred to some psych ward, where they'd force-feed me drugs! Fortunately I managed to gain full-time employment as a shop assistant in an organic bakery. I'd collect the wares in the morning and drive them to one of their shops, where I'd sell them. Their vans even had rapeseed motors!

I prayed for miracles, but things weren't happening fast enough. Feeling guilty about so many things all the time was very tiring and unpleasant. Not just that, but seeing everybody else I cared about making even less of an effort to live harmoniously was tormenting too. Perhaps Peter had been right? Some of us might just be here to overcome our bodies? I implored the heavens to just take me out of my body; surely leaving a little debt behind was less deplorable than being partially responsible for animal testing and other atrocities… I prayed not to wake up in the morning, but you guessed it, I did.

I could have jumped off a building, but I figured the spiritual forces would be capable of arranging an easy, natural leaving of the physical body for me. Even if my Ultimate Good helpers were disappointed with my continuous failure, I was certain they would not let it out on those poor suffering animals. Furthermore, just jumping of a building might not kill me, but just leave me disfigured and paralyzed. And who knows what chemicals doctors would use on me while I was unconscious. Was I missing something, was I supposed to show the Divine I meant business and commit suicide myself? The voices in my head called me a wimp and a coward. I decided to take action.

I had read that nutmeg ingested in high doses, like two or three ground up whole nuts, would be fatal. This seemed a reasonable way to go. I was not afraid; I was certain I would go on, just in a different form. Another benefit of 'the nutmeg alternative' seemed to be that in case I was, for whatever reason, not supposed to leave my body, Spirit should be able to prevent it from happening, neutralize the nutmeg toxins.

On my next day off I ground up 3.5 nutmeg nuts and drank them with a glass of water. I meditated and prayed that should I leave my physical body, Spirit should make sure I did! If not, for my divine helpers to please protect me and keep me in my body. I lay on my bed and meditated. There was a lot of energy and if anything it seemed to try to keep me in my body. I fell asleep at some point and… I woke up again! Nutmeg is a hallucinogenic. I was nauseous and very dizzy. It took a couple of days to get back to work. In the meantime I just slept, drank water and went to the toilet. For weeks I had the taste of nutmeg in my mouth. It seemed I was supposed to stay. I started to think about where the guilt feelings and ideas came from then. Were they inside me? I asked for them all to be removed please. Their strength did not seem to abate though. Were they from the outside? Was Peter sending them, because he was pissed off about me disrespecting him in front of the group and leaving?

While working in the bakery, I got in touch with an anti-animal testing campaigner. I helped her distribute leaflets at a home show exposition. Animal testing can be quite gruesome, but I started to think about numbers. Back then it was 20 million animals killed annually in testing worldwide. Bad enough, but how many animals were suffering in industrial animal rearing? On a drive in the countryside I passed a cow field, I stopped, walked over to the cows and talked to them, "You are big and strong. Look at these flimsy gates, you can run them. Even if you get hurt during your breakout, is that not still better than captivity. Try to get out and then organize any other cows you find. Start a cow revolution." The cows just looked at me with their big brown eyes, but their interest soon diminished. Were they stupid – or what? (I obviously do not speak 'Cow', but I did try to communicate telepathically too, sending them images and asking the angels to translate (in spirit) where necessary.)

I had an idea. One could organize the billions of discarnate animals in heaven, who had suffered at human hands, and lead them to strike back. Not revenge, but surely with the spiritual power of billions of discarnate animals some clear signs could be given – a stop to animal abuse. I prayed to their departed spirits, but did not get any news of animals coming to haunt farmers... Perhaps the animals' souls needed a general to organize them? I was willing and was prepared to leave my body to do so. This time I got myself a 50ml bladder syringe and injected three lots of air into my right arm. The first injection missed the vein, but I was confident that the next two, in quick succession, went in – 100ml! But my heart did not stop. Why? I figured I really was supposed to stay here, and humbly conceded the fact that out of a trillion enlightened animals' spirits, they would have found a general amongst themselves by now. If anything I had been pretty arrogant, to believe that they needed me to come and help them.

My next problem was plants. So I read up about them. The first book was called *The Secret Life of Plants*. When I 'Google' it today, I find that it is widely regarded as pseudoscientific, but back then it was right up my street. The book portrays plants as sentient. In one experiment a scientist attached a polygraph to his office plant and noticed that there was an impulse when he approached it with a pair of scissors. The plant seemed to know even if he simply intended to cut off a bit! I believed that plants were conscious already. I had not thought too much about the welfare of plants yet though. Sure, I felt sorry for some, like trees in cities. Trees could not move; get up and leave in the evening, like the employees in that monotone, ugly, characterless office building, going home at night. If I was reborn as a tree in my next life, there are a lot of unattractive man-made places I would wish to avoid.

Not to offend anyone but the German countryside, in the north around Hamburg, is not exciting. It's very flat and highly organized – Germans are good at that. The countryside is mostly divided up into square fields, with few trees or hedges to make it more interesting for the eye. When out in the country there, I'd feel depressed. Now that was where the crops grew which made the bread, which I mainly ate and earned a living from. Each loaf I ate needed say 100 blades of wheat. One loaf a week would then equate to 5200 blades per year. Each haulm would have to grow for say four months. If Karma applied, and I were to have to come back, and be such wheat for future human generations, one wheat spear at a time, I'd have to spend 1733 years in boring, unattractive wheat monocultures. And that is just for a single year's worth of bread. I lost my appetite.

Could we not do something to improve the happiness of wheat and other crops? My organic farmer friend, the one I had worked for on the market, actually confirmed some of my suspicions. There is economic benefit to hedges around fields. More hedges and trees on and around fields does mean an increase in small animals and birds, which in turn can help prevent certain pests. Hedges can prevent wind damage to crops and diminish soil erosion too.

I found that the most 'plant friendly' way of growing food, in my opinion, seemed to be Permaculture – a system where multiple species of plants would be planted on the same plot. These plants would be chosen by their heights, seasonal growths and for reasons of benefitting each other. So if one plant attracted certain pests, but there are other plants which deter that pest, they'd be planted together. The higher growing plants e.g. would lose their foliage and mulch and fertilize the ground for the lower growing plants etc. According to the books I read (sorry, I forgot the titles), the per hectare yield in crops increases (in comparison to monocultures), plus one will save on herbicides, insecticides and fertilizers. It might be a bugger to harvest though. But I figured that humanity is spoiled by modern huge harvesting machines, and I for one was willing to put in the manual labor.

It all sounded super to me; the only problem was that there was no permaculturally grown food in the shops. I went out and searched for farmers that practiced permaculture. I went to see two, but it was a disappointment. One farm had dedicated ¼ of an acre to try it out. The farm was a commune, with no more room for another loony like me – even if I had wanted to join. Also their motives were anti-capitalist and self-sufficiency from industry, close, but not all mine. They still lacked a thought about plant welfare. Not only was the area they had dedicated to permaculture a fraction of the land they had, but they had only just started. All we got to see at their permaculture seminar were tiny seedlings in the ground – they would not be feeding anyone any time soon.

The other permaculture group I visited pretty much just had a corner of their garden dedicated, and there was not much to see yet either. These guys were eating out of supermarket bins though – a lot of food being thrown out by supermarkets, just expired, but still perfectly alright. An interesting idea, especially as I was no longer happy with the organically grown food in the shops. Even organic farmers mainly still used monocultures. This had left me in a dilemma. I did not want to hurt plants (and earn myself more bad plant monoculture Karma), so I tried to just not eat at all! But I got hungry and ate. I heard some Eastern monks manage to 'overcome' hunger and eat next to nothing. I kept on 'handing-over' my hunger to Creation, but it was a fix that lasted a few minutes only. Every time I ate I felt guilty. I let the plants and myself down. I managed to lessen my bad-plant-Karma footprint by collecting the crumbs falling off the shelves in the bakery. I'd sweep them together with my hands from the works surface under the shelves. I would take them home at night and cook a crumb-water soup out of them. They were whole-grains, so I got some nutrition. There were organic crois-sants in the shop though, oh the temptation! I succumbed more often than not. For good measure I was vegan by now too.

I got myself a list of the charities that distribute food, collected from supermarkets and restaurants, to soup kitchens or the like. If it was throwaway food, perhaps there wasn't any Karma attached to it? I went to one place, desperate, hungry, set up for junkies. There was a large buffet, laden with loads of goodies, tons of pastries – I was salivating. The junkies kicked me out though. They considered it their food, and if I did not inject drugs, I would not be admitted! I tried supermarket bins in the end. I had not eaten that well in months. Good stuff, but it is pretty nasty to fish the good stuff out amongst the rotten fruit, and they don't wash those bins regularly either… Now I hope the plants will forgive me, but for them I did not attempt any further assisted body-leaving ventures. I had decided to live my life as if it would be a going concern.

There was one good thing that came out of that period. I

really started to appreciate sex. The best things in life are free! Sex was pretty much the only thing left to me which I did not have to feel guilty about. If mutually desired, sexual encounters were enjoyable for all parties involved. I used to have a monogamous outlook, but I soon discovered that my eccentric, if not extreme, spiritual outlooks were not considered very sexy. On the other hand, if I just let potential suitors talk, they would talk about 'petty' problems like the photocopier not working in the office or dramas with their ex, which in turn would really put me off. There is a way out of having mood-killer conversation though – anonymous sex, just don't talk before. I mostly hung out at the public park, the cruising area, where gays meet at night.

It seems that a benefit of casual sex is that not looking for a relationship can free a sexual encounter. There is less of poten-tially having to impress a potential mate with monetary or intel-lectual achievements or feeling like one has to potentially commit to being with a person for a long time! It makes me less critical and lets me be more in the 'now'. I had also started to believe that Creation is more promiscuous than monogamous anyway. If we are 'All One' then everyone loves everyone, unconditionally – monogamous coupling did not make too much sense to me anymore. Everyone should be free and not owned by anyone; jealousy has nothing to do with Divine Love. There was also the hope that merely my energetic presence, wherever I went, might trigger a few enlightened ideas in people around me. If there was a sexual connection, might this transfer be even stronger?

Not sure what exactly my thought processes were, but one day sitting in the bakery and thinking about something – things clicked into place. I had thought about homeopathy and its foundation theory – similar heals similar. The theory that if one has an illness that is in its expression similar to e.g. arsenic poisoning, then by ingesting highly diluted arsenic – so highly diluted that physically there are no actual arsenic atoms left in the remedy – one can cause a healing effect. Now if something as potentially poisonous – we humans might even call it 'evil' – as arsenic, in its core essence, can be healing – perhaps that proves that in its essence all is good and divine? I know arsenic is only a lifeless substance, but homeopaths also use e.g. snake poisons and tuberculosis bacteria to make remedies.

It strengthened my belief that at the core of every being is 'good' and made me ponder the possibility (again) that actually all beings on this planet must have chosen their suffering – and that is why dead eaten animals and bored out of their mind monoculture plants do not come back to haunt us. If there are beings that want to experience suffering, then there have to be beings willing to take on the role of perpetrator though! And there are benefits to experiencing suffering at some point in one's eternal existence. Once one has experienced the opposite of happiness and love, the rest of one's eternal existence, in happiness and harmony, should be even more appreciated and enjoyed! I suddenly started to appreciate the beings that take on the role of the sadist/perpetrator/villain! They are all-loving, divine beings too – it must be a big step, if not sacrifice, for them to become 'bad'.

If, as I believe, all of Creation is good – in its true form, perfect love and happiness – then no being can hurt another in such a loving state, unless it is pre-agreed. Just like a sadist-masochist couple meeting to 'play'. The masochist is not going to turn around after their meeting and sue the sadist for assault (generally). Thinking about the world in such a way suddenly made more sense to me than believing that all is good – but out of itself good has gone bad, has lost control and is now stuck in a near endless spiral of (ineffective) Karma. Suffering seems to have been pre-chosen before we incarnate, just that we forget about this and it then seems 'real' and random or unjust.

Suffering comes in all shapes and forms, and most beings seem to choose a mix of being both perpetrator and victim. I understood though that all beings can still pray, and that there are copious amounts of spiritual help to alleviate if not to stop suffering (which has been pre-chosen). Alternatively one can obviously make choices and influence one's current and future affairs through one's deeds. A doctor might attract less violence than say a gang member. Prayers and good deeds are a bit like our 'safe words'. I understood though that we have to make clear (to Creation) that we do not want to suffer anymore. As long as we do not do this, just praising the Divine and trusting it is going to look after us might result in them simply respecting our pre-chosen suffering plan... Being divine ourselves, the original suffering plan is divine too...

I put the theory to the test. I gave the 'Good Spiritual Powers', including all deceased animals and plants that might be in the heavens and pick up my prayer, free rein to stop me by any means necessary (including dis-carnation), walked over to the next discounter supermarket, bought some conventional grilled chicken wings and ate them! I did not drop dead. Believe me I made sure I made my intentions clear to the Ultimate Good powers before going to bed that night. I told them the chicken wings were not just a slip in my behavior. I intended to go back to 'normal' life. A normal life including eating food I liked and could afford, buying fashionable clothes etc. I also would not care about where I worked (as long as I liked the job).

I intended my compass to be happiness, to do the things I liked and enjoyed. I chose to be perpetrator to some degree as well, potentially against animals, plants and the environment. Not that I would enjoy or get off on that role, but at least some seemed unavoidable! And maybe there is huge queue of beings waiting to incarnate as a battery chicken? And I am sure they do get briefed thoroughly beforehand. I would not complain or demonstrate if meat was suddenly outlawed and out of the shops, but I would wait until the masses made that decision. Or until there were clear irrefutable signs, such as all cows breaking out etc. If the environment required healing, because we humans damaged it, I told Spirit that they were more than welcome to heal anything/everything that needed healing. In my name, where necessary!

I asked the Divine to please remove me from my body if I was wrong in my assessment. I told Spirit that they could take me out whenever I might go too far! But I would henceforth work and live under the assumption that I was here to stay. I asked Spirit to cancel all future suffering I might still have pre-ordered, laid back and expected a wonderful 'normal' future! I was both excited and apprehensive. I liked the potential of normal life – especially the bit where I did not have to demonize my family and friends anymore for their 'normal' behaviors. There seemed enough fun potential to be had on this planet, regardless of it being a ghost train, with suffering all around me. I was honestly willing to leave there and then as well though – should I be wrong in my understandings…

But my radical decisions did not just make my guilt demons shut up. Their suggestion when waking up the next morning was that ever-loving and hopeful Ultimate Good knows I will repent and come back to my more righteous ways of the last three years. That I would achieve even more harmonious living, they know I can do it, and they aren't giving up hope just yet! I disregarded such suggestion! Ever all-loving, just and fair Spirit would not leave me in my body on the off chance I might change my ways again. They would consider all the beings I inadvertently could harm until then.

I don't believe that a just, loving divine force would prioritize humans over animals or plants, as in our essence we are one and equal. That would make the Divine unjust and cruel. Consider your child going to school, having anger issues and stabbing other children. Your child would tell you it thinks its behavior is alright and that they have no qualms about stabbing more kids again. It would be enough if they just looked at them funny. Now I would not let my child go back to school the next day, just because I believed they are good and should have another chance, a few more chances even. I would not give up on my child either; rather I would try and find them the best help available, to help to change their thinking. As long as I would not be certain that the other children are safe – I would home school though, send them to a special school (with metal detectors) or get a private tutor.

As with many realizations, an internal ripple effect followed. My mental, emotional and spiritual innards are shaken until a new equilibrium is found. Every time I have a spiritual epiphany, there is the hope too that this is the 'one' (revelation) that answers everything – from now on it will be plain sailing. The next morning I will wake up totally psychic, see auras and everything, three times as beautiful and find I have won the lottery! But no. Changes are subtle and best recognized retrospectively. After having gone through that rigmarole a good few times and finding that hoped for abilities and money blessings just have not materialized, I try to keep my expectations lower these days. No expectations, no disappointments!

I was tired of handing over suffering at a time, so I had prayed for Creation to take away 'The Lot'! So why was I still cash-strapped and still good bedfellows with doubt and guilt? We are talking God here – surely God can organize a lottery win? I had forgiven myself and everybody else with whom I might have some relationship Karma, so everybody should love me uncondi-tionally, right? It appeared I would have to give it time. As for the lottery, perhaps there are others in line before me... What if they had pre-chosen the joy of winning the lottery and ending their financial constraint with that draw, how long might that queue be... anyone willing to share their jackpot with me?

Initially there was a fear that I had been cleverer than antici-pated and 'survived' my pre-chosen sufferings, including suicide attempts. Maybe Creation now had to build a glorious life for me from scratch. That thought sounded like it could take a long time.

Today I am confident though that as soon as we choose a less suffering path we don't need to worry. Creation does not have to rebuild the Earth because of it. It could rather be seen like removing a stumbling block to a more natural flow of things (which is always just behind each suffering). It might just take some time until the suffering/stumbling blocks have been dissolved.

The ideas in my head argued that if I had decided to be a potential villain against animals and plants, I might as well become a villain against humans too. I should really do something to become a valuable part of the ghost train. Anything negative, even terrible, I could think of, if I did it, it must have been pre-chosen by the person(s) I would harm. Might I even be letting them down if I didn't go through with it? It took a bit to think myself out of that trap. As for the letting potential victims down, it is a two-way street. If a crime is pre-arranged, both the victim and the perpetrator can cancel that contract if they do not want to go through with it anymore! Else one might just as well argue that future suffering cannot be cancelled, as the villain might have fun tormenting one, and one is a spoilsport to take that experience away from them.

Perhaps I am legitimizing everything horrific. If a person with murderous tendencies ever reads this book, they might take it as a free pass... Well I am writing this book for all the good people I have met who are plagued by fears and feelings of guilt for 'normal' things they do. For those who want to move on, but cannot forgive themselves or others for things they have done or that have happened to them. Someone who is hell-bent on committing some atrocity might not be stopped by this book, but I do not think they can use it as an excuse for any misdeeds they commit. Secondly once you understand that everything is pre-chosen, you might just reconsider murderous rage or anger towards another, as you always only have yourself to blame for any (past and present) suffering experienced. With any conflict it is best to forgive and ask for healing and happiness. There is still a lot of 'guilt' in the world – it might take some time to rid us of it, so I would not be able to guarantee that a delinquent would go guilt free. And I can tell you, guilt is no fun!

There is a good chance that horrific deeds will energetically isolate an individual – you might just lose your peace of mind. Having been involved with wars and battles, even if 'just' on the spiritual and emotional level, for the last 17 years, I really cherish my peace of mind! Peace of mind is a good thing and I would not recommend risking it. Even if one might feel (or be told) that one will get away unscathed with some crime, that feeling can't be trusted; it has a tendency to be unreliable and untrustworthy. Furthermore one's family, partner, friends will often not approve of horrific deeds either. The only people which one might still be able to hang with will be other villains, who I doubt will be too much fun to be around and, in the long or short run – trustworthy.

How would things work though if I had pre-chosen to live through an earthquake? Would Creation cancel the earthquake, because I had chosen to not suffer anymore? I believe that if just one of the to-be-earthquake-hit players prays the right prayer, makes it clear somehow that they don't want the experience anymore and Creation cannot rehouse them before the event, the whole event would be cancelled (if there is enough time to remove all energies that cause the earthquake). The conscious decision for non-suffering always wins.

Now it was time to face my 'professional' calling: my desire or requirement to 'help' others. Could my reluctance to go back to medicine have ill effects? What if there were patients that were suffering an illness which I had been pre-chosen to find the cure for? Would they now be stuck with that illness if I did not go back to medicine? It's a real nasty dilemma. My solution was (and still is) to hand the situation into divine hands and ask that other avenues of healing or help be found and activated. Surely something as awesome as Creation has a backup plan. For good measure I apologized to Creation for any extra effort potentially created. (I might have become an incompetent doctor too, and may have actually alleviated suffering by not finishing my studies. But then I do try to think of myself as capable, not incompetent.)

Around that time I also asked for Spirit to please take me out of my body again. I had grown into a bit of a suffering-phobe. I was not in this for an extended masochistic ride! I might have to battle 'guilt' demons, telling me I should bear some suffering for longer because some human somewhere was hoping to save a whole bunch of people (including me) with some Hollywood style heroic act. They were really looking forward to feeling the adrenalin rush and the satisfaction that comes with having saved the day. It's nonsense of course!

That also works the other way around. These days, being a healer and masseur, I sometimes still get energies trying to tell me that I'm just after the rush of having helped to free a client of some disease or stress energies. The energies then imply that subconsciously I am in league with some negative forces, which keep people diseased, as it would not be in my interest if everybody would suddenly be stress-free and healthy. Well, sometimes you just have to let the voices babble along; I'd be the last to stand in the way of someone's attempt to heal. I have told all humans (telepathically) that if they are holding on to suffering, so that I can help them heal it (and get a healer-hero kick out of it), they are welcome to let that suffering go... now!

One more interesting point might be that my mind – ever trying to think people good – tried to keep finding explanations as to why Peter had done to me/us what he had done? Perhaps he had had the same enlightenments and was just trying some shortcut path for his disciples? Perhaps he figured that extreme pressure would get our asses in gear, make us work real hard and achieve results in record time, which in the long run would safe us a lot of suffering?

In the weeks after my epiphany, I was still bombarded by the same old guilt regarding food, animals, and plants. I had been under the romantic impressions that big understandings (coming out of true divine love and wisdom) just melt away all resistance, instantaneously! So was there some foul play involved; why was I still not 'free'? Was it Peter? There definitely seemed to be some intelligence behind the attacks exposing my old weaknesses. They were coordinated and I could have intelligent conversations with them.

I wrote Peter a letter. I re-explained the Mengele scenario. I let him know that I understood now that we all pre-choose our suffering and that I had forgiven him fully. I had made the conscious decision not to suffer anymore, but that it felt like there might still be psychic attacks coming from his side. I asked him to please stop. A few months later I met him on the street. He just smiled and referred to the 'silly' letter I had written. He obviously did not understand or did not want to understand, nor did he apologize. I mention the apology bit because for years, every time I was considering taking action against him, I would be 'attacked' by strong emotions of sweet forgiveness, as if everything is okay.

I have been in Hamburg twice since, and met an old friend (still attending the circles and having sessions with Peter) for coffee. I had to fight hard to not succumb to fluffy energies trying to convince me that Peter was the good guy. I had visions of going back to him. It was like having a haze around my head, like being under the influence of some mind-altering drug. These energies came up with some convincing arguments. There wasn't much 'head space' left to myself to think myself out of the situation. What I held onto at those times was that if Peter was a good guy, if the Mengele incident had in fact been a misunderstanding, perhaps his intuition had been tampered with as well. After my letter I would have expected an apology; I would have expected him, like a normal person, to get hold of me and clear the air – personally! Needless to say, as soon as I left Hamburg the 'convincing' arguments fell in on themselves, like a house of cards. The feeling of being in a haze lifted and I had the feeling as if I had just woken up from an unpleasant dream.

Over time more notions fell into place. I had the epiphany that carrying Karma across 'lifetimes' was illogical. I already thought it somewhat 'unloving' that one might be served with the bill for something done in a previous life, without being able to remember having done it. If one knows one has done something wrong, one can repent and possibly try to make up for it somehow.

Supposedly you can dissolve Karma through forgiveness. It is enough if either the perpetrator or the victim forgives to dissolve Karma between the two. Now allegedly between incarnations we are enlightened again. We meet our divine helpers, angels etc. and we 'know' again about our eternal all-loving being. If my last life ended because someone murdered me, then between lives I would 'see' that I only got murdered because in that or a previous life I was a murderer myself. As I see it, truly understanding this 'in-between' existence would automatically lead me to fully forgive myself, as well as the person who murdered me! I would dissolve any Karma there and then. Nothing ever carried over. All of Peter's endless regression therapies could therefore be seen as needless.

I can see that past life events can have entertaining or possibly educational, historic value, but Peter used it as a sadistic tool. Still reincarnation theory has its positive philosophical conclusions. Even if a 'proper' human lifetime would be, say, 500 years and we would reincarnate on Earth a few times to reach that age – it teaches us to let go of one-lifetime illusions and arrogances. For example racism is obsolete, as we might well reincarnate as different nationalities and races across our lives. We'd just be holding stereotypes and prejudices against ourselves. Just as absurd is sexism. One might have been of the opposite sex in a prior life and will be again. Same applies to sexual orientation. Even arrogance about being smarter than anyone else or other 'selection of the fittest' arguments become senseless. Even the smartest human will probably be stupid compared to say an angel, and a genius in one life might have been the village idiot in their last incarnation. We might have forgotten everything when entering our fertilized egg cells and have to 'learn' most things in childhood and adolescence, but one might have been a professor in one's last life.

The above is academic though, as I came to understand one more thing about reincarnation. Now if, as many teach, there is an evolution of souls, meaning we are maybe rocks first, then plants, next insects, then animals and finally humans and then angels – what then? What will happen to the beings that are rocks now who are gagging to become 'more advanced' beings? By the time they are ready to move on to plant form, there won't be any beings left to be rocks for them to grow on etc. I therefore willingly accept that after having been human now, and then having taken a holiday and review of this life in heaven, I might spend some time again being a rock, an oxygen atom or maybe just a ray of light, so that other beings can enjoy their incarnations 'using' me as such. I am sure that all beings have fun, whatever shape or form. Maybe I am a bit nostalgic, maybe just grateful, but it is also one reason why, even with potential suffering around me, I try to make the best out of this life. Who knows when I might get the chance to have a human body again! All beings should cherish whatever (reasonably healthy) 'bodies' they have and get, for as long as they have them!

Other guilt traps fell in on themselves too. I had felt guilty about living in a city. Did humans not take away all the room for plants to grow by asphalting the ground, and building houses? Now I allowed myself to be an Earth dweller as well. We need shelter and we need to build it somewhere. In a way living in a multistory apartment building is, if anything, economical. I also saw that, whereas plants had been the dominant ground covering species in the past, maybe we as humans now gave rocks and other minerals a chance to come to the surface in more places. I had also felt guilty that by cultivating land we, as humans, had taken away room from the trees! I then saw a program professing that over the last millions of years there has been a 'fight' between grasses and trees already, without human interference. Grasses came to be the dominant species in some areas of the world, where it was trees before, because they burn easily and at high temperatures (at which trees die), but retain their fertile core. In turn herbivores such as buffaloes and horses had then come to depend on these grass plains for their survival.

I also felt guilty about human grown grass monocultures, be they crops or decorative lawns. I had forgotten that there are natural (almost) grass-monocultures too – think of Mongolia. Furthermore humans could only become farmers because some ancient wheat mutated a few thousand years back. Wheat could now be cultivated, cut, collected and then thrashed. Before that mutation wheat grains would just drop off the haulm, as soon as ripe, and touched or shaken by wind. I would argue that there is a good chance that wheat used us humans to become a more successful plant.

But back to events in my life back then. All my epiphanies had not served me with financial abundance (yet). I'd been brought up on the notion that one has to work for one's upkeep, so that was what I had to do. The organic bakery sales job, as delicious as the bread and cakes were (and which now all could be consumed unimpeachably), was not enough. I had had some run-ins with management there as well, and with my newfound philosophy I could think about my well-being for once – so I quit. It soon found a job in a really funky shop, selling designer furniture and knickknacks. This was more of where a fashionable gay guy would work. On the side I did some bar keeping work and waited in a gourmet restaurant.

I was aware though that, in the long run, I would have to find something a little more challenging. Not to be arrogant, but a busy brain can easily get bored, plus if I could use it to get jobs with higher earning potential I'd be stupid not to. I was thinking about a business career. I was 29 after all (and had little to show for it, except philosophical enlightenments); time to do some catching up with the rest of my peers. I could go back to studying medicine, but for now I just wanted to make some money and have a bit of fun – my nerves, battered by three years of cult trauma and nonstop guilt pangs, needed a bit of a holiday. A change of scenery, perhaps even countries, might be just the thing.

Chapter 6

Civilian Life

London was my first choice. I figured that my language skills would get me a job there and I could work myself up the career ladder. It would have probably taken another year or two to save enough money to move, but fortunately I met a Londoner on holiday who, after a bit of a holiday romance, invited me to stay with him and his family. I had no regrets leaving Germany. In Great Britain someone might study Biology, go work in a bank and after some years there change to working in Human Resources. The system appeared more flexible than the German one. It was just what I was looking for.

After a few months of intense job hunting and doing a computer course, I got a position as an International Payroll Administrator for an IT recruitment company. Six months later I started a correspondence bookkeeping course. I liked it. I find a certain peace in numbers. Accounting seemed relatively straight-forward. Either the bottom line balances or it doesn't. After the introductory course, I decided to stay at it. I kept studying and sitting exams through a professional accountancy body. I even managed to get a job in the accounts department of the company, which meant that the company then paid for my studies. I stayed with that company for over five years – before being made redundant.

Except for my health, everything seemed to be on track. I never got an official diagnosis, but from my research I seemed to suffer from IBS (Irritable Bowel Syndrome) and CFS (Chronic Fatigue Syndrome). The only diagnosis I ever got from a GP was depression, but prescribed antidepressants, at first attempt, really did not make any difference. Physically I felt like I was suffering from a nonstop flu: I had stomach cramps, felt achy and was generally utterly exhausted.

I developed all sorts of theories and tried every therapy I could find which promised some potential results and which I could afford. Just showing up for work was a huge effort. Going to the gym (I was not going to lose my athletic looks because of some stupid illness) and studying in my free time often felt impossible – but I forced myself to do it. Since my blood seemed alright, my GP and family seemed to attribute my symptoms to 'just' being in my mind. At times I almost felt jealous of people who were sick and had a 'proper' diagnosis to show for it, like a tumor...

I did as much spiritual self-healing work as I could manage. I even started a two-year spiritual healing course with the NFSH – National Federation of Spiritual Healers or Healing Trust. The Healing Trust was then the biggest organization of spiritual healers in the UK and I liked their nondenominational approach. No one was telling me what I had to believe in or what I had to call the source of energy I worked with.

After being made redundant during a company restructure, and not getting the desired position I reapplied for, I decided that accountancy might need a break. I was 35 years old. Working as an accountant had been good for a few years, but in my heart I wanted to work as a spiritual healer. Perhaps now was my chance? So I took another risk, created a Web site, did some advertising and prayed for a thriving spiritual healing practice. There was an empty bedroom in my house I could rent as a treatment room, so I rented that too and waited.

But it was not all that easy to break into the alternative complementary therapy market. Initially I only got a couple of clients – not even enough to cover the marketing costs. My redundancy money soon ran out and I resorted to a bit of escort work on the side, to pay for the bills. Not my favorite occupation, but I wasn't just going to give up on my dream. Luckily I was guided to do some massage courses, and after a year I started a practice as a tantric masseur. I have not had any problems finding clients since. I had feared that I might end up just massaging and not doing any healing work, but those fears seemed unfounded. Most of my clients are very happy for me to include healing/energy work with their massage.

The last few years have been very fulfilling and educational. Regularly working as a healer, and feeling my clients' energies, has given me greater insight into the nature of energies, especially the negative ones. I still don't claim to be a reliable psychic and would be careful about handing out any diagnosis about a client's energy affairs on a first visit, but over the years many have come back again and again. This enabled me to sort out, with greater certainty, which intuitively felt energies were client-related or just potential cross over effects from my private life or other clients. Doing regular healing work has given me greater understanding and deeper peace of mind than before I set off on my spiritual journey; plus I mostly look with excitement and fearlessness to the future.

Being self-employed also has other benefits. I am able to organize my time after my needs. I can book clients afternoons or evenings, which is handy because I am not a morning person. I can also look after myself better by working within my physical, emotional, mental and spiritual capacities. All the continued spiritual help and finding a few food supplements (that work for me) have helped to improve my health immensely, especially in the past three years. No more fluey feeling and extreme exhaustion.

So since 2007 I have been working as a masseur and spiritual healer. Tantric massage includes erotic elements and usually for men a lingam (Sanskrit – phallus) and potentially prostate massage; and for women a yoni (Sanskrit – vagina) massage. I only see male clients though.

Happiness (here in connection with triggering sexual energies) is one of the pillars of true divine life and existence to me. Sex and happiness do not just make us generally feel good, but I strongly believe are very healing too; a healing that goes beyond a bit of a physical immune boost, through endorphin release. Sex is one of the most profound tools of helping us to connect to the Divine, to experience oneness with another being and beyond this – to feel 'One with All'.

There is still some stigma about this kind of work. However, I am happy doing it. Most of my clients need plenty of healing, including sexual healing (healing using erotic tools, i.e. lingam and prostate massage; I do not usually have sex with them). It would not have been my first choice; I would have preferred to work as a healer only or just do 'regular' massage, but there wasn't the demand. So do I mind or resent working as a tantric masseur, having to connect the erotic to healing work, to be able to do healing work in the first place and live off it? Admittedly initially there was a bit of resentment, but it soon passed. Since I wish everyone that they receive all the healing they require, including the healing they need for a fulfilled sex life, I am happy to help here as well. I used to work in nursing; I have washed and cleaned people's bottoms in the past. Compared with diapering an adult, giving someone a tantric massage is much more on the side of health and life-empowerment, than sickness and fear of death.

The steady flow of paying clients was there, but the first two years or so I frequently ended up having to cancel work, as my health was still a roller coaster. I figured that my clients came for relaxation and healing, they paid good money for it – I did not want to give them a cold. Especially as I was doing healing work, I did not want clients to subconsciously start associating spiritual healing with getting sick after…

At times I worked even though I felt borderline. I made sure I burned some antiviral eucalyptus oil in an oil burner at least. Something inside was telling me too that with all the healing energies in the room, even if I truly had some viral infection, the likelihood of transferring anything was minimal. (My GP agreed; as long as I did not cough on my clients she saw no reason why I should not work.) 'Strangely' with that I started to make the observation that often symptoms would disappear halfway through the massage or straight thereafter. In all my years of working, only two clients ever called me up after their massage describing something that sounded like a potential healing crisis, including flu-like aches. Statistically two out of hundreds is very low though; those clients might have been incubating some cold or flu before they came to see me – it might have just been coincidence!

I get much more positive and immediate feedback working as a masseur than in my office jobs, where I usually had to wait for an annual appraisal. I am fascinated as well with the things I feel and experience during each healing session. I always remind myself (and if necessary the client) that I am not a reliable psychic though. I pretty much trust my intuition with regards to how long I might hover over a chakra, until it is time to move to the next one; I am much more skeptical with regards to 'explanatory' intuitions though like, *this client's heart chakra is blocked because he is a cold hearted lawyer.* Such intuitions can be interesting bits of information, but I won't share them with my client. I find that an 'innocent until proven guilty' approach about judging people (and their energies), even just in my head, often serves me well. Still, over the years I could not help but start to see more patterns to some of my intuitions.

Some clients were more pleasant to work with than others. There seems to be a stronger, healthier and happier flow of energy with such. I would often discover during the massage or afterwards that these clients already did some spiritual or meditation work. Most clients, however, seemed to create some adverse reaction in me. With one regular client I might tend to sweat a lot, with another I would feel cold, I might get a pain in a specific joint or another would cause me to feel nauseous.

Many clients come with a certain lethargy or latent depression, but it is the varying strength of the symptoms or the combination with other physical, mental or spiritual symptoms that make them more memorable. My 'reactions' did not only happen during healing sessions. Frequently I started to detect particular emotions before clients even arrived. With some clients these could be very specific. With some clients I would be bombarded with hefty thoughts and energies apparently trying their utmost to get me to cancel my appointments. They would usually start a few hours prior to their arrival, sometimes the night before.

I could not help but think that all 'fault' for all these sensations did not lie with me. Could my clients' (negative) energies influence me even before they'd arrive? Was I experiencing some kind of backlash effect from their energies (if feeling destroyed after) or even a prelash effect, if starting to feel more unwell before seeing a particular client? I had read once or twice about healers getting sick after giving healing to a particularly ill client. It seemed to be an exception to the rule though. I though was feeling stuff with most clients. I struggled for quite some time with accepting that my clients' energies might be influencing even attacking me before or after a session.

There was a concern. My thoughts are a potential creative force, so negative impressions about my clients, especially if untrue, might influence them negatively. If I think negative thoughts about a client like *oh, he feels very depressed*, I may actually only be projecting a depressive feeling from inside myself. He might actually be hit by my false negative belief and walk out of my studio with depressed energies he did not have before... I knew how uncomfortable negative energies could be; I did not want to inflict them on anyone, even if for a few minutes. With clients it would be even worse; they would have paid for my services. And it could not be good for business either if clients walked out of my studio feeling worse than when they arrived, even if only for a short while.

Still I continued working. I hoped that in the end more healing would be effected, through my channeling Ultimate Good energies, for my clients and life in general – as opposed to not working. I also considered the alternative. If my clients did not get healing from me, they would have to go to another healer (or masseur, most of which do not do any energy healing work). I know plenty of nice healers, some colleagues of mine. They are good people and competent healers, but when talking to them, I still felt that I probably meditate and pray more than most of them, i.e. potentially I could well be a clearer channel than many of them.

Plenty of the energies that 'hit' me before, after or during a healing were quite severe, vile or viscous, especially during the first 2–3 years. But I've thus far only had four clients who felt as if they were actually contemplating murder. With others though I thought/felt as if they were contemplating other nasty things, including a handful of child molester visions. With one regular client with an old burn scar and whose presence always brought out the strongest resistance in me – I was told that I had such strong, resistant emotions against him because, in a previous life, he had burned my children alive. I.e. in this life he received the burns as karmic retribution. He also had cerebral palsy. This client was though, at least towards me, a very nice guy. I am not a qualified psychic, if there is such a thing, and from my healing organization's Code of Conduct I am not allowed to diagnose or speak of intuitions to my clients anyway. But even without that Code of Conduct stopping me, I was not going to turn around and ask a client: "By the way, are you a child molester?" "Are you thinking about murdering me?" "Did you burn my children in a past life?" I.e. it was often impossible to verify my intuitions with a client.

Sometimes my hand would get 'stuck' on a client's body. There seemed to be a particularly strong need for healing there. Again, especially in the first two years of my massage work, I'd sometimes get the intuitive feeling that it might be cancer. Again not an intuition I would spring on anyone lightly. I would probably have to feel a distinctive lump too etc. Unless I was very, very certain I would not share my intuition. Even today, after about 17 years on the spiritual journey, I still do not trust my intuitions enough to tell a client something like, "It feels like you have cancer." Of course a correct spiritual cancer diagnosis might save lives, but one should not forget the potential stress and fears one might trigger in a client with a false positive diagnosis. I also try to think about myself. I am not allowed to diagnose, I could be kicked out of my healer organization for doing so, and if a client would go to the doctor and find that I was wrong, he might, rightly so, sue me for emotional trauma or misconduct.

Another problem I faced was that some clients with the 'heaviest' energies were really nice. I could not picture them with a voodoo doll to psychically attack me before seeing me. They appeared to really enjoy my work, so it was unlikely they might be having negative thoughts about me. Why would such clients come back in the first place? Could their (negative) energies attack me without my clients' knowing or being aware of it? That would imply that their negative energies were self-aware and capable – little black magicians!

I do approach tantric work with thorough professionalism, but I am aware that the industry carries a certain stigma. Many clients appreciate my discretion. And not all of my clients would be happy if I asked them too many questions about their life, relationship status and health. Regarding client's health – I do have a list of contraindications for massage treatment on my Web site, and always double-check that my clients do not have serious heart disease or other contraindicated illnesses before commencing the first session. With my tantric massage clients I do not take extensive notes though, as I want them to relax and not worry about what information I might glean and misuse later.

Clients with particularly heavy energies could be psychiatric candidates, plagued by nasty thoughts and dreams. If they do not tell me of their own accord though I am not going to pry. Most of my clients primarily come for the massage bit and see the healing work as an additional benefit – not the other way round. I would be put off if a massage therapist tried to conduct a little psychotherapy session before we started a massage too. I might be more sensitive here than most, with my cult background, but I do get suspicious if people try to extract sensitive information from me when it does not seem appropriate or necessary. Such sensitive information could be used to attempt to manipulate me afterwards. With a massage therapist I would possibly be even more wary, as straight afterwards I would be at their mercy on their massage table, in semi-trance and intimately exposed!

Considering the latter, I often only know a client's name, their profession and possibly regional or national background. But even with that information, I made some observations. Clients with very heavy energies often seemed to be connected to certain professions. It also seemed to crystallize that clients from certain parts of the UK or particular countries seemed to come with a higher chance of having loads of negative or particularly strong negative energies. Furthermore there seemed to be a possible connection between me experiencing heavy energies and clients having severe handicaps or illnesses – which I could see or was informed about.

For the first three years I blamed myself for my reactions to clients during healings – with growing suspicions though that my clients' energies had some part in it too. I thought I was pretty unconditional in my love and willingness to help people. I thought I had proved that already, especially with all the work I had done to heal myself, others and the planet – but according to my reactions, I potentially was an arrogant, superficial prick, reacting adversely if a client was unattractive, old, obese or handicapped. Funnily though some large clients would not trigger any uncomfortable feelings massaging them, whereas some lean, handsome clients did! The other big question was – if I did not know what a client would 'look' like before they arrived, how come I often reacted to their energies before I even saw them?

After about three years I booked a two-week holiday, starting off with an excursion to a renowned sacred site in the UK. On the day a healer friend and I were supposed to drive down to this spiritual place, I woke up in the wee hours and experienced very strong resistance. I was full of voices, thoughts and emotions, all trying to convince me that going was a bad idea. The excursion had been planned for several months – I really could not see any reason why I should not go – so go I did.

There was a lot of traffic that day and we arrived two hours late. The energy there was very palpable (apparently warm and comforting) and at first I was happy. I might actually get a rest, maybe let down some of my energetic guards a bit and heal. I sat down to meditate. Perhaps because of the resistance I had experienced the night before and because I had learned in my cult years that a sugarcoated, strong energy in a place can be positive only on first glance, I kept all my protections up though. Prudently I attuned to Ultimate Good in pure Ultimate Good places first. I watched what would happen.

I was open to connect to Ultimate Good energies at the location, should there be any. A bit of a battle seemed to ensue. My very strong feeling was that I was not connected to any energy nearby – quite the opposite. I started to feel very constricted, as if the energies were trying to smother me by lying heavy on my whole body, constricting my chest. The energies seemed hell-bent on getting inside me, but were kept out by my Ultimate Good protections.

It was a very reminiscent of my last days in the cult, when I had started to ask for perfect protections against any potential negative energies in the cult. The energies 'attacking' me seemed very determined to break through my barriers and they felt as if they had an agenda that went beyond the benign of Ultimate Good – true wolves in sheep's clothing. They seemed quite affronted that someone dared to question their holiness too – and not just drop all their protections! I could understand that other spiritual people, perhaps still naïve, as they never had a destructive cult experience, might fall for the energies in that place, rejoice at feeling something so strong, and fully open up to them.

I started to ponder whether the energies that had kept me awake the night before, and which had tried to fill me with so many doubts and fears that I should cancel my trip, might be connected? Why would they not want me to go there? Were my energies, the energies I connect to Ultimate Good and what I believe in, a threat to them? How did they even know I was planning to go? When I was with Peter and had very strong resistance against going to Maui, he consoled me and explained that it was just my subconscious rebelling. My subconscious was rebelling because it would know that there would be a lot of healing work happening. Maybe the resistance to go to the healing place was from negative energies inside me who wanted to stop me going?

But this was some twelve years on now, and I had countless more hours of healing and cleansing meditations behind me. I could not really imagine that I had so much negativity left inside me to be able to kick up such a big fuss. Also any meditation I do would be a strong threat to my subconscious, or whatever negative energies left inside me, but I do not experience strong resistance before sitting down to meditate, nor feelings of being smothered by outside energies. Furthermore, in all my healing experiences before I never felt as if a divine energy would try to break into my energies with force. I usually experienced Ultimate Good healing energies as comforting and they would make me feel calmer and stronger – this was the opposite. Still, if my suspicions were correct, it would mean that there is some kind of 'negative energies information network' that pre-warns about the presence of lighter people and healers. It did sound rather paranoid and I was not sold 100% on the idea yet.

My next holiday destination was a gay Mediterranean cruise. Even though I had looked forward to this trip, here too it was a huge effort to get myself to packing the night before. The morning of the flight it was near impossible to get out of bed. I could obviously blame nervousness. I think I have mostly overcome nervousness by now, but this one could have been due to going alone on a ship with 3500 other gay guys. It meant potential sexual and romantic encounters, but also rejections. I think I have had gay-holiday-nervousness in the past, but that usually meant that I was more hyped than usual, would be packed days before, and would be excited and not able to sleep. Here though I was drained and joyless – inexplicably so.

I contemplated whether my travel resistance could be resistance from the energies of the country I was going to? But could 'just' my physical presence in a location be a threat to negative energies there? Could I be a threat to negativities in a larger place, such as Venice? Or was it the negative and confused energies of the guys or staff I'd encounter on board that resisted? I wasn't even planning to work on board, or in Venice (just my regular healing, meditation work for myself, maybe send some distant healing to friends and family).

The cruise started off with me pretty much on my own, not meeting many people. I never was one to just go up to guys and start chatting – I do need a bit of eye contact and a sense of the other's body language confirming I won't be rudely rejected. But before my spiritual journey I would go on a holiday alone and have a bunch of mates by the end of the first or second day.

The ship was full of Americans, they are pretty good with small talk, but that was all it usually was – a few sentences of polite chat when sharing a table in the restaurant. At the evening dance party, on the 2nd or 3rd night, I had enough of blaming myself for the lack of contacts. What if the blockages were with the other cruisers – not me? I started to send healing into the dance crowd, then extended into everyone on the ship, the ship itself etc. Uplifting music, exercising and moving while being in healing mode in my experience helps to stay connected, in the 'zone' and in strength for long periods. If I would try to meditate for six hours, just lying on my bed, I would probably fall asleep. If I channel healing during exercise, I can potentially power through more stuff and/or overcome greater resistances. I kept on doing healing, whenever and wherever I could, but nothing much happened for the next couple of days.

Three nights later it felt as if a huge chunk of resistance lifted/dissolved. For the last few days of the cruise I felt 23 again. Confident, handsome and flirtatious, and more importantly suddenly people started smiling at me and approached me again. Somehow the ship now seemed to be an oasis of happiness. We still stopped at different ports every day. Just stepping off the ship (or even intending to) brought up great amounts of resistance. I.e. on shore there was like an invisible barrier around me again that blocked the happy energy flow between me and others. As soon as I stepped back onto the ship, the energy barriers lifted and I was pretty much all free again though.

One could argue that over the course of the trip everyone had relaxed and de-stressed more, so naturally it was more likely to meet more guys towards the end of my journey. People had tanked up on sunlight and good food etc. – but I argue that was the case on the three cruises I had been on before as well, as well as on all other holidays I had been on in the last 15 years for that matter, yet then I did not get the same effect. On all the other recent, prior holidays there was a slight improvement with each day I spent on them, but nothing as dramatic and as palpable as on that cruise.

This experience was my 'light switch' moment, the last big missing piece, propelling me into a state of awareness where all my experiences would now start to make sense and form the basis of my own conclusions, answers and coping strategies for living. Now it's time to share with you different spiritual concepts, teachings and tools I find work in achieving an ever more happy and successful life. I hope what follows will help you to find meaning, answers and inspiration too.

Book Two

Strategies & Cures

Chapter 7

The Powers That Be

I believe that visualization and imagination are an important part of healing work, so over the years I have tried my best to address the Divine with titles/descriptions which made sense to me, which had meaning and triggered the best and most suitable picture of these healing powers in my mind. Since Peter's teachings were mainly Christian, I initially started with the word 'God', then after a while 'Our Father' or 'Holy Father'. Both 'God' and 'Holy Father' felt restricted. I believe that the Divine is in everything and that everything is created by and as a part of Creation. Saying God or Holy Father paints an image of a single, distinct entity though – the old man with the long white beard.

The father/child relationship has its benefits. It helped me to embrace my divine core nature – being a son of the Divine I should have all the Divine's abilities – I just need to rediscover them. But this did not make up for certain shortcomings. The logistics of the heavens are just too mind-boggling for me to be able to contribute all of creation (Earth and all its beings, our solar system, the Universe etc.) to one single entity. And that is not even considering the ongoing support and help provided when any being prays.

To create a being out of clay would require a very skillful artist, which could be attributed to one being. It becomes more difficult when speaking of millions of species, from single cell to multiple cell organisms. Every cell alone is a miracle in itself. It would take more than seven days and the concerted effort of many creative beings to manifest a planet like Earth. I feel more comfortable believing that there are a huge number of divine beings that help all Earth dwellers.

For a while I prayed to the Universe or Creation, but that

possibly includes both positive and negative powers. I did ask to only get hooked up to the good guys, but found I had to reaffirm this plea again and again, fearing that some bad guys might still think I was inviting them too. I did not want some crooks to answer my calls when trying to reach the police. Some other spiritually minded people call on specific named entities, but I figure that getting 100% accurately channeled information, like names, is tricky business. Even if we pray to departed humans (whose names we know), maybe they have reincarnated into another physical body already or are still in Helper school, to become truly ultimate good again? I didn't want to offend by calling my Helpers by the wrong names. Nor do I want to restrict the beings helping to a certain number. Also, who says angels, for example, don't do shift work, deserve holidays or even fancy retirement at some point? I apologized for being somewhat vague and kept my addresses (to the Divine) more general.

The 'Divine' seemed a good choice for a while. I have had my years of spiritual paranoia though. What humans describe as the Divine has so many names and attributes, some mutually exclusive. Over the centuries quite a few atrocities have been committed in the name of the Divine. Considering that I believe that humans pre-order suffering before incarnating, is it possible there are some forms of suffering connected to the spiritual realms one might be able to select? I hoped it was not so, that our prayers ended up at the right address straight away; but what if there were rival Gods? What if some heavens did have an agenda of their own? Peter did seem to have some powerful spiritual backup; what if the Christian Heaven supported Peter and not me? It seemed too horrific to consider, but bearing in mind my ill health and lack of improvement for years, was it possible that I had been forsaken by the Heavens?

I still believed that the sum of all Creation is ultimately good, but what if the heavens, the God and angels that most humans believe in were part of the suffering illusion? It could explain a lot! I found that contemplating such scenarios was maddening. To believe it might be me against the Heavens is too daunting. I did not feel like I could ask anyone (human). Even if I asked a vicar and they would tell me that the Heavens are all good – might they just try to comfort themselves? I knew how disconcerting these fears were, so I did not want to risk infecting anyone else with them either. Even if I was right, what help would it be for humans to find out? One would require great powers to heal tainted heavens; getting a bunch of humans to believe me would not cut it.

I started to pray to 'Highest Possible Good', at times preceding it with the word 'True'. Even if our (religious) heavens were tainted and part of the suffering, Highest Possible Good would be 'behind' those and infinitely stronger than any tainted God(s). 'Good' will always prevail. I did make sure to let Highest Possible Good know that living a life, fearing the Heavens felt too stressful!

I don't want to tell Highest Possible Good its business, but I begged them to clear out the Heavens, should they be tainted, and protect me (and whoever else necessary; especially my family and friends) against any possible energetic backlash during this cleansing process. These days, I think I was most likely attacked by spiritual paranoid concepts/ideas. It has been years since these prayers, so even should there have been 'suffering/tainted Heavens' – I strongly feel they'd be fully healed by now. Any imperfections humans attribute to their God(s) and Heaven(s) is much more likely coming out of human projections of their own faults. And maybe these projections create and support beings/entities sitting in between us and the heavens? Beings which then interfere in our communication with the true Heavens?

The term 'Highest Possible Good' made me think 'up'. When the world was still believed to be flat, that might have made sense (on a round planet everybody's 'up' goes somewhere else though). Who knows where the Divine really resides? I feel there is a great amount of help coming from Ultimate Good Powers from below our feet too. 'Highest' keeps on implying that the one-and-only true and pure energy comes through the crown chakra, but I believe there is a pure ultimate good Source for each chakra or energy system, from all directions. I changed 'Highest Possible Good' to 'Ultimate Good'!

Since becoming spiritually aware I had believed that everything is conscious and alive. It is the shamanic way of looking at life. A shaman believes that everything has some consciousness: a rock, a plant, a mountain, your kitchen table, fire, wind etc. I believe there are divine, spiritual, nonphysical beings, such as angels. Furthermore I had allowed for some negative spiritual beings, but had never really thought too much about them. I had seen movies such as *The Exorcist* and as much as I thought such possible, my life path so far had not made me come across any possessed people (levitating or speaking in tongues), so I figured such demons must be rare. Obviously spiritual worlds are not all just black and white; there must be countless spiritual beings which could be called grey, and which may or may not support a human. Whether such energies interact with us, positively or negatively, might depend on circumstances, but overall I guess that the spiritual realms are much like humanity: some good, some bad and some a mix of both.

As a healer I believe that love, health, happiness, kindness, empathy etc. are energies which we would call 'light'. One might call such energies Life Enhancing Energies (LEEs). On the other hand there are also Life Limiting Energies (LLEs), such as stress, anger, fear, guilt, envy, pain, illness, which can be visualized as grey or dark and which depending on their strength or number can cause suffering. Talking about this side of the energy spectrum is often seen as unsavory, to say the least. If you start talking to other Lightworkers about LLEs they might make the sign of the cross and change the subject, so as to not attract such energies. (When I pray, I often just call LLEs 'negativities' or 'baddies' – less scientific. In colloquial language I might talk about 'demons' too. I try to avoid the latter term as much as possible though, as it can conjure strong religious imagery.)

In talking to skeptics about LLEs you run the risk of being branded as a lunatic, and it is not just these external reactions that constitute a challenge. For years I fought energies suggesting I seek psychiatric help whenever I delved into understanding more about the murkier sides of the energy spectrum. But simply ignoring LLEs does not make them go away. Especially as a healer or Lightworker the chances of encountering LLEs are increased. After all we channel Light for our clients' benefit, to help them get rid of grey or dark energies and to improve their well-being. To refuse to think about the nature of LLEs at all is a bit like a doctor refusing to conduct research into a disease, fearing that more knowledge about it will make it worse. Usually the opposite is the case; understanding a disease often removes some of the fear associated with it. Understanding more about LLEs has definitely helped me to be more imperturbable about mine or my clients' suffering. And more importantly, understanding an illness can open doors to finding tools and mechanisms to combat it.

For the first few years, and in my darkest hours, I would get doubts about whether there is a spiritual realm at all, let alone divine powers. Was I just imagining things? Was I totally wasting my time and resources staying on the spiritual path? There was one book by Dr. Elisabeth Kübler-Ross, *On Life After Death*, about her near-death experience research, which gave me strength in times of strong doubt. If you are not aware, Dr. Elisabeth Kübler-Ross was a renowned psychiatrist and author, who gained international fame for her landmark work on death and dying. I had even learned about her and her postulated 'Five Stages of Grief' in my medical psychology lectures. I guess most Western doctors and medical students will know about that part of her work. That she conducted research into near-death experiences seems much less commonly known.

Dr. Kübler-Ross talked to blind people (who had had sight up to some point in their lives) who had near-death experiences. Their experiences matched those of sighted near-death patients. Remarkably blind patients could see again during their near-death episodes. They reported the common phenomenon of floating above their bodies and observing all that happened in their hospital rooms – how nurses and doctors attended their cardiac arrests etc. They then potentially went on to see 'The Light' or dead relatives. If near-death experience would just be 'lack of oxygen-induced imagination' these patients could obviously have 'heard' stuff happening around their hospital bed, but they could not have 'seen' (being blind!) who was in the room and especially what they were wearing. Could the patients have heard what people were wearing? Someone remarked on the chic blue-red striped tie of the doctor attending the resuscitation? I would think that in view of a patient's heart failure and the ongoing resuscitation attempts, doctors and nurses will probably have better things to do then to exchange pleasant small talk about each other's attire?

To me these stories prove that we as humans are more than just a physical body. Our soul seems to be able to exist beyond and outside the physical body and hence likely beyond death as well! Every time I read about remote viewing or out-of-body experiences, it helped me further consolidate my beliefs. If I add books about scientific experiments on telepathic and telekinetic human abilities to this list, extrasensory perception becomes very viable too.

That begs the question: if spiritual realms exist, is there some higher power? Are there Angels for example? Well I argue that if a remote viewer can accurately tell you (to significant detail and with statistically significant correctness) what a remote location looks like he/she has never been to – that proves that they can connect to a place and see it (outside their physical reaches). So if a healer, sensitive, psychic or even 'normal' person sees angels at times, there is the potential that they are not just imagining them either! I know I have no hard evidence that Ultimate Good exists. I have done shamanic journeys into the angelic realm, where I usually experienced a greater sense of peace and happiness, with occasional images and impressions in front of my 'inner' eye. These impressions are very fleeting and more of a knowing than a 'seeing' – so without a camera which I can take with me on such travels solid proof eludes me.

Nowadays I always experience healing energy when I work on others or myself. To me those energies have become a part of my life. I believe them to be 'all good'. If I meditate, the energies usually make me feel better, happier and more peaceful and that is the effect my clients usually report as well. This too is proof, to me, that there are benign powers. Even more so these days, as I hardly do any visualization during my healing work, but try to just be an open channel for the energies to do their thing. I know one could argue that my clients just feel better because of the massage I perform on them. I might just be a good masseur?

I do get clients though that have had massages all over the world and who report that mine is one of the best: relaxing, refreshing and the most intuitive they have experienced. Furthermore most note that my hands can get exceptionally hot and that there can be a strong urge to 'nod off', which they don't get with 'regular' masseurs. If I were barking mad, one might also expect that reasonable people, such as most of my clients (mostly all higher educated and professionals), would have a hard time relaxing in my presence.

I used to go out and look for scientific studies to affirm my beliefs, and help alleviate doubts, but hardly feel the urge for this anymore. I usually found plenty of studies affirming the value of spiritual healing or meditation; they can often be matched by the writings of skeptics, who tell you that you are deluded and/or simply experiencing placebo effects. Regular meditation seems to produce visible changes to the human brain, as do other regular activities, e.g. dancers diminish their vertigo center in the brain and can hence spin more. An obvious difficulty with conducting studies into spiritual activity and effects is that they might not appear from one day to the next. Most scientific studies expect to see results relatively quickly. What if connecting to the Divine, feeling beneficial effects and losing one's doubts is a skill, which has to be 'trained', potentially over years? No one would argue for example that a violin cannot produce beautiful music just because it is in untrained hands...

There is something else too. The following reasoning works for me, because I believe that I experience LLE resistance. Obviously if someone thought I was 'mad' and that the LLE resistance I report is just a figment of my imagination, the following does not count. If I am right and I do experience LLE resistance – negative energies attacking me before, during and sometimes after I see a client – then that indirectly proves that I do channel benign healing energies. Why else bother to attack me? If the energies I channel were no threat to a client's e.g. stress energies, they would just ignore me or laugh at me.

And I am not the only person that experiences energy resistance – many people might just be scared to talk about it or admit to it. It is pretty unsexy and sounds rather crazy to say that one is so light and/or spiritual that more confused energies seem to see one as a threat, and attack. I know that some would argue that I have been deluding myself for so many years, that today I feel energy resistance regularly as part of that delusion, that I might need it to make myself feel important or such. It is an interesting line of thought but, I feel, unlikely.

I never really read about energy resistance before. Perhaps some healers might report backlash effects when exorcising spirit possessions, but I have not read anything about experiencing energy resistance with 'regular' clients. As mentioned, I actually rejected this theory for a good while, as it seemed too crazy. After working for a while and observing my clients and the thoughts and emotions that went through my mind before, during and after my sessions with them, I was 'forced' to deduce that there is such a thing as energy resistance, attacks and so forth. Perhaps my mind was frantically searching for theories and constructs for why I was not performing miracle healings? And so it came up with the elaborate LLE structures and resistances? Possibly – but then again it would be remarkable that my mind could just do that, without my direct conscious input.

I believe that Ultimate Good has created everything and guided evolution. I doubt that negative forces, which innately want to suppress and destroy, would have had the patience to create anything as complex as the living creatures on this planet – we'd be blobs of mud continuously bashing each other's mud heads in. If the Bad was stronger than the Good, if Bad was at the core of everything, how could any Good ever have come to be? I am saying Good created Neutral and Bad (as a temporary experience), while others might believe that Neutral created Good and Bad. It could be argued that it is highly unlikely that Bad created Neutral and Good. Even if our universe started off as 'neutral', I cannot believe that it would take billions of years for some souls to decide for themselves that spending eternity in Good is more fun than in Bad, or with the potential of Bad. Call me naïve or romantic, but a few billion years is a very long time to learn that Good makes one happier than Bad!

I know it is hard to agree with this if one is stuck in some major suffering at the moment, or if you generally tend to just look at all the ill in the world. But if we step back a bit, the world is truly remarkable. All this sums up my belief that there is Ultimate Good and that I am not crazy to believe it. Believing that Good is eternal, and Bad an artificially created temporary illusion, gives me greater peace, than to believe that my (and everyone's) core might be neutral and hence the 'fight' to stay good potentially eternal. I believe that Ultimate Good is indeed ultimately good. It has taken me years to relax into this belief and I believe it wholeheartedly. I do not intend to go back to making uncertainty an option. I have also seen enough good – relaxation, healing and happiness – come out of channeled healings, for others and myself, to back up my beliefs.

Chapter 8

Understanding the Enemy

Understanding LLEs and LLE structures has helped me become more serene and confident. More importantly it allowed me to understand why some healings seem to be easy and effortless, while others take more effort and time to work through. The more I observe and analyze why I might have felt bad, fallen into a specific trap or believed LLE propaganda – the greater a chance I have for it to not happen again. More knowledge can help to debunk paranoia, which in my experience is a common tool utilized by negative energies.

At a basic level I believe that LLEs are born, forgetting their previous Ultimate Good self, and die at some point. Looking at the Christian model, demons are fallen angels. I see these stories as humanization of the Divine though. Humans project their own fallibility (illusions) onto Ultimate Good beings. Alternatively some prophet might have been told, with apparent divine authority, that it is so. Well I had powerful voices talk to me, but what they told me just made no sense when I thought about it. Or some such prophet just was not ready to hear the truth, namely that the Divine created evil for our 'entertainment'. The 'fallen angels' theory fails to consider that this planet is a pre-chosen 'suffering' planet too. Furthermore LLEs come in all shapes and sizes. A fallen angel would be a formidable demon and possession would be like that of a horror movie. What about 'little' negativities, a feeling of sadness, a bit of envy or a touch of stress?

I believe that all suffering and the LLEs enabling it are 'artificially' created. The whole suffering system is so complex and well thought through in its creation though that, living in the middle of suffering, suffering becomes 'normal' and 'real' – even though it is just a temporary illusion. It is a suffering theatre production, where the audience is part of the play and the players have forgotten that they are only acting… In this illusion it 'looks like' we create evil by thinking, feeling and enacting negative thoughts, emotions and deeds. It also looks like we as humans are 'new' when we are born, and 'gone' when we die, yet I believe that we are eternal, individualized divine spirit.

One way for LLEs to be sustained, grow or multiply is to get humans to think negative thoughts or feel negative emotions. In our 'creational' capacity as divine beings we use 'neutral' energy and turn this 'neutral' energy (Prana, Chi?) into either 'good' or 'bad' thoughts, emotions etc. Both saint and tyrant breathe 'neutral' air and eat 'neutral' food, which enables them in their physical bodies to think, feel and do either good or bad things. But even this 'neutral' energy like air or food is part of the illusion. In a truly Ultimate Good world we might still breathe and eat, but air and food would be fully self-aware as well and refuse to sustain and strengthen our bodies if we just contemplated to use them for 'bad'.

Do we enable LLEs to multiply like bacteria by giving in to them, by continuing to think or feel negative about something? When I am in a room with others who have certain beliefs, especially less enlightened ones, I will often start thinking similar thoughts or feel similar emotions – as if being 'infected'. Similarly, if I read an enlightened book or attend a seminar on healing – it will be easier to think about healing and believe in its power. Is that how mobs work – via energetic infection? But one also might have to consider that some people might be more sensitive and susceptible than others (already).

I don't feel like going out and killing after watching an action movie, but have to admit that there is some 'infection' that can come through watching TV, especially if strong emotions are involved. Therefore I much rather watch a feel-good movie, than a downer (and I cannot watch horror anymore). I would not propagate the prohibition of action movies though. I don't feel their influence is strong enough to a 'sane' mind. Where would one stop? Even the radio, books or just verbally told stories can potentially influence one's mood, beliefs etc. Vicariously experiencing some suffering through seeing it on TV or such might help or teach us to not live it ourselves too.

One other aspect of LLEs is their size. How big or small are they? I am not 100% sure. Again I can only go from what I feel. Mostly when meditating and going into specific emotions (which I intend to rid myself of) they feel like (heavy) patches inside my aura, sometimes inside, but mainly 'outside' and pressing onto my physical body. A typical patch would be 20 centimeters in diameter, whereas the actual emotion might fill most of my being. The only problem with this observation is that it seems 'physically' impossible for every emotion we have to be that size. There are so many emotions that I experience every day – my emotional body would have to be humongous to make room for all of them.

When clearing negative emotions, I at times get a different picture, that of fine-grit particles, a bit like clusters of bacteria or a lump of sand. This makes more sense rationally. If there is an accumulation of LLE clusters inside or before a chakra, this could also explain the feeling of a chakra being 'blocked' when trying to cleanse/heal it. The best allegory I can come up with is atherosclerosis. Fatty cholesterol in the human bloodstream can lump up, get stuck on our artery walls – which can lead to inflammation of our artery walls, with cholesterol plaques settling in them and over time literally clogging up whole arteries. Plus our arteries become more brittle and less flexible. So perhaps the 'actual' body of a negative thought or emotion is as big as a grain of sand (probably even smaller). Each grain perhaps has some more 'auric' bodies around them, so they feel bigger? Or perhaps they can project energy, puff themselves up and make themselves feel bigger than they actually are?

Unless you cleanse your auras regularly, these grains of negative emotions can accumulate. The bigger these lumps become the more negative energy they accumulate. They might be more connected to LLEs on the outside too, all of which can give them more and more power to manipulate and make us forget that in fact we are unconditional loving and eternal beings. I try to understand how big LLEs are, how they look, to help me remember that at times small things can have great impact. For example if I step on a needle, the pain can be intense, but mostly calms down when I see it is just a tiny red dot. Equally if I realize that an LLE might just be a small patch of energy, even if it feels terrifying, I'll get onto removing it rather than feeling sorry for myself and indulging the fear.

Clients who do little to cleanse their own energies frequently feel clogged up. Trying to send healing energies into them can feel like hitting a brick wall. The solution is to treat these encrustations with some spiritual solvent, bit by bit. Understanding that LLE encrustations are likely an accumulation of small LLEs also helps me feel better about dissolving them. I am not cutting up a large LLE body to remove them. I am not killing them, rather dissolving the plaques into their original elements of a multitude of tiny-bodied LLEs.

At some point I tried to understand how Ultimate Good can create evil or confused energies/beings out of ultimately good energies. My initial thought was that the LLEs might just be playing 'bad'. If they were consciously playing bad, asking them to stop being bad would put an instant stop to whatever suffering they are causing. I asked them to please just stop making me suffer, but that did not do much. I had to conclude that LLEs must be more complex than that. The next idea was that, as every being – however bad – has an ultimate good core, maybe that core could influence the evil energies surrounding it? I asked the cores to get their mantles to stop their evildoing; but again, not much of a (quick) result. Perhaps the negativities just act bad because they have forgotten that they are good? That would mean though that there is some energy making them forget, blocking their memories. Maybe that energy is still conscious? I asked that energy to unblock the LLEs' memories – no result. Maybe there is another energy that is conscious above that? Nothing. I could go on like that forever.

I imagine that perhaps a single little negativity, say a bit of envy, is probably created out of say a million Ultimate Good energy parts – each just the tiniest fraction 'off' its ultimate best center – to an allowed degree. If one adds all those tiny degrees of twistedness, 'the whole' is so twisted that it creates an abnormal behavior. Fuse multiples of such twisted parts and have them re-enforce each other, and one gets more and more of an LLE that thinks it is 'real'. It appears that when Ultimate Good creates something, even LLEs, it is quality work and not all that easily dismantled. Well, I assume they have special tools in heaven, not available to us down here, to dismantle or rehabilitate LLEs more quickly. For whatever reason we cannot get these tools yet, so, for now, we have to bear with the slower healing processes.

Considering that I can feel 'attacked' by a client's negative energies before a client arrives or before I travel somewhere, LLEs could be argued to have (varying) degrees of self-awareness and self-preservation mechanisms. They could be either psychic or receptive to mechanisms/networks that 'warn' them in advance against potential healing threats. Some 'warning' mechanisms might be quite straightforward, e.g. when a client reads my Web site, I openly explain that I work with healing energies – I presume that client's LLEs might see a potential threat coming that way.

What though with the resistances and attacks I experience just planning to go abroad? I am filled with thoughts of *Oh, I don't really fancy going anymore* (when clearly I am looking forward to my trip), and the closer I get to my departure the more violent the attacks will get. My vegetative nervous system will be in upheaval, e.g. I'll have to pee every five minutes. I will be hit by procrastination, apparently trying to make me miss my flight, but I also used to get visions of my plane crashing or exploding, and that everyone will die because I selfishly wanted a holiday. Now to date I and all my fellow travelers have survived all flights, yet it was often very uncomfortable, and naturally I do pray for sufficient Ultimate Good protections.

If I ignore these threats, the LLEs might try another approach, alerting me to the fact that the resistances I experience to stop me travelling are because the flight is 'scheduled' to crash. They just want to save my life! They pretend to be Ultimate Good intuition. I pray to Ultimate Good and ask that if they do not want me on a particular flight, they either have to get me to book another one initially (surely they know far ahead if a flight is scheduled to crash) or really incapacitate me for travel.

A few years back, when scheduled to go to Croatia, I got bronchitis four days before flying out. This had me running to my GP trying to get antibiotics. The antibiotics gave me such bad stomach cramps that I had the cab driver, on the way to the airport, turn around and drive me back home. Needless to say the flight did not crash! I changed the antibiotics and flew the next day – it was my grandma's 90th birthday after all!

How do LLEs know I am coming and that I am a Lightworker? Do they check all flights booked to their destination against a list of known Lightworkers? Am I famous in LLE circles, a Lightworker celebrity, a Van Helsing for LLEs? It sounded all too far-fetched and paranoid, but after years of experiencing it and considering other experiences of mine – it started to feel more feasible. The most fitting conclusion I can come up with is that there seem to be LLE structures and hierarchies, some of which operate independently and outside of humans. Like the Mafia, there will be little guys, the runners then middle-management right up to the Dons/Godfathers.

Lower levels will look to higher levels for instruction and protection – but they will likely have to pay their dues to receive these. So each city, each country will have their LLE Dons with systems in place trying to keep Lightworkers out. Or if Lightworkers are there already, they will try their best to push them out.

I now understood why at times I might have been attacked so strongly and consistently with apparently nice clients. I most likely had been attacked by energies inside their bodies and also LLEs on the outside – backup LLEs. If a certain kind of debilitating energy or negative emotion gets removed during a healing, then as soon as possible it might be replaced with more of the same kind. And if a healer attempts to remove an LLE from a client's body he/she might get hit by outside supporting LLEs, trying to stop the removal.

I understood that not just illnesses, negative emotions, countries, regions or places might have their Godfather LLEs and collective subconscious LLEs, but so might certain professions and other structures which can cause suffering – political associations, religious beliefs and so on. Potentially I am a targeted not just for the client's energies, but by higher-ranking (outside) LLEs, who have a vested interest in the client not being enlightened or healed.

The stronger a suffering, the greater the interest of the LLEs to keep it going, and the more likely a higher level LLE structure is behind it, therefore the more healing energies and effort it will take to defeat them. Perhaps it is one of the reasons why acute illnesses are often healed more easily than chronic ones, because acute illnesses create suffering for a short period, chronic are more 'lucrative' for LLEs.

The healer vs. illness-energy battle is obviously a very clear cut and strong example of an energy conflict. I believe that such 'battles' do not just happen to conscious Lightworkers though; wherever lighter energies come in contact with greyer, more confused energies, a conflict may arise. In a relationship for example where one partner is messier than the other, the messy energies might try to resist the tidier energies of his/her partner. Or the unpunctuality energies of your friend might resist your punctuality energies etc.

LLEs seem to have a great PR system to stay 'hidden' too. One of the reasons why it took me so long to fully acknowledge LLEs was that I was scared to be seen as a paranoid psychotic. I guess Carl Jung – the collective unconscious he describes – might have described similar LLE structures as I see now. I am not sure if he took another step though to allow these collective unconscious energies self-awareness, intelligence and the potential abilities to grow or defend their reign too. Another reason why LLEs might have an interest in staying hidden is because as long as they are unaware, healers and Lightworkers might not pray for their removal and keep on blaming themselves or their clients for everything negative they feel or apparently unsuccessful healings.

Sure it sounds scary (and paranoid) to be surrounded by negative energies out to get us. But life just makes more sense to me if I add them to the equation. Initially after the discovery of bacteria and the theory of infection, some people became consumed with paranoia. Suddenly they 'knew' they were surrounded by ubiquitous, invisible (to the naked eye) organisms that had the potential to kill. It might have taken a few years to get used to these new realizations and remember that life on this planet had survived and thrived thus far, without being eradicated by bacteria. As a healer I already believed that the healing energies I channel have their own intelligence and that they will do what is necessary, go where needed etc. So why should negative energies not have some intelligence too?

I consider any energy that is confused or negative, and tries to make me feel, think or act in ways that are not Ultimate Good, an energy that should be removed. If it is in my body, I kick it out and ask for Ultimate Good to take that energy for safekeeping, or rehabilitation. Strictly speaking I am almost constantly exorcising LLEs, but then I have a high standard for my well-being; every grumpiness, sadness, loneliness, undue tiredness, irritability, anger etc. that I notice I expel as soon as possible. I do not believe that every LLE has to be consciously banished though. We probably have some kind of 'immune-system' for all our bodies, not just the physical – by that I mean systems and mechanisms which fight negative energies, defuse them, kill them or expel them – without ourselves being consciously aware of this or having to control it in any way. I postulate that our auric bodies too have receptors which make it easier for some LLEs to influence us than others (like some people might have physical, genetic dispositions to certain diseases). Vice versa some people's auras might have better self-defense mechanisms than others' to fend off the negative influence of some LLEs.

My 'conscious' exorcising efforts might sound like a lot of work, but I have prayed for 24/7 Ultimate Good support, so whatever my aura-immune-system cannot handle is dealt with automatically by Ultimate Good. At times I put more awareness into the process, to support it with my own energies, but I have not actually 'verbalized' the handing-over tool in years anymore. That still leaves an increased level of awareness to cut off unsavory thoughts or emotions as soon as possible, which has become more and more a work of love and hence requires less and less energy.

The great thing is that humanity already has most tools necessary to combat LLEs – there are the principles of leading a sensible healthy lifestyle, with decent food, some sunshine and exercise. In addition one can cleanse one's aura with incense, smudging or salt baths for example. These basics are good and might be enough for some. For larger scale or more intense attacks, one just has to ask (Ultimate Good) for help and it is given! I find prayer, meditation, visualization and other spiritual tools can be very effective to heal and excrete LLEs, as well as increase our protections against them.

I suspect that some LLE structures often go much further afield and are much more complex than I might imagine. I do believe that however extensive healings have to be and however many Ultimate Good helpers it may require to heal something, if you pray for 'perfect' help it will be delivered. For all suffering in existence there is an abundance of Ultimate Good help just waiting for someone to ask for their assistance. Should you still be worried by all this potentially new information, I am still here; I have survived thus far!

Today I am a clean channel; my chakras feel clear and flowing. Before, I often saw them as my enemy and/or conspiring against myself. They seemed to either be full of sheer endless amounts of negativities and/or incapable of expelling these negativities. Now I am confident that Ultimate Good loves and helps me. I am not forsaken.

I asked years ago that if the rest of my life would just be suffering (especially as bad as during my CFS years) could I please be taken out of my body ASAP. I did not see any good reason to hang about for such a masochistic experience. Still being here and having improved in my general well-being – I conclude that living on this planet and truly wanting to be free is a cause worth fighting for. There is abundant happiness and love still to be experienced.

For now I am more of a Lightsoldier than a Lightworker. I try to be vigilant about my thoughts and emotions, to make sure that they are not in fact invading LLEs, trying to twist me into living, thinking, feeling and acting the way they would like me to. Still the overall happiness bottom line seems to get greater and greater. I believe that one day either there will be no more LLEs that attack me, they won't be strong enough anymore, cannot attach to my energies anymore or they will have learned that attacking me and my life costs them too much. This I believe wholeheartedly.

Being a 'Soldier of Light' is the safest kind one can be. Ultimate Good can always place its helping troops as strategically and wise as ever possible, and there is never a shortage of troops. So far it has not been a fight that has brought me much fame or even respect. I have plenty of very grateful clients, which is great! But most of my clients' knowledge does not stretch as far as to know that I might get attacked by their accumulated negativities or associated LLEs on the outside. I would think that most healers will experience healing resistance from their clients' energies to varying degrees. Healers do not just stand there and hold the hands over the clients' bodies. Most masseurs I talk to report that they have 'experienced' clients' negative energies.

Whenever I get a massage, I ask my masseur if they ever get 'negative' clients and feel their energies. Usually the answer is a resounding, "Yes." One masseuse reported that she gets pains in her (hand) tendons, even before such clients show up. Even doctors and other therapists express an understanding when I ask them about their patients' negative energies. Usually I have to be the one who mentions these phenomena first though; I would not be surprised if many of them are ashamed of feeling their clients' negative energies and scared that there might be something mentally wrong with them. I also ask clients, who seem/feel spiritually advanced, if they experience 'resistance' – and usually they appear to know exactly what I mean. One such client said very nicely, "That is the thing with the spiritual path, resistance increases; but the good things become more and more intense, better and better too!"

Again, some skeptics would argue that my mind has created all the above negative constructs to make me feel better about some psychosis, transforming myself from a mentally challenged person to a potential healer hero. With many humans come many different opinions. As with all mental and emotional experiences any e.g. psychiatrist will only be able to observe their patient from the outside and rely on their patients to share what they are experiencing inside. The psychiatrist will then extrapolate these narratives and observations with their own beliefs founded on their own socialization, education (medical and other) and observation of their own personal minds and mind mechanisms.

In the end how we 'interpret' our thoughts and emotions is a question of belief. There are few tools available to objectively measure the mind. My beliefs are based on my conviction in Ultimate Good, as well as observing my thoughts, feelings, experiences and sensations over the last 17 years. This belief in Ultimate Good and my observations have led to my conclusions and theories. For an atheist and skeptic (of all things spiritual), their beliefs are founded on scientific observations (which, I believe, with regard to emotions and mental processes are hard to quantify) and often the premise that there is no Ultimate Good.

My beliefs give me peace of mind, help me improve my well-being and most importantly give me hope for an ever-improving quality of life. If I were an atheist and skeptic, and believed I was say schizophrenic, the only hope I would have would be in drugs (and their potential side effects) to suppress my condition, or that one day some brain surgeon finds the right nerve to sever or implants some microchip, suppressing or bridging supposedly defect processes in my brain, which in turn would make me feel more whole again.

I believe that there are many people who go through similar experiences. They too might suspect that they are battling outside forces more than inside ones, but are still not confident enough to admit this. My experiences and theories might set them free too, especially if they have not already allowed Ultimate Good (or whatever they call it) to act on their behalf in the outside too. I strongly hope and believe it is going to help them as much as it is helping me.

I have to admit there is one, more selfish reason... I believe that the more people who read this book and in return give Ultimate Good free rein to heal them, their bodies and their lives, the quicker my life should improve too. (Not just from book sales, but energetically!) I am confident that in time I will be able to heal my life completely. But there are certain big projects which need as much 'Light' input as possible – like preventing climatic meltdown, I really prefer a nice environment to live in to a catastrophic one; a stable enough (world) economy or, what I am personally interested in, ridding humanity of HIV and other STIs. All these goals will be easier and potentially quicker and more effortless to achieve the more Lightworker/soldiers face these challenges and ask Ultimate Good for their perfect healings.

In retrospect I realized, that for a few years, I lived in research-like conditions. Being self-employed I scarcely left the house. I would only head out to the gym across the road a few times a week and go to the supermarket and bank about once a week. I wasn't a loner, I used to enjoy being around and working with people, but there were still certain resistances about going out to town or to e.g. pubs, bars and clubs. If I planned to have a night out, I often had to prepare myself energetically before – meditate and exercise against the resisting/opposing LLEs who rather I didn't go. The only other (main) factors (on my energies) were regular phone calls to my family and usually long-term flat mates, i.e. both relatively invariable.

By just being at home and having the one or two clients a day, it was easier for me to identify certain energy patterns with certain clients. Again, there might be the fear that if I start to see patterns and associate certain clients with heavy energies, I almost expect them to come with loads of negative energies. Might I project my expectations onto them? For one, as said, I have a continuous prayer placed with Ultimate Good to protect my clients from such energetic mechanisms, but I have also had clients in the past that surprised me and did not fulfil my energetic expectations of them. For example I had a client from Europe. His phone number was from country 'A'. A country I had started to associate with usually tons of negative energies. When I gave healing to said client, his energies were refreshingly normal though. It turned out that he only lives in country 'A', but stems from another European country. Another time I had a client who came every few weeks for a while and during his first four sessions had terrible energies. When he came the fifth time they were gone. Loads of negativities must have dissolved in between sessions four and five. I was still bracing myself for a turbulent healing ride when he arrived for session five, but it turned out to be a breeze.

At times I wish that my realization about LLEs was just a figment of my imagination. I cannot guarantee that I am right, but I have learned that admitting to their existence and facing them head-on has actually improved my well-being and given me increasing peace of mind. Obviously I do not want to create more suffering with my theories; I simply want to explain the suffering that exists already. I had strong fears in the past that committing myself to a worldview including LLEs I might just help create them, bring them into existence. If anything though, my life is better than before I had this idea.

Understanding that sufferings have a negative energetic component too and engaging positive energetic measures (like prayer, meditation and healing) to counter them can help heal or protect oneself. I know that I am not the first to make these discoveries. I am not sure that had I read about LLEs myself years ago, I would have believed what I had read! It might have speeded up some of my thought and conclusion processes though. I was only able to start to understand (and accept) the LLE/LEE-systems myself through my experiences, my self-healing journey and giving healing to others.

Chapter 9

Tricks, Traps and Weapons

Not all LLEs will try to trick a healer; many probably just leave when they encounter the Light and understand that their presence is not wanted anymore. I have encountered others though who did attempt to harm or trick me. Preparation is key, so to follow are some of the tools, tricks and weapons in their arsenal.

When holding a healing meditation I will usually get several explanations as to what energy is currently attacking me. Some of these intuitions may be correct, but others might be coming from the LLEs themselves. I will try to keep an open mind to whatever 'intuitions' come through, but stay aware and not totally disengage my rational thinking. Most attacks seem to be 'prelashes', i.e. attacks from the LLEs and associated LLEs of clients scheduled to come see me that day or the next. The intention behind these attacks seems to be to have me cancel that client. With backlash the intention, I gather, is to not see a client another time.

Prelash or backlash is hard to describe, sometimes just resulting in a few aches to feelings of being punched in the gut. Often there is also a feeling of my energies having been contaminated; they are no longer 'clear' and bright. Sometimes this can manifest in a flu-like feeling, but it will yield to a thorough cleansing meditation. Emotionally it can range from just being grumpy to thoughts of suicide. There can be a feeling of malice and sometimes the connected threat that I (or my loved ones) will be attacked again if I dare to send healing against these forces in future. There might be feelings of fear, increased runs to the toilet, or general tiredness and weakness. I recently had a client whose LLEs managed to almost completely cut me off from

Ultimate Good energies. My legs ached and I felt nauseous. Fortunately such 'heavy energy' clients and long-lasting prelashes are less and less common. Remarkably once such clients are out of the door, almost all of these attacks cease completely. So even if some LLEs will have tried their best to disconcert me – before and during a healing will have tried to convince me that they are unbeatable, as too strong, too big, too well protected and supposedly having access to unlimited amounts of negative energy reserves – in the end when they are not immediately threatened anymore, they lay off attacking (if they haven't been removed with that healing). Their energy reserves are not inexhaustible and you can overcome the negative feelings.

Some LLEs can be quite clever and intuitive. They'll try to exploit anything they might think a weakness, including strong fixed expectations about their behavior. For example – I read in a book about dealing with negative entities that one can communicate with them to find out why they are with you or a client, find out where they came from, who potentially sent them and how long they have been there. The LLEs might obviously talk balderdash when asking them anything, but supposedly – according to some 'universal law of three' – if one asks repeatedly, three times, energies are compelled to answer truthfully.

I tried all that. It seemed to work for a while – until I almost gave up all doubt that this 'universal law' was infallible. But at that point they clearly started lying again, regardless of how many times I repeated my questions. I have since cut down any potential communication to an absolute minimum again. There are still LLEs trying to tell me they have been sent by Ultimate Good, that I am cursed for all eternity and that I will never be rid of them etc. These thoughts, emotions, intuitions can be very convincing. But once the client leaves or after a good night's sleep they are no more, so I am calmer when such like happens these days.

I have heard about or believed other 'rules' e.g. if one uses a particular color light or visualizes some symbol one's energies will be impregnable. I have also read that negative energies will always attack from the left – through one's emotional, female side. I ask for perfect protection on both sides of my body though. I have plenty of clients too where the right body half is more tense than their left, and the energies are heavier on the right! Furthermore I stay away from certain expectations as to what takes how long to heal etc.

So my rule is... there are no rules! It is best to stay alert, as well as, as protected as possible and to expect the unexpected (without skidding off into paranoia). I know this might sound exhausting, but it has become ever easier. Furthermore if I compare myself to the majority of my clients I have seen so far (and who do not do any spiritual work) – my muscles are more relaxed and my energies clearer and better connected than theirs. I must be doing something right? I am not saying that my clients cannot be happy and have a good time too – many probably have better social standing and income than me. From what I remember about my 'pre-spiritual' times though, it was quite exhausting to be a slave to my emotions, exhausting to be naïve and be game to disappointments or disappointing situations hitting me. Also then I did not have the knowledge that I can access incredible, all-powerful Ultimate Good forces to come and assist me whenever I need their help.

I find that if LLEs try to weaken, demoralize or hurt me, they will use whatever opening they can find and exploit it. When I believed that all emotional problems might stem from my childhood, I would get visions of how I did not have many friends or how friend so and so one day did not want to play with etc. When I believed in regressions they gave me fears of having been Mengele. When I contemplated I might have food allergies, I got gut cramps when eating all my favorite foods. With consistent and honest observation and what I see as a good bit of divine intuition, inspiration and support, I have debunked any such false beliefs. It appears that once I do not fear something anymore, LLEs will use that suffering tool less and less.

Still there are patterns, LLE behaviors, types of attacks, which come up again and again. I guess it is a bit like fencing; the more you practice the more proficient you become at protecting yourself. These days I believe I can say that my mind has become much quicker. A lot of LLE traps I don't fall into anymore – usually by recognizing them as traps quickly. At times it feels e.g. as if I already know what a negative energy is trying to tell me, which fear it attempts to trigger inside me, before it has even verbalized it. I can hence sometimes 'gag' it and commit it to healing light before my peace of mind has been disturbed.

This does not mean that many LLE attacks and resistances are not still uncomfortable, but it does save me from panicking and falling into despair or hopelessness as often as I used to. A common trap I watch out for, for example, involves LLEs trying to make me believe Ultimate Good has forsaken me, because some years ago I was not entirely truthful or straight with someone. Usually, if I rethink the accusations, I find I acted reasonably, plus I do not believe that Ultimate Good would forsake anyone and especially not with a lag of a few of years after something happened. Guilt seems to be one of LLEs' favorite tools in trying to weaken my resolve. To give LLEs as little ammunition as possible, I would therefore recommend to live as straightforward a life as possible and to forgive yourself for anything in the past that might have been, however dodgy. I know self-forgiveness can be tough, but I find it gets easier with time. You have to love yourself unconditionally too, not just others.

LLEs make some suffering look and feel more powerful than it actually is – trying to increase my fear. If a single robber broke into your home, threw a black sheet over you and held you down, they could easily convince you that there are ten more robbers in the house. I find trying to stay as calm as possible and using visualizations helps. I work a lot with Ultimate Good Earth energy. Some LLEs will try to cut off my connection to Ultimate Good Earth energies and pretend they are stronger. I try to remember that there is some distance between me and the pure Ultimate Good Earth forces. Living in a big city like London I need to reestablish the connection to Ultimate Good Earth energies several times a day anyway. But in my view there is a lot more good stuff than can ever be accumulated from negative energies! It is a question of proportions – LLEs might reside in the Earth crust = ca. 70km thick, whereas the Earth radius is over 6300km thick. Add the Divine Ultimate Good energies that are in the Sun and other 'heavenly' bodies and dimensions, and all bad energies on this planet are hopelessly outnumbered.

During a heavy attack LLEs will try their best to either block my memory and knowledge of such facts though, or emotionally try to warp my intuition in such a way that it feels as if there are more destructive forces than positive ones, and it can really feel like that. If you are lost in a swamp for days, it is easy to 'forget' that there is plenty of 'dry' land in other places – forgetting the dry land does not make the dry land disappear though! Or some LLEs have in the past suddenly filled me with doubts about my favorite healing crystal(s) with which I have had loads of successful, comforting and 'good-feeling' healing meditations. Suddenly it felt as if my crystals have just been pretending to be good and are in fact in cahoots with the LLEs. If LLEs are stronger they may even try to make me feel as if Ultimate Good Earth energies and Ultimate Good Sun energies are in fact allied with LLEs affecting humans. I might then have to get other (holy) stars in, exponentially bigger than our Sun, and remember that etheric Ultimate Good worlds, plains are virtually infinite. I usually also pray to the Ultimate Good in the Earth and Sun and inform them about the LLEs' claims; strangely attacks then cease quite quickly.

I have a strong suspicion that at times strong feelings and illusions of 'all-powerful' LLEs can be the way a client's belief that something cannot be healed manifests (especially if they do not have any higher beliefs). For example a client may believe that a character weakness, physical imperfection, illness etc. is genetically 'fixed' and can therefore not be healed. They believe that genetic forces are stronger than the spiritual healing help available to us.

Besides some LLEs trying to make me believe that they are too big to conquer and defeat – some LLEs come with other apparently insurmountable problems. With some very strong LLEs I have seen very thick, very solid, pitch-black protections around them. A bit like black Obsidian – shiny and blackest black – but where Obsidian is natural volcanic glass and can chip, this black stuff was solid and felt absolutely impregnable. Shining a bit of healing light on such a solid black wall did not really do anything. I did have to remind myself then though that Ultimate Good has created LLEs and whatever weaponry they possess. Ultimate Good would be stupid (which they are not!) if giving weaponry to the LLEs for which they do not have some remedy or tool to defeat it.

Solid black walls such as the above do take a lot of energy and time to dismantle. Waiting for something to happen can be quite unnerving. But nothing is impossible and Ultimate Good does have endless amounts of energy at its disposal. Ultimate Good can also go into the smallest of the smallest. Even in the blackest of blackest particle there is some light. If one finds that light in every spiritual atom of the black wall, and pours more light into these, the blackness literally unravels and the most solid, blackest wall can simply crumble into dust.

A common result of illusions of insurmountable negativities is self-pity. Self-pity can be an easy trap to fall into. With it one might even be able to emotionally bind others to you – who feel sorry for you. Being stuck in a self-pity hole you have to watch out that you do not forget that you chose all this suffering and that, even more importantly, there is an abundance of Ultimate Good help out there which can heal any suffering. Self-pity might make us forget too that we are individualized divine and as such actually perfect. Overall it will likely take less time to heal anything if one works on one's adversity, rather than if one wallows in self-pity. Self-pity is just LLE energy. If I ever fall for it, I just forgive myself, hand it over to Ultimate Good and get on with my healing work.

LLEs can attack with an array of negative emotions. With one client I might get lethargy and feelings of dislike about seeing him plus self-pity about being attacked by such; with another lethargy, self-consciousness plus anger about being attacked. LLEs might also have me believe that the emotional responses I feel are 'normal'. When I believed that all such negative emotions would come from me, I would spend hours clearing them, in the hope that I would never feel them again. The LLEs then tried to make me insecure about my decision to 'never feel anger again' though. They reasoned that if I remained happy after an upsetting event, I would use upsetting events to make myself happy and hence be a masochist, or worse I would become a sociopath, incapable of relating to 'normal' people's feelings! But who says that just because you decide not to be unhappy anymore, regardless of what life throws at one, you forget what it used to feel like? You would choose empathy not anger.

Then there is revenge. LLEs that prey on this emotion can be very convincing. If I get hit by anger or revenge energies, I usually just go with the flow. I find it can be more useful to have some adrenaline pumping during a fight, than to start to feel small and sorry for myself. So I will usually just take the energy and use it to power Ultimate Good energies against my attackers. The Ultimate Good energies channeled against my attackers will be free of anger and revenge desires in their actions. For example even if my head is full of thoughts such as *Oh, I hope that bastard hurts when it is being removed by Ultimate Good, at least as much as it hurt me!* I am confident that Ultimate Good sees that these thoughts are not my true heart's desires, and ignores them. Obviously some LLEs will try to convince me that I am giving in to my lower self and living the anger or acting out of revenge. They will try to make me feel guilty. I remember in the *Star Wars* movies how Darth Vader or the Sith Lord would goad the Jedi, "Good, give into your anger; live that hate – they are the path to the dark side." I have learned though that some anger energies are so powerful, I cannot just switch them off. I therefore believe the sin is not to feel the anger, but rather to grab the knife and 'live' the anger. If I utilize the anger instead to fuel my meditation or a good gym session, I can use it for good, and funnily the anger energies are then usually quite quickly withdrawn too.

There is another LLEs ploy to weaken my resolve – threats. The first few times they happened they were very unnerving. I felt under threat that attacks would be made on my family or other loved ones if I went ahead with a particular healing or wrote this book, for example. I know how uncomfortable and unsettling some LLE attacks can be, so the last people I wish them on are my family or loved ones. Initially I did my old self-sacrifice stunt and asked Ultimate Good to take me if my work as a healer jeopardized those I loved, or if Ultimate Good could not simply protect my loved ones against such threats. Well I have not left my body yet, and my family has its shares of dramas, but compared to other families we are still in the 'norm'…

I also understood that from everything I know about LLEs' behavior they can be pretty psychotic and sociopathic. There is no guarantee whatsoever that my family would be safe from attacks, if I were to pass on. If anything, might I be drawing off fire from them by staying incarnated? Furthermore giving in to such attacks is like giving in to terrorists' demands. They'll keep the hostages anyway and make even greater demands or take even more hostages the next time. Or just because the Mafia threatens the families of the police or the judge, one should not abolish the police or the judiciary. In our world those families might be rehoused and get a constant police escort. Well in the spiritual world I expect nothing less. There are probably a number of formidable angel bouncers and warriors around all my loved ones, whenever there might be some danger… One would not say, "Do not befriend a policeman, they are the main target of the Mafia." That might be true on the surface, but not befriending that policeman does not make the Mafia go away! The Mafia is a threat to everybody. Just because they have not tried to extort your say business yet does not mean that they will not do so in the future. If one does not befriend policemen/women and they all get depressed for not finding friends and quit their jobs, it is bad news for everyone. The Mafia would go totally unchecked and unopposed. Some friends might forsake the policemen when the going gets tough (it can get scary), but I doubt they'll condemn the police for doing their job.

When I entertained more of the classical healing philosophy, that any dis-ease I experience is somehow self-generated, I was terrified that these 'bad' energies, still residing inside myself, could somehow 'infect' people around me. I prayed for the outside to be protected against me, but if I could apparently not be protected within myself I was uncertain if other people could. Again I offered to leave my body. Even after years of sitting next to my colleagues in the office, and them not succumbing to mysterious illnesses or going insane, it proved to be an easy fear to fall for nonetheless. I meditated and prayed for my colleagues' protections. From what I knew, few of them had any higher beliefs, or did any spiritual work, so who was actually the greater threat to whom? I could also argue that, if the negativities were inside me, my symptoms would probably be diagnosed as some mental illness by Western medicine. And I never learned, during my medical studies, that mental illness can be infectious.

I have become more sensitive with the passing years. That is great if I have a good day, I'll be happier, really feel my connection to Ultimate Good – the love and compassion; but there were times when just going down to the shops, I seemed to be hit by all the negative energies from the other shoppers. It was exhausting and painful and left me wondering if I had made the right choice following the spiritual path? Maybe if I had stayed ignorant, I would have remained less sensitive and hence happier? Today, however, I believe that what feels like heightened sensitivity is not the result of me becoming thinner skinned and potentially less resilient. I rather believe that by becoming lighter, I have become more of a threat to LLEs. As a result they invest much more energy in attacking me now than they would ever have used years ago. I have not forsaken the hope that one day I might be so perfectly protected and whole, that all my healing work is an effortless breeze – I'll be pretty much invincible, I'll be able to work 24/7 etc. For now there might still be things in my being that enable LLEs to affect me unfavorably with their resistances, pre- and/or backlash attacks.

E.g. I had a client recently who lost his capacity to ground – connect his bodies, through his heels, with Ultimate Good Earth energies. He is South African, of Indian decent. It felt as if the previous generation (let's say his grandparents), who left India and immigrated to South Africa, left their roots behind in India. It felt like the inability to ground was then passed on to future generations. Until I saw this client I wasn't as aware, that our light bodies might also pass on defects, just as our physical bodies do through gene defects. In other words the bodies we enter, when incarnating on this planet, might have defects, due to events happening to past generations. In this example it implied that my client needed a new set of roots. In case there was still any LLE influence on his grandparents' roots, which may affect him today, he had to be disconnected from this effect and his grandparents' roots etc. needed to be freed from their LLE captivity.

After I saw this client I lay down and meditated. I asked that any past-generation defects, on whichever level and in whichever energy system, be healed. There might well be other defects I still haven't uncovered/understood; and until I have, my work and life might be harder than it ideally could. Now I could get depressed that after 17+ years of self-healing I still find 'new' stuff that might need healing, but what is the use of getting depressed? I still believe that I do not necessarily have to know why something is wrong and Ultimate Good will, wherever possible, fix defects, even if I am not aware of them yet. Furthermore there is no use fretting about stuff that simply needs more time to be healed. In the above example, missing soul parts must simply have been protected so well, by the LLEs 'causing' it, that it took that long for me to debunk that healing necessity. The only choice I really have is to move forward and not get frustrated about the tougher days – and especially to not see myself as incompetent, blame myself in any other way or start to feel unjustly treated by Creation.

I do believe that any healing can have far-reaching consequences. Any healing or prayer can help remove suffering energies from this planet. I guess there is a tendency for humans to hope for a limited number of villains. If we naïvely believe that all the ill of a nation is due to its evil dictator, there will be the hope attached that if one manages to topple or kill that dictator all will be well. Perhaps why conspiracy theories talk about the power of the twelve – that supposedly there are 12 mega-rich and powerful individuals on this planet who influence and dictate all worldwide politics and who in turn, indirectly, get blamed for all social injustice globally, the exploitation of resources etc. If only one could find those twelve individuals and 'dethrone' them all would be well. Would it?

I am not so sure if there is a council of 12; however, I am pretty confident that there is still enough greed and hunger for control left in this world that even if the 12 existed and were toppled nothing much would change. I guess as long as people think, believe and feel negative emotions: jealousy, envy, anger, fear, loneliness, greed, revenge, arrogance, superiority, inferiority, self-consciousness, hatred, possession, distrust, misery, disappointment etc. they help to feed and multiply suffering. But if enough people ask for complete healings and non-suffering for themselves and their lives things might change/heal faster (and for the better) than ever thought possible…

The main recurring battle is to reassert my beliefs in Ultimate Good. The LLEs try their best to convince me that they are either bigger, stronger or in greater numbers than Ultimate Good helpers. They try to blame the suffering which they create on Ultimate Good, filling me with doubts like: "Ultimate Good is testing your devotion." "Ultimate Good has better things to do than to help you." "Ultimate Good is all-powerful and could heal you and your life, but do not care to." "This matter cannot be healed, as it is too big (e.g. an incurable disease, the climate or the economy)" etc. Call me naïve; I say they are wrong!

Chapter 10

Sense in Suffering

Could it be LLEs serve a divine purpose; is there any sense to suffering? Is it a learning tool? Does Ultimate Good make us suffer or want us to suffer? I often ponder – when do I have to bear suffering and when should I rise up and fight? Generally I believe that Ultimate Good does not want us to suffer, full stop. Obviously we are allowed to suffer on this planet though, as we have chosen such for ourselves before we incarnated. But I also believe that we can choose to have our sufferings stopped, by asking Ultimate Good for all current and future sufferings to be abolished as soon as possible. Abolishing/healing suffering can come in many forms. We might be taken out of a suffering situation where the situation goes on without us. A suffering might be healed and disappear. Or we might reach higher understanding/enlightenment and our view towards the suffering changes; we either do not see it as suffering anymore and/or it doesn't bother us anymore.

I would say that I am less of a wimp than before I embarked on my spiritual journey. I have learned to ignore certain discomforts, to bear them without letting them get to me – but it took years to get to this stage. I do not believe that Ultimate Good would expect such skills from a Lightworker novice or that Ultimate Good helpers do not bother helping a novice with problems, which, for someone further along the path, might be banalities. I believe that Ultimate Good knows which suffering is bearable at any point of a person's development. I am certain that my Ultimate Good helpers did not mind if I ranted at them in the past, because I was in the middle of a heavy attack and felt forsaken or the like. I cannot claim that, regardless of my asking for the abolishment of all sufferings, my life has been plain sailing. At times I feared that Ultimate Good had forsaken me, that they are hard-hearted or even conspiring with the enemy. Someone less enlightened might still pray for rather selfish and disharmonious endeavors too, and suffer if their objects of desire do not come to fruition, but even then I believe that Ultimate Good will be comforting and help that individual understand and find more harmonious desires. Today I am confident that Ultimate Good does whatever it can to help.

Some ideas in the alternative and complementary therapy scene border on the masochistic; masochistic for the patient and potentially sadistic for the therapist. In many an alternative or complementary therapist's view, painful healing processes seem the norm, healthy, unavoidable or generally caused by their patients' noncompliance. Some therapies are impractical or masochistic in themselves, like diets that take all the joy out of eating, or are so elaborate or frequent, they become unaffordable. Often such therapies are described as 'break-through therapies' though, and not utilizing them is, in turn, marked as ignorant or self-harming. One of the worst culprits is to make clients believe that the persistence of their symptoms is linked to them still not having let go of x, y, z conflict or facing their demons. They might have done so already, and the persistence of their symptoms is due to more practical factors. These clients need help and support, even if they require lengthy healing periods. Not constant attacks on their self-confidence and self-healing abilities.

As a therapist one should very much keep in mind that many a client might have read books, browsed the Internet or seen other therapists before coming to them. Many clients are not total novices to complementary healing, and even total novices might be more enlightened than expected. New Age books have not invented concepts of forgiveness and other 'healing' acts. Some clients might just intuitively know about them! It can be tempting to just blame the client, if they are slow to respond.

Especially if clients have strong insecurities or even self-loathing programs, I too have to watch out that I do not take on their projections, but remain understanding and patient with them. We have to remember though that everybody is individualized divine spirit, and aberrant behavior is always due to LLE manipulation and never due to a conscious decision of the divine part of that being.

In the middle of my chronic fatigue years I read several books which claimed that as long as one suffers, it is due to the patient not truly letting go of their suffering. The sufferer is actually holding on to their suffering because they still need it. Perhaps the sufferer seeks pity and/or attention from others? As a result it took me a while to even voice my troubles to friends and family, fearing that I might just be attention seeking. I begged Ultimate Helpers to break my spiritual fingers or even cut off my spiritual hands – if they were still holding on to my sufferings. In meditation I'd spend hours travelling into the deepest parts of my subconscious to face my demons. None of it helped though and today I am confident that my suffering was unavoidable at the time. Perhaps knowing about probiotics, vitamin D3 and LLEs would have helped, but I just did not have access to that knowledge back then.

Every time I discover and/or activate a new chakra, subchakra or energy system the energy I have available increases. For a little while I will feel this marked increase in power and I'll start dreaming about all the things I might accomplish with this increased amount of energy. I might finish this book quicker, do more clients per week (and with it earn more), get up earlier in the morning etc. Quickly things go back to normal though. It is as if LLEs have caught onto my increased abilities and upped their resistance too. I believe it is the LLEs upping their resistance, not Ultimate Good shoving more work (suffering) my way, thinking I can take it. If I decided today that I had enough of healing work and could afford to change my profession, Ultimate Good would let me. If I won some jackpot tonight and retreated to a Pacific Island that would be allowed (I might just get bored quickly).

I do admit that some pain is 'healthy'; if you cut yourself deeply or broke a leg and didn't seek help, the consequences might be dire! Pain in such cases is the signal of the body that something is wrong and needs urgent attention. Perhaps some emotional pains work along the same lines? They are often much harder to understand and interpret though. I concede now, that if you let your bodies slip into imbalance, you cannot really expect to feel balanced and well either. I would think it is sensible to inform your clients along these lines. I think it becomes damaging, though, if you neglect to tell them that there might be 'outside' forces involved too.

Not all suffering can be attributed to a client's poor behavior, and as a therapist or lecturer one should make sure that clients do not needlessly end up blaming themselves for things they do not directly cause! Sure, they will have pre-chosen to get into whatever suffering they experience – but that ideally just requires one big blanket self-forgiveness – and then one makes the best of it. No need to rub it in again and again and/or make someone believe that they have to practice forgiveness for each iota of their pre-chosen sufferings separately.

Or, as I did when suffering with CFS, patients start to mistrust their own body. I wanted to love my body (physical and all my aura bodies) back then, but it would not heal, regardless of how much healing time and other efforts I put in. Were parts of me conspiring with suffering energies? Being pretty certain today that the onus for the attacks on my well-being was mostly external, and it was simply overwhelmed, I can now love (and trust) my body again.

Another popular suffering reason in alternative healing circles can be 'healing crisis'. If a body is out of sync, it might be more effective if large chunks of suffering are removed in a short space of time. Yet it feels insensitive to potentially scare a client, who likely never had any healing work done before, by shaking things up too much and making them very uncomfortable. If one shakes things up too much (and with it potentially triggers LLE booby traps or resistances) the client might be scared to have healing work done ever again. This might be more detrimental to his health than a buildup of intensity from session to session.

In a physical detox, for example, if one mobilizes toxins, which had been stored away in fatty tissues, one's body will be confronted with these toxins again. Having these increased amounts of toxins whirling around can make one feel pretty crappy. In the same way removing mental, emotional and/or spiritual toxic energies might make a client experience them again, even if just briefly and in a mostly 'safe' healing context. Most of my clients do not show any signs of healing crisis though. I do not believe that this is just because Ultimate Good handles them with velvet gloves and/or tries to prevent me getting into 'litigation' trouble, because a session was too uncomfortable. The main reason, I believe, is that when leaving healings to Ultimate Good forces they will do all in their power not to trigger any healing crisis. Ultimate Good finds no joy in seeing us suffer needlessly.

Ultimate Good might defuse toxins before mobilizing them? Apply a bit of spiritual anesthesia? Healing crises might at times be unavoidable, but if they happen a lot it might not necessarily be a badge of honor for a therapist. There are many ways of healing something – some are more sadistic (or masochistic, from the clients' view) than others. Some clients may seek out more harsh healing modalities, because they have, for whatever reason, feelings of guilt. Subconsciously they may think that if they suffer plenty during a healing process, this may act as some form of penance – after which they deserve to heal. If the result is a good healing, fine. The danger for the therapist and/or client is that they generalize their experience and try to project it onto everyone else with similar symptoms, giving them doubts that their chosen, more painless healing avenues are worthless.

Take detoxing; there are drastic means such as forced vomiting or induced diarrhea. Colonic irrigation might be more comfortable. Plenty of detoxing can be done with cleansing meditation exercises as well though. Or one can try charcoal capsules or zeolite powder; these substances then simply bind more toxins in the gut and one excretes them (more) effortlessly. There might be occasions where forced vomiting is the most practical. A hard-core drug addict might not believe in meditation or zeolite powder. I would always try more comfortable and effortless techniques first though.

Many of my clients have heavy energies on their liver, probably because the liver is one of the organs responsible for digesting (heavy) emotions. I know there are diets to cleanse the liver. The ones I read about did not sound like much fun though. And just trying milk thistle capsules (a strong antioxidant herb for the liver) is so much easier and more effortless.

Ideally healings should be effortless and joyful, but that is not always practically possible – it is more about potentially finding those avenues which are most effective, and prevent or placate LLE resistances as much as possible. I.e. where *easy does it* does not work anymore, *no pain no gain* is sometimes unavoidable, but that pain should be kept as small as possible. For good measure I do not generally expect pain with any of my healings and leave its potential necessity up to my, and the client's, Ultimate Good helpers!

In my professional experience, with clients who do spiritual work already, healings often feel more intense – which could be due to the fact that with less blockages in their energy systems energies are simply able to flow stronger and faster. I know from work on myself that some of my healing meditations are nice, relaxing and almost ecstatic, whereas others are hard work and more uncomfortable. I might just lie there on my bed, but I'll feel like I have been in a spiritual battle when I come round. Still, these days, even uncomfortable sensations are usually easily bearable, as I also feel my connection to Ultimate Good and I trust that they look after me and that all is for the best. Again Ultimate Good does not want us to suffer, but some healings are battles – a few scuffs and grazes might be unavoidable. Every healing is different. I want to avoid people starting to think that only a 'tough' healing is a good healing though. What I want to convey is that tough healings might be necessary at times and one should not be scared of them. The fear element, if one experiences uncomfortable healings, is probably what makes such discomforts the most uncomfortable. The more we advance on the spiritual path the less we will be shaken by such discomforts.

I had regular, uncomfortable side effects with just about every complementary healing method I tried, for years, before starting to feel better at all. This is supposedly quite common with people suffering from ME. I believe that my healing journey was not painful because Ultimate Good wanted it to be, but rather because I stirred up too much LLE resistance at once. So if you constantly suffer from healing crises or uncomfortable side effects, you might just be very bright (energetically) and not necessarily have tendencies towards healing masochism.

As mentioned before, Peter used to say that with spiritual growth and changing to healthier behaviors – one always gets tested first. If deciding to start meditating regularly, one's workload might suddenly increase or one gets more invitations to parties etc. He made it sound as if Ultimate Good was testing the resolve of its subjects. I object. I believe it is LLEs trying to make one forget about one's good intentions. If something tries to stop me in an endeavor (spiritual or otherwise) I just pray for as much Ultimate Good support as necessary. Sooner or later the time, motivation or behavior patterns to enable that endeavor will emerge – LLEs cannot hold up again Ultimate Good forever.

Embarking on 'new' ideas or healing modalities can be uncomfortable occasionally. Recently I have started working more with Hara energies. They seem to harmonize grounding and different level chakra energies. When increasing the amount of energy in some such energetic system, this has been at times accompanied with some form of growth pain. I might feel muscle aches, like after a gym workout, loose bowels or soreness of the spinal cord. If one tries to go with a natural Ultimate Good-spiritual-development-flow though, as best as possible, I do believe that Ultimate Good will always do its best to not develop energy systems prematurely, and to activate them as pain free and effortless as possible.

Personally I did not work much with Kundalini energy until 2012. I was pretty sure it was mostly up and running before. I had read several reports about Kundalini release traumas though – supposedly very uncomfortable, painful and/or psychotic experiences when Kundalini energies had been forced up too prematurely. I heeded these warnings to a degree and definitely still do not force my clients' Kundalini energies. On the other hand Kundalini energy is often described as one of the most pure, divine energies in our bodies. Sometimes it is described as 'the' divine essence of our being. As mentioned before, in my experience Ultimate Good energies always try their best to not cause healing crises, therefore I wonder if Kundalini releases or other spiritual emergencies are more of a life limiting energetic conspiracy trying to deter people from embarking on spiritual development journeys?

Some suffering can turn out to be a blessing. As my grandma always said, "You never know what it is good for." For about two years I had mice living in the house. I knew I could just go into meditation, connect to the mice-in-my-house-spirit and ask them to leave. A healer friend of mine had successfully used such a technique to banish ants from her kitchen. So I talked to the mice-in-my-house-spirit and asked them to leave, but there was no change, they kept bouncing around happily. We made sure no food was left out and sealed all cracks we could find, but the little critters are very flexible and kept on finding loopholes. It was exasperating.

Next thing they started to ignore chocolate and nuts too. I tried 'talking' to them several times. I told them how unhappy I was, especially about them defecating and urinating everywhere. Funnily shortly after telling them that, they stopped doing so. They still ran about, but when moving the fridge, we did not have to clean away mouse droppings from underneath anymore. After two years of do it yourself help I asked our landlord for help, but he pleaded ignorance, blaming it on all the 'food stuff' we must have in the house. Did he expect us to live on dust? That really infuriated me. I told the mice they can move into my landlord's house next door and they disappeared apparently overnight. There was another part to the story though...

Around the same time my housemates moved out. It was time now for them to get closer as a couple and find a place of their own, though. Also they had expressed concerns about me seeing healing clients in the house. They did not want strangers in the house. Since this was my newly chosen profession though, and having been made redundant from my accountancy position, I had no real choice. Only after they left was it possible for me to build up a successful healing and massage practice. It could all have been coincidence, but since the mice did not listen to my pleas or threats during the years before, why did they disappear around that time? It has taught me that some adverse situations in life can have their place and may help make future positive situations possible! Today I live more by another of my grandma's wisdoms – *Nicht aergern, nur wundern!* Loosely translated, *Don't get angry, just wonder at it!*

I used to get really upset about my financial dependency on banks, overdrafts and credit cards. It is a slow process getting out of debt. I have affirmed financial independence and abundance for 17+ years now. I have wanted to leave London for years too, to move back to Germany. From my regular visits back I can see now though that a move back might take more than just a few savings. It might take a few weeks, months if not years before German collective subconscious LLEs would stop attacking me, trying to make me move away again. I have established my base here in London and I think contributed to healing some of its energies. And it appears – even if there are still plenty of LLEs around – they mostly leave me alone, unless they feel majorly threatened or suicidal. Had I moved away before starting on this book, it could have taken several more months, if not years, before I would have carved out enough of a Light-space for myself to have the strength and energy to commence with my writing. Or had I won the lotto jackpot seven years ago, I might not have ended up working as a healer and masseur, which has been of major benefit to me, as it really has helped me to understand more about energies and life.

I am not suggesting that one should not tell Ultimate Good about things one does not like or appreciate. If I do not like something I tell my helpers, guides, protectors. If I need to moan at someone, I moan at them – they can take it. Also, if there might be any chance that they did not consider one of my desires in their healings, then it is better to get it off my chest than find out afterwards that all I had to do was ask. It is not about finding excuses for Ultimate Good and giving up on my dreams. I am still confident that financial independence will happen in my life (if required and creating more happiness than suffering). I just become more and more aware what *all in good time* really means.

So yes, at times suffering might be unavoidable and actually help us learn (or rediscover) something or help us to suffer less in the long run. However, to resign to suffering believing it is creation sent, in order to learn something, is misunderstanding Ultimate Good. Sure most of us are here to experience suffering, we have pre-chosen it. But once we have had enough of it (and some people might not be bored of it yet), we are allowed to ask for its abolishment. From then on, I believe one has a right to and should fight for happiness, and you will get all the necessary spiritual help to gain (or regain) happiness as swiftly and effortlessly as possible – always.

Chapter 11

Ethics of Healing

Channeling healing energies per se is easy. You just ask Ultimate Good for perfect healing help and tell them that you are willing to be a channel for healing energies, for yourself, who- or whatever else. Furthermore you ask for perfect protections and grounding and off you go. To then just step back, be fully trusting and let the healing energies do their work is the real challenge. One's inquisitive and querying mind might come up with some questions about ethics and moralities for our healing work too and it is good to have the answers to them, so that our healing is and remains working for the highest purpose of the recipient. The more we understand about healing and life, the less likely we will be shaken and the better we can advise our clients.

It is important to use healing sources that are as unconditionally loving, pure, enlightened, capable, considerate and as wise as possible. I have long ago told Ultimate Good that I only want to work with them and on their behalf. I pray to 'Ultimate Good' and 'Those trusted by Ultimate Good', i.e. if e.g. my dead grandma would like to help, but is not a fully qualified angel or helper yet, and it is 'okay' with Ultimate Good, she is welcome to join in too.

The only physically embodied beings I consider working with are Earth, the Sun and the Moon. I am pretty certain that there are Ultimate Good forces inside the Earth, the Sun and probably the Moon, which I frequently include in my healings. The Earth as I see it has some confused energies in the crust, but the mantle and core is Ultimate Good and that is where I probably get most of my help from. Furthermore I do like crystals, so after vetting them I keep them around me and use them to help me focus and channel healing energies too.

Generally I am not a big fan of working with nature spirits. In the past I followed the advice of Pagans who work with nature. At first it made sense to me that if Ultimate Good is in everything, it will be in Nature's beings too... A few trees I tried to hug, even after asking for their blessing, seemed to tell me to 'F-off' though. A few places I have been to out in the country felt uncomfortable, even malicious. The majority of all beings incarnating on this planet, be they human, animal, insect or plant, perhaps even rocks, seem to forget that they are individualized divine spirit when incarnating, so there is a chance that not all trees are gentle, enlightened giants for example. And if there are any nature spirits that do fancy helping out with my healings, and who are trusted by Ultimate Good, they are welcome to chip in.

A further benefit I find in working with Ultimate Good energies is that they are available 24/7. Especially during my chronic fatigue years I was pretty much constantly in a state of spiritual emergency; when then reading books telling me that I might have to wait for an e.g. particular moon phase before I could work a healing was pretty exasperating. To keep the source of my healings as pure as possible might at times be overly cautious and even borderline paranoid, but it saves me feelings of guilt or panic should a client ever complain about a healing crisis or otherwise be unhappy with a healing outcome. Furthermore when encountering strong resistance I can be confident that the energy sources I work with are not going to be limited and potentially insufficient to help, worse that they might not be strong enough to protect themselves against LLE backlash triggered. As for perfect protections – I ask for my protections to be totally permeable to all Ultimate Good energies, but to keep out any confused/bad energy, so when connecting to a 'clear' Ultimate Good being, there should not be any feelings of separation.

I believe that working in such manner keeps the healing energy I channel as pure, loving and effective as possible. I cannot guarantee a client that the energy I channel will always come through 100% pure, but it should be near as pure as we can get on this planet and we'll just have to make do with what is possible at any given time. With ever more Lightworkers active on Earth, LLE resistances and interferences should lessen and the energies we can access become ever purer.

One of the great questions of morality with any kind of spiritual work is probably – where or when does spiritual work start to go murky? I think it is usually when we insist on a particular healing outcome or a specific way to get there. There is an anecdote in esoteric circles, which I have heard more than once... A woman really wants a house she sees on a walk. She knows about visualizing and affirmations, and so she sets out to fervently visualize owning that particular property. Supposedly she gets the house, but for her to get it, the previous owners perish in an accident. One could argue that the previous owners pre-ordered that they would perish in that accident. Maybe it is coincidence and the accident was not triggered by her visual- ization, which could else be classed as black magic; still it is not something I would like on my conscious. If I pray for money, I won't insist on it being a lottery win and especially not an inher- itance. I leave it to Ultimate Good to find a way for me to receive funds. Of course we are allowed to pray for good things in life, like a good job or happy relationships, and I believe that Ultimate Good will do its best to get them to us then, but as we are not alone on the planet we should not insist on working for that particular company or going out with that one specific person – that will only happen if is the best for the other party too and there is no one with just as good or stronger a claim.

All my knowledge and desire to not harm anyone does not mean that LLEs don't try to tempt me. Their argument is usually that if I asked LLE energies for help, and even if they in turn hurt someone to fulfill my desires, that someone would have pre- ordered that suffering. So there is nothing that can really go wrong, is there? I don't get any happiness out of screwing people over though; it's not what I am, or what I want to be. Harmonious ways might take longer at times, but the results are so much more enjoyable. I am not very versed at the black magic ways, but I can imagine that those energies would want a hefty price in return for their services too. Ultimate Good help is unconditional and requires no payment; a simple *Thank You* is usually enough.

Does that mean though that I do not assert my position and desires at all? That I forever step back and let the person behind go in front? No, unconditional love is about giving unconditionally, but I don't believe it is about giving to such an extent that you are forever deprived. It is about giving what can be given effortlessly – 'You shall love your neighbor as yourself' not 'love thy neighbor more than yourself'. If in the supermarket cashier queue I kept letting people in front of me, I would never get to pay myself. And does everyone else have more important things to do than me? I happily let the frail or pregnant woman skip in front, but that's about it.

If sending healing to a terminally ill person, the question which will likely arise is whether I am giving healing to try to save this person's physical existence, or to help them pass over/transition into spirit more effortlessly. The honest answer is I do not know. I really don't want to play God! I trust that the Ultimate Good healers, helpers and guides will have much more information than I, as a human, can ever have. The information Ultimate Good helpers will base their decisions on will be clear and unbiased and enable them to provide healing help, which will alleviate the patient's short and long-term suffering the most.

I am aware that even LLEs, as evil as some might appear, are still Ultimate Good beings. They too are miracles of creation. I don't think I, in my Ultimate Good essence, am worth more than any LLE in its Ultimate Good essence, but that is not the 'game' we are playing down here. I believe it is a divine law that no Ultimate Good being can hurt another without prior consent. In our divine form we would not dream of hurting another being. If I withdraw my consent to being hurt, harmed or suffering, LLEs have to yield otherwise they will have to suffer the consequences!

I believe that one day (after I have left my physical body) I will meet some of those beings who have tried (and managed at times) to make my life hell. They might all be rehabilitated again though. We will recognize each other for what we are – individualized Ultimate Good beings. We might even be old friends. We will embrace each other in love, joy and happiness. We will go off and have a drink together, or whatever else one does in spirit to have a party.

Right now many a time it feels though as if LLEs try to make me feel sorry for them or to make me feel in awe of their incredible existence too. Ultimately they don't want me to go through with a healing. They try to weaken my resolve when healing. Their argument is somewhere along the lines of: if one goes to the fairground, rides on the ghost train and gets really frightened, because one is scared, it would be unfair towards all the other ghost train riders (who enjoy the ride) to sue the ghost train owners for criminal scared-my-pants-off-and-almost-gave-me-a-heart-attack damages. Damages which would lead to the ghost train owners having to close down the ride. One would be a real spoilsport. I or my client have pre-chosen the ghost train ride and by now asking for its dismantling no one else is going to be able to go on that particular ride. How selfish!

If I ask for my (or my client's) ghost trains to be demolished, there are plenty of other trains left for others to go on. Though I definitely do not want to be forced to have to go on the ghost train rides anymore! I don't insist on all ghost trains to be shut down, I am happy to coexist – I just refuse to let the ghost train operators spoil my fun-and-happy-rides. In real life this translates to that I am certain that I can insist on a happy life and all that it entails: sustenance, perfect health and energy on all levels, a good body, proper comfortable housing, a good and interesting job, family and a decent amount of good friends, clothes, interesting hobbies, financial independence, good sex and maybe some nice holidays. If these great-life-essentials are being blocked from myself or from whomever asks me for healing help, I don't and should not have any qualms to bring in the Light and clear them away.

The general rule might be 'live and let suffer', but it is not always that clear-cut. Frequently large-scale events influence my life, like the 2008 recession. I can ask for a good job, even if there is unemployment, but it might be 'selfish' if I insisted that all economic recession be healed, especially if it does not affect me directly. As soon as a recession would become so strong, or threaten to become so strong, as to have unemployment and general suffering rise to such a level that I would start to feel threatened by it (my job might constantly be under threat of becoming redundant) or there might start to be poverty and homelessness at every corner, and I would feel guilty for still working and having a normal life, I don't see anything wrong with asking for Ultimate Good help with the overall state of the economy. I.e. I am allowed to ask that indirect suffering influences on my life are abolished as well, not just direct ones.

I have learned to be as sensible as possible about my energy capacities and how much I can spare too. Ideally I believe that helping should be effortless. If I am too weak or ill, I will look after myself first and not feel guilty for not being able to help others at that time. Sometimes, I believe, it is about trying to find the path of least suffering though. E.g. when my mother developed cancer, I sent her as much distant healing as I could, even though I was still in the midst of chronic fatigue myself. There was no argument there. Not helping could have had far more painful consequences than to sit down and send some distant healing her way. I also feel that as long as certain resources of mine are limited I am allowed to spend them wisely.

My (physical) energy is often limited, so where I can I choose which battles I fight and which to avoid.

I have stopped trying to proselytize others indiscriminately. I do not have a Peter on my back anymore, telling me that if I do not spread the word of God, humanity will perish and their souls be doomed for eternity. I now believe we have free will to believe in Higher Powers or not while incarnated. Both choices come with different challenges; still I believe the faith route will be the far happier choice. I know though that telling a client with religious or spiritual fears and doubts that he should believe in Ultimate Good can create a lot of energetic backlash too. On the other hand, the more people pray or lightwork effectively, the potentially quicker my life will become more effortless. It is a balancing act, so since spring 2012, I started explaining some easy energy cleansing visualizations to some of my clients – but I make sure to not mention the 'G' word, 'divine' or the like, unless I know they have higher beliefs already.

I have found again and again that besides potential time and energy expenditure there is the backlash effect to be considered when helping. Depending upon the strength of the LLE system I am dealing with or up against, I can get energetic backlash for having helped. When helping spiritually I have observed some differences in the immediacy and strength of such potential backlash, between helping through 'just' prayer and actually channeling healing for someone. When channeling energies the backlash seems potentially greater. Which makes one wonder if channeling healing energy is more effective than 'just' prayer? Also when I channel healing for someone with very strong negative energies e.g. when someone suffers from cancer or has a severe handicap, the backlash will be greater than when giving healing to someone that is 'just' stressed out. But again – overall I experience fewer and fewer backlashes, which might mean that there are fewer LLEs, I am evermore clearer and energies cannot stick anymore or do not dare attack as much as they used to?

When I first understood what was going on (re backlash) I was pretty upset and felt unfairly treated, even forsaken by Ultimate Good. I prayed for more protections, angel warriors or whatever else might be necessary, but nothing changed. I needed to remind myself that Ultimate Good is ultimately good and perfect and will always do everything in their power to help (those who have asked for help) as thoroughly and effectively as possible. For whatever reasons some backlash is unavoidable for now, and it is best to just get on with it. I am quite happy (for now) to live with the backlash regarding my clients (they pay my bills) and when sending healing for someone that is dear to me.

When I watch the news and there is a war, I will still feel empathy for all involved, but will usually just send out a helping prayer and not get in the middle of it channeling healing for that nation. Even for my prayers I ask for as much 'incognito protection' as possible. Ultimate Good can feel free to help in my name – on this planet (or further afield) and where and for whatever they see fit – but if possible, please, in an around-the-corner way, so that their help cannot be traced back to my prayers. If I had to list in order of priority I guess first I look after my own well-being and safety, then that of my family and friends, colleagues and clients, the United Kingdom (because I live there), Germany (because I am from there), the gay scene, humanity, other species and beings.

Another factor I consider is whether I have been asked to help or not. I will be more inclined to help if asked directly than if not asked. If not asked and I help, I am confident that if my help is inappropriate, it will just not be delivered by Ultimate Good, or maybe it goes to someone else who wants it, or goes into some Healing Energy reservoir. Last but not least it is the urgency and severity of someone's problems. I'll probably be more eager to help someone that is battling for their life than someone battling a heart ache (I know they hurt, but they can be survived and are usually caused by having wrong expectations in the first place). I hope this does not sound too calculating, but on a planet like this one, where there is suffering most everywhere one turns, it is impossible to help everyone and everything. The healing energies I channel are inexhaustible, but my physical capacities are not. I would not want any being to give up all their time, energy and fun to help me either.

I don't want to stop anyone who reads all this from sending healing to wherever they would like to. Not all healers I talk to seem to experience backlash. I am not sure if that is because they don't identify backlash as such (they might just think it is normal to feel exhausted and grumpy after a healing) or if there are other reasons (a lot of healers might 'just' give healing to people, without considering or asking for associated LLEs in the outside to be removed as well). I have survived all backlash so far and if one starts to feel that one might engage some entities which are too threatening and dangerous (for the time being!), one can always stop channeling and/or pray for (more) help.

I don't have any qualms to bring in the light and clear the way, to heal myself, my clients and so on. How Ultimate Good heals and clears the way I leave to them though. I trust that, wherever possible, Ultimate Good will remove LLEs in the most efficient and pain-free method possible (for both myself, my clients and the LLEs), but I do not insist on it having to be pain free for the LLEs. If someone were to attack me with a knife, and I had to punch them to incapacitate them and defend myself, I do not feel bad about it. I might have in the past, when I thought that unconditional love was selfless and necessarily non-violent, but I believe now that it is selflessness exclusive of self-destruction. I am individualized divine too – if I get hurt, a piece of the divine gets hurt, just as much as the other (very confused) divine being I knocked out in self-defense.

I pray that Ultimate Good protects and defends me as 'fairly' as possible. I think my aura is probably tattooed with countless warning messages, signs and/or symbols of "do-not-attack!" I trust all LLEs have been warned before they attack me that they really should not – a Mafiosi does not have to be a lawyer to know that extortion and theft is against the law. LLEs seem to see any 'capture' by Ultimate Good akin to a death sentence though. I frequently got them arguing that I am 'killing' countless LLEs every day (I feel attacked by or am attacked by), but that their crimes were 'just' minimal. The LLEs try to make me feel like a despot. They try to make me believe that I would shoot someone dead just because they scratched my car – well I would not. I trust that Ultimate Good will use adequate force where necessary, no more, no less.

I am quite thorough. I ask for healing for any energy that is not happiness, unconditional love, abundance, effortlessness, joy, beauty and so forth. Ultimate Good is not bound to help me though and I have told Ultimate Good that they have my permission to just ignore me if I am simply whining about nothing. Feeling a little down or depressed might be so common-place for us that it does not seem all that grave – but from Ultimate Good's perspective something might just be trying to 'murder' our absolute happiness. A small infection in our body might not kill us, we might not even get a fever, but any infection still means that there are cells dying – so if we are depressed, maybe there is spiritual-cell infection in one of our light-bodies and light-body-cell death. So removing energy, which might be smaller than the cell killed, does not look like excessive force anymore if we think about it that way.

I have never experienced refusal of help when trying to make myself feel better, even on relatively good days. Most times when feeling pretty content and good, I'll just end up sending healing to others anyway. When I concluded that, when it came to battling a nation's collective subconscious LLEs, it might require armies of Ultimate Good helpers, I was stuck with another fear. *Am I worthy of an army of angels to fight on my behalf?* For one, I trust that the angels love their job. Their love for us humans is probably greater than we can feel for family or best friends. They will have endless supplies of weaponry and be perfectly protected and so forth; still I do not take their help for granted.

I also believe that keeping up a system of suffering must cost immense amounts of energy – more than it takes to dismantle it! I also consider that even LLEs have pre-chosen their existence, which also means they will have chosen a get-out clause. Suffering is always temporary. Like if I'm asking for continuous healing and I get countless LLEs taken into Ultimate Good's custody, which is likely their pre-arranged get-out clause, which they may have forgotten, just like we 'forget' so many things when we enter our human bodies. Therefore if I require a spiritual army, or even armies, to heal myself or a client I choose to think the armies are there to help the LLEs to 'get out'.

In a way LLEs are somewhat 'suicidal' to attack me in the first place. If the LLEs just respected that they were not wanted, left without resistance and desisted from any potential 'revenge' attacks against my clients, myself and/or our friends, families, colleagues then they would not have to be taken into Ultimate Good custody. They might not be allowed to make anyone else suffer 'more' on Earth, but they would likely not be taken in for rehabilitation.

Maybe some LLEs cannot communicate with anything else but what they inflict, a bit like a baby crying for food? Maybe they are actively seeking me as a channel out? They might make me feel tired, depressed, frustrated or else, but is it their way to communicate and ask me to get them out? Still realizing that LLEs need a way 'out' does not mean that one has to give up on one's own life and become a 24/7 channel out for LLEs! Thinking about it this way does help me though to turn potential anger into pity for the LLEs, which in turn takes less of my energy – and I change from potential victim to possible helper hero. At times I ask for pillars of light on the Earth's surface and inside the crust to work as a portal for LLEs who want out too, so they don't have to use Lightworkers for it.

When in 'healing mode' I am a channel in and out, but I would not recommend intending to function as a channel out for every negativity one can think of. Too many might prove too e.g. sticky to pass through, without at least causing strong discomfort. I generally tell Ultimate Good that I am willing to be a channel out, but only please where absolutely necessary or unavoidable. Obviously for energies which might be too strong or big for my bodies, Ultimate Good will have to find other 'out-channels'.

I also pray for preemptive healings, be they a potential climate meltdown or civil unrests, or more direct planned attacks on my body. Similarly as we humans might arrest and incarcerate someone that is only planning a crime, especially if they are planning anything grave, like murder or terrorist attacks, I am okay that Ultimate Good 'arrests' LLEs that consciously plan or even just support attacks on my well-being. If I watch a movie and the villains buy the gun before the intended crime, I will keep hoping that they might still change their mind, before they actually go through with the murder. The intention to do someone harm is hard to prove. Buying a gun might just be for sport. A psychic might get a feeling that someone has an ill intent, but I doubt anyone would be convicted upon such a psychic's suspicion.

All these considerations are academic though, as Ultimate Good helpers and protectors do not have these problems. They will know if an LLE is planning to attack me (and would go through with it), so if it does not create too many problems elsewhere they will 'disarm' the threat before it strikes.

In the past I have done everything 'by the book'. I tried asking LLEs to just leave me alone; I even thanked them for the experiences they had created and told them that it was my choice now to discontinue the experience (I was aware that I might be dealing with different LLEs after a while, so I asked frequently – again and again). I tried to argue with them, explain to them why what they were doing was not right, and why they should stop what they were doing. I cannot say that these 'polite' methods had much of an effect. Perhaps many LLEs cannot feel any empathy for their 'victims'. Arguing with those kinds of LLEs or asking them to stop is likely just going to get you a laugh. They might stop with what they are doing, if it serves them a purpose, but they will not do it because they are experiencing remorse or have learned to be good now. (There might be some 'better behaved' LLEs, which actually do leave when we ask them to. It is a viable method of cleansing out negativities. You just talk to all the energies in your bodies and tell the negative ones to please leave – in an orderly manner. I am confident some will adhere.)

After a while all that got too cumbersome though. These days I assume that LLEs I might find on a body scan are new and should not have invaded my bodies in the first place anymore. Hence I do not feel guilty if I just bring in the light and kick them out without much fussing about with pleasantries. Should I be too rough handed in my approach, I have asked Ultimate Good to please apologize to them in my name.

I also used to try to converse with the energies; surely they were just there to teach me something about myself? So I'd ask why they were there, where they came from and the like. I got usable answers at times, but as soon as I would start to half trust these answers many LLEs would soon become malicious and, with their answers, would try to convince me that e.g. the root of all is Evil (not Good) or that my only salvation is suicide.

If I seek an answer, I will put it out there by asking Ultimate Good. I find that the answers I seek will then usually just pop into my head at some point. Any necessary communications or negotiations with the LLEs I leave to Ultimate Good though. I have found it is much better for my sanity this way. I don't mean to be callous, impolite or lazy if I just 'hand-over' a negative emotion or thought as soon as I notice it. I don't get the feeling that Ultimate Good minds me doing so. They understand that it is not because I cannot be bothered, but because I cannot see what is attacking me, how many, where it/they come from, how they might be supported and because I cannot trust my communication with them.

Ultimate Good also knows that most times there is no time for niceties and that at times I'd be spending all day trying to argue with LLEs and would not get anything else done anymore. Besides having to earn my keep, I have already spent loads of my time in the last 17+ years being in healing and meditation mode. It is not really my first choice to spend most my free time, at home, working spiritually. I too would prefer going out, meeting friends, travelling, reading, studying a new language, doing a course in naturopathy or else. Again I trust that my Ultimate Good helpers will be their Ultimate Good selves and be loving and polite enough to well make up for any potential rudeness towards LLEs on my part.

I also ask Ultimate Good to do all energy cleanups for me. I have heard of healers who actually visualize spiritual bins in which they neatly place all negative energies and then call in the spirit waste-disposal when the bin is full. Since my spiritual vision is not 100% reliable though, I have asked that spirit just 'sucks away' whatever comes loose in a healing session. Practically it is impossible to always conduct proper disposal of removed LLEs anyway, especially when distant healing (and most in situ healings probably have some distant healing elements with them too, taking care of outside negative influences on a recipient). At times I will do a general cleansing visualization for my house, but I never get the feeling that my healing room accumulates negative energies.

One question of morality faced when giving or receiving healing is: Do we deserve to be healed? I have found that there can be feelings of self-doubt or guilt that try to insinuate one does not deserve full healings or divine help. I find that those are the times when healing is most in order. Many feelings of guilt might be irrational, but even if you feel that you have done wrong, remember you are still an individualized part of the Divine and each part of the Divine deserves full recovery to wholeness. I recommend changing your life, where possible, so as not to act in a manner that will just invite guilt in again; there is no use beating yourself up over spilt milk though. I honestly cannot remember ever having had a client where no healing energy flowed, so I am confident that Ultimate Good would never withhold their help.

Obviously if I know that someone is a 'bad' person, it is easy to fall for thoughts of *he does not deserve to receive healing*. Also I might be hit by fears that the client might have more energy after a healing session (than before), as is mostly the case. Could he potentially use that energy for ill? Most criminal or psychopathic people will probably not seek the services of a healer in the first place. Whatever energies are making them 'bad' will do their best to keep them away from spiritual healers. It is not impossible though. I do pray for personal safety too and that dangerously-minded people are kept away; still in six years I did have a handful of clients where there was a strong energy in the room trying to convince me that they were contemplating doing me harm. I also pray that the outside be kept as safe and protected as possible against unsavory clients.

We can but hope that healing energies are going to increase the chance of criminals or psychopaths to see the light and change their ways, but I am confident that healing with Ultimate Good energies is always for the good, and that the overall suffering bottom line will become smaller with each healing we give. If a villain does something evil after having received healing, it will be despite the healing not because of it! Considering that LLEs (so I believe) survive on negative energies, there is a higher chance that a cruel dictator changes their ways with time if one sends them healing and love than if one does what many do, which is send hate and fear. Any hate and fear energies might just strengthen the LLEs that create and sustain the dictator in the first place.

From the above-mentioned clients, who felt like they actually intended me harm, only one came back for more sessions. As the energy did not improve, I simply told him at some point that our energies do not match every well and that I would prefer to not see him anymore. I think that healers, like doctors, are obliged to help if asked, but obviously if you feel your personal safety is at peril you can refuse a client! One could still give distant healing, or maybe organize sessions in a clinic, with other therapists around.

When I learned about spiritual healing, I was told to ask Spirit for 'permission' before commencing a healing. Well, I thought about this one a few times and could not come up with a scenario where that makes sense, so I don't do it. Obviously we live in a free will system and e.g. my clients are allowed to refuse healing. I only had three or four clients in six years of massage/healing work who did so. I did not take this personally and asked Ultimate Good to adjust their healings accordingly. I did stay in healing mode for myself though and kept on fighting whatever client energies attacked me. Self-defense takes priority! If that caused collateral healings for the client, so be it!

As for permission when sending distant healing, if a recipient should not receive healing because they might refuse it when asked directly (there might be issues of pride or atheism), again I am certain whatever healings I channel will simply go somewhere else or try to help that person indirectly by e.g. clearing obstacles in their life. If I send distant healing to a being that would cause me more suffering (and not just the 'hurt ego' kind) if the healing would not take place, I am sure it will, even if the recipient would have refused it when asked directly. Again it is an issue of self-defense and suffering having to yield to happiness.

That leaves the argument that Spirit might tell me to not go through with a healing because the backlash generated would harm me too much. There are a couple of reasons why I ignore that argument. For one, most resistances in my practice, if they happen, happen before a client even shows up. I need to earn a living and especially in my early healing years I would have had to cancel most clients. Last but not least I just cannot tell a client that his energies are too nasty for me to give him healing. What if my intuition is wrong? I rather live with the potential backlash, and it has served me well so far. Heavy energy clients are often the most grateful after a session – and often very loyal too! In the long run, with healing becoming more mainstream, I could imagine that there might be more and more options where healers work together in groups though. In that way heavier healing resistance clients will receive healing from more than one healer, so as to spread out potential backlash generated.

Once we understand that our health is not just connected to physical factors, like diet, exercise, lifestyle and so on but that there can be emotional, mental and spiritual factors causing illness, it is but natural to start seeking for the source of one's problems in those areas too, especially if one's health comes out of balance. I do not deny that many an ailment will have emotional, mental or spiritual elements to it, but from my own experience I can only recommend to stay grounded, rational and try to keep things in perspective when searching for one's 'problems'. Illness can be a (very) complex equation, there can be inside factors – self-generated or acquired, but also outside factors, over which we may have limited to no direct influence. I believe one has to be careful as not to conduct one's search too unbalanced or in a way that causes more harm than good.

Some alternative therapists teach that if one wants to heal completely, one has to consciously work through all the past, unresolved traumas in reverse order, back to birth or even through past lives – forgive and dissolve them. I am all for learning from past mistakes, forgiving and letting go, but I strongly doubt that I have to go through each uncomfortable childhood experience to heal myself. (I'd probably get paranoid too that I might have left a few out which I just cannot remember!) When I realized that I had pre-chosen all my suffering, I forgave myself and all others associated in one go. There was no need to go through every non-invited birthday party! It might take time to 'clear' our bodies of all energies, stemming from past traumas and which have accumulated, but I prefer to do such cleansings in an abstract manner, rather than going through specific past details. I might e.g. just concentrate on healing a chakra and keep my healing intent on it, until it feels 'cleared' and the energies 'flow' again. This, I feel, is much more effortless and probably quicker too. It might be compared to rewinding a video tape. If you do it with e.g. regression therapy or hypnosis you rewind and clear the video in real time; if we just concentrate on the energy being released we rewind at many times the real time speed. Hypnosis or regression might initially teach us that we can store negative energy from past events, but once we have learned this I think we can get on with just releasing such energies.

I saw this documentary on TV about a woman in psychotherapy. She had 'trust' issues. Under hypnosis she supposedly 'saw' herself in her crib, alone in her nursery crying. She felt abandoned, a fear that carried into her present life. There was no more information about her general childhood though; were there siblings who needed attention too, was the mother an only parent and had to work from home? Just that one hypnosis session seemed to prove the documentary's point: leaving your baby alone in a crib and not attending to it immediately when it cries can cause severe emotional scarring for the future. Well, I feel sorry for all children who are neglected by their parents. Without a lot more information, I feel we cannot simply judge this 5-minute excerpt of her life as parental neglect though. I hope that the actual psychotherapist did conduct a more balanced and fair therapy, but have to admit that when I first saw that program, before my Peter time, I thought it made sense too. I used to be a bit of a drama queen.

With the years I have toughened up though. Working in hospitals, studying medicine, my cult experience and years of ill health have taught me to cherish the good things in life and to not get hung up on everyday little annoyances. I have also learned that humans can be quite tough and resilient. If unresolved trauma and forbearance would be the cause of all ill the e.g. European populations after the World War II would have been totally incapable of pulling themselves up again and rebuilding. Considering how many people lost loved ones, got wounded, lost all or some of their worldly possessions, were uprooted, raped, tortured etc. If such trauma would breed all criminals and emotional cripples, post-war Europe would have been one big jail or nut house. Obviously one does not have to be a war victim to warrant a visit to a therapist, but I find it is good to remind oneself at times what humans are capable of and have borne in the past, before becoming depressed because one might still be driving the same car after two years (and the neighbors bought a new one already). I know such depression LLEs can be convincing, but with some practice it becomes easier and easier to not fall for them anymore, up to a point where we laugh inside when any such might try it on.

For me it often is not all outside circumstances that create happiness too; i.e. my life is not perfect yet, there are still plenty of things I am working on, but on a good day none of the short-comings really bother me. Whereas on a bad and depressed day, I find 1000 reasons why I should be depressed – but except for the depression LLEs, nothing is really different.

With the above lonely-baby-in-crib example we have to keep in mind too that if a therapist were to tell a client that such a one-time short-term neglect can be the root of complex issues in adulthood, that adult might become oversensitive, paranoid and therapist-dependent. Next time she is supposed to meet friends, and they are ten minutes late, she might believe that she will need at least another three therapy sessions to overcome that 'trauma'. I would think too that most (more) lasting emotional problems, unless triggered by a very traumatic events, are due to a buildup of smaller unhappy events, not just the one.

There is a German proverb, *Wer heilt hat recht*, meaning *He/she who heals is right*. You will probably have gauged by now that I do not stand wholeheartedly behind that anymore. Just because a healer might (at times) effect good healings does not necessarily mean that their whole character is impeccable, or that their healing method is solid. What they do effect might just be placebo; it might be ultimate good, regardless of the healer not being all clear about the Ultimate Good message yet (but having prayed correctly), or they might even be backed by unsavory LLEs. I would recommend to be grateful for any healing we might experience, just not accept any confused teachings or conditions attached to them. If the healings are then reversed it is a bummer, but attached conditions would most likely have caused even more suffering in the long run. If one asks for perfect protections before any healing one receives, it should help to not be infiltrated by the confused elements of a healer's being and beliefs. I have found it gets easier with time too. Whereas it can be nice at times to get some outside support, and sometimes we really might not have the confidence or strength to help ourselves, in the long run I would also recommend to become your own healer by learning to pray and meditate effectively – build up our own understanding of life, healing and higher powers.

Chapter 12

Patience and Passion

When I first read about spiritual healing I was enthralled by the prospect of healing serious illnesses (vanquishing LLEs/suffering) without side effects. It sounded fabulous. However, rarely (if ever) were any timescales given, like how many sessions a cancer would take to heal or how many sessions you would need to rid yourself of a disease or overcome a particular affliction. As I understood, even if humans had the 'same' illness, the reasons why they have it, the root causes, are individual and hence the spiritual healing will be individual, so the duration of the healing processes might vary.

Still, it came across as if the Divine could theoretically heal anything almost instantaneously. Procrastination would be down to the sick individual for example 'not allowing' a speedy recovery by simply believing it takes time to heal and therefore 'creating' a lengthy healing process. Or the sick person does not believe strongly enough, is unable to forgive themselves or others, cannot let go of something or someone, and so on.

I understood that it might be an emotional (and potentially even painful) path, the path of self-discovery and healing. But surely a severely ill person should be strongly incentivized to heal. I felt that most people should have the common sense to recognize that any shame about admitting to some erroneous behavior cannot be any more painful than cancer or a severe chronic disease. I believed that understanding or even just hoping that such journeys of self-discovery and self-healing promise full recovery should be incentive enough for any half-rational person. I might have been somewhat naïve back then. I did not yet understand the power of 'guilt' nor had I met that many really nasty people (or energies) at that stage.

Still considering the amount of really sick people there are, they cannot all be sick because they feel guilty? Most sick people aren't drug barons, crime lords or mass-murderers. I never clearly rationalized all these thoughts back then, but I seem to remember that I was pretty confident that there should be few occasions a healer might have problems helping someone effectively within a few sessions. I would not have seen why it should take months or years to help someone heal.

If, as I read, supposedly some healers help clients to heal malignant cancers in just one or two sessions, and do so quite regularly, then how hard can it be to heal anything less severe than cancer? I recall the example of a man who apparently broke his back in a plane crash and was told by doctors that he would never walk again, yet he managed to do so in less than a year, by healing himself through positive thinking. Again if one can supposedly heal a broken spine in less than a year, then I surmised most illness should be curable even sooner. Back then if someone would have told me they were suffering for five years from psoriasis or were depressed for over ten years, I would have felt sorry for them, but I would (somewhat arrogantly) have thought they had failed to try spiritual healing or were self-sabotaging their healing process in some way.

Today I have the experience of having been at the mercy of CFS myself – and I did use spiritual healing, forgiveness, spiritual self-discovery etc. to assist my self-healing, but it still took years to improve my health. I know now that some healing processes can be extremely difficult and you might need sheer endless amounts of tenacity, brawn and above all patience. I have also discovered that such procrastinations did not fit any of the usual esoteric models of illness and their causes which I had come across.

To consciously or subconsciously expect healing success within a given time frame and then it not materializing on cue can lead to all sorts of additional problems. Many will probably 'blame' themselves, potentially opening all sorts of doors to fear based speculation, such as being forsaken by the Divine, or having accumulated incredible amounts of negative karma (in past lives?). All of which in turn can create unnecessary guilt and further emotional turmoil, which does little to help someone heal, emotionally or physically.

I am not saying that swift and miraculous healings are not possible; a lame person might walk again, a blind person might see again after just one healing session. However, from my observations having been involved with spiritual healing since 1996, such successes are the exception and not the rule. I am confident that some healing always takes place if you ask for it or seek it out, but I know too that not all healing will necessarily have palpable results, and some may even trigger a healing crisis. I would always recommend giving healing a go, even if time seems to run out; you might just be one of those where healing has miraculous quick effects. In my experiences of receiving and giving healing, many people do report increased peace of mind, relaxation, better sleep and numbing of pain during and after sessions. That may not sound like much, but to someone who might be chronically ill or in grievous pain 'just' such effects might be more than miraculous already.

So, if not (all) down to the client's mindset, why do some healing processes take so long? At some point I understood that there must be some Ultimate Good helpers for everything – every human, animal, plant, rock, but also every thought, emotion, disease etc. I understood that to heal a disease it might require not just an angel for every human who suffers from that disease, but also at least one divine being each for all the other associated LLEs who create, support and strengthen that disease. To heal myself of CFS, I would have to ask for help from my angel(s) and the angel(s) responsible for looking after the chronic fatigue LLEs associated with my condition, plus any associated outside chronic fatigue LLEs who still have access to other chronic fatigue sufferers and can feed off their suffering. There might be even more layers on top of the associated first line outside chronic fatigue LLEs, so one would need to draft in the Ultimate Good helpers responsible for their safe removal too. So to heal myself, it might not just require one or two personal guardian angels, but an army of angels, maybe even several armies and other Ultimate Good helpers. These armies will have been on standby, happy and ready to help when asked. So to cut a long story short, I asked for as much perfect healing as it would take! I felt some strong energy there and then, but almost immediately I was just stuck again and nothing much seemed to move in a positive direction anymore. What was I to do now?

All sorts of worries surfaced. Should I have meditated longer? Would further meditation be respectful or disrespectful towards my helpers? If there are armies of angels moving about now, do they really still need my meditation? Would, by meditating, I offend, because I could be seen to doubt their awesomeness, and that they have the situation fully in hand? There might be nothing left for me there and then but to go to sleep and hope that, waking up the next morning, it will all be different... Potentially, it won't be just me that wakes up rid of chronic fatigue; might chronic fatigue just have disappeared from the planet?

Usually with such scenarios, I will wake up the next morning and not feel any better; though possibly I'll feel particularly bad. I'll hope for a few more days – but then it becomes clear that chronic fatigue seems to be there to stay in my life for a good while longer. Did I misunderstand? Were all the angels on holiday somewhere – Mars is supposed to be lovely this time of year. I will realize (again!) that I let high hopes get the better of me. I'll forgive myself though and try to not fall for a similar trap again. There is simply more to be done still, more to be understood – before I will be completely healed.

Obviously a complete recovery would have been nice, but the

good thing now is that I can meditate as much as I like again. It feels good to fully partake in my own healing processes. I realize that the angels never asked me to stop meditating in the first place – they understand that I do not meditate to disrespect them, but that I seek to feel as if I am doing everything possible and in my power to help my own healing. Also my doctor friends won't be coming round my house just yet to beat me up because they are out of a job. For now there are plenty of diseases left to treat on this planet. I'll discover again that patience is a virtue. I understand again that since I have asked for it Ultimate Good is already moving at maximum speed. Some healing processes just take more time than others. I am not being negative, just realistic, which helps to avoid unnecessary disappointments.

Reading some esoteric literature you might believe (as I did) that our spiritual/energetic bodies are rather simple blobs of colored light. Sick energies could be seen as grey or black light inside the healthy colored stuff. One might be guided to just pump in some more healthy colored light to 'flush' out the grey, which should take care of one's sickness. One problem why this might not work is natural bottlenecks in the energy flow, like one's chakras. If someone has for example accumulated stress energies for years, there might be too many, or they might be so compacted by now that if one tries to flush them out in one go they will simply pile up behind the relevant chakra and squeeze off whatever little amount of energy still was flowing. Plus little-used and neglected chakras might be slow and sluggish as they are. Accumulated energies will have to be removed bit by bit; compacted ones might have to be softened first. More importantly though I have come to believe that our auric layers are no less complicated and complex than our physical body. They cannot just be soaked and flushed out. Processes of healing are far more complex. Take atherosclerosis on the physical level for example. As described before, over the course of a lifetime fatty deposits accumulate on someone's artery walls, actually grow into them. Cholesterol plaques will have been generated and organized that sit on top and within the artery walls. These plaques in turn can irritate and inflame the artery walls. You cannot just simply connect an atherosclerotic patient to a heart-lung machine and pump some healthy, low cholesterol blood through their body to 'dissolve' and flush out the cholesterol plaques though. You would actually have to avoid this. Higher blood pressure might loosen some deposits, which if they swim free can end up causing heart attacks, embolisms or strokes further down the cardiovascular system. I have heard of Tibetan medicine herbal mixtures which can help restore artery health, and there might be other things that work, but again they will probably take more time and be more complex than a simple flushing through of the system.

Luckily Ultimate Good beings helping are – what we for our physical bodies could possibly compare to medical professors, renowned experts in their field – the best help money can buy, and then some! Ultimate Good helpers help for free, regardless of creed, sex, race, sexual orientation or social standing. Still just as even the most specialized surgeon would not perform a liver transplant that usually takes ten hours within ten minutes – Ultimate Good helpers will need however long it takes to help us too. I believe they have to go through a sequence of actions – first fix x, then y, then z – to heal us metaphysically and our lives, which after all are anchored in time and space. (I am sure our Ultimate Good helpers do what they can beyond the confines of time and space, but this work still has to be translated into our time-anchored bodies and lives). This sequence of actions will take time. The next time-consuming factor is that we do not just have one auric body, but at least seven. Some problems might affect multiple aura layers, i.e. they are even more complex. One might have to keep to certain sequences to heal such ills or coordinate healings on multiple-levels etc. Plus there are further energy systems like Hara and Kundalini or the consideration of healing energies in transit, coming from far away, other people or beings we are connected to etc. Our lives are mostly quite complex, so there might have to be a lot to be considered.

Another problem, especially when removing darker energies, is that some of them come well protected and even booby-trapped. In deep meditation I was usually happy to find any dark energy, as its removal promised relief. I guess my Ultimate Good helpers needed to teach me a lesson here – they indulged my impatient desires and removed some such buggers hey presto. This then seemed to trigger some other dark energy elsewhere to 'go off' and start causing pain, fear and other troubles. Like in the movies, where the hero goes against the mad bomb technician and has to beware that he stays calm, does not cut the wrong wire to trigger a secondary device. Again this takes time. As mentioned though, I feel that Ultimate Good will try its best to keep any Spiritual healing as pain free and effortless as possible.

Then there are external 'booby traps'. At some point I felt that if I continued to ask for healing for myself or clients, my family and/or other loved ones, or the loved ones of my clients, they could suffer. I touched on such threats before. Again, I feel that there is always enough help available to defuse outside booby traps or protect loved ones from backlash; still any such outside 'complications' will need more Ultimate Good help to be dealt with and might be time-consuming too.

There are other ways LLEs may protect themselves against an easy, quick removal – not just booby traps. Some might be invisible or impalpable, some might have very solid protective shields, others might be (like malignant cancers) extensively grown into healthy energies, i.e. removing them quickly might cause too much damage to surrounding healthy energies.

In the beginning of my journey I also believed that in a loving universe reaching a higher state of understanding meant that the lower prior state of understanding, and all associated fears and other negativities, would be dissolved within hours, maybe days. The truth shall set you free! Today I accept that it might well take days or even months to cleanse out some fears. Today I seem to understand that just because I reach a higher state of understanding about something does not mean that all LLEs will just leave. They might actually kick up a fuss and try to convince me that my enlightenment was wrong and try to get me to go back to the old state. Or they might cling on and it might take more active efforts to expel them. And that is not even mentioning that I might be hit by outside LLE backup of such energies. I kept on cussing my emotional bodies for always lagging behind my rational healing understandings before I understood this phenomenon.

Since these realizations I do my best to stay calm and patient during all my healing work. Whereas I still do not ignore that collateral damages elsewhere may happen when healing myself or someone else – just because I do not panic as easily anymore, when I receive threats, that alone seems to have diminished the number of them already. To put things in perspective, I have never felt that, during a healing session, the flow of healing energies stop or diminish, either for myself or for a client. Energy flow might grind to a halt at times, but it feels like this is due to (local) blockages, not because Ultimate Good turns off the tap or does not have enough personnel to help. It can be exasperating if one suffers and one's healing feels slow, but just because Spirit might heal stuff far away does not mean that they help less where you are. I also get happiness out of the understanding that any healing work I do, even if it only has small palpable effects for myself, might have several, far-reaching collateral healing effects elsewhere. There is so much spiritual, energetic muck on our plain, and the more that gets removed, the quicker the state of humanity will improve. Perhaps it's the ultimate BOGOFF effect? Do one healing; get a million other healings free! Usually when I get such sparks of understanding how extensive some healing can be, I feel both empowered and overwhelmed. The overwhelming feeling dissipates quite quickly and I just get on with my work again.

There are different scales of healings. Some are more complex and far-reaching than others. Perhaps that is why some healings appear to have immediate and impressive effects, where others just drag on. Depending on where an LLE resides in our bodies, even a tiny thing can have resounding ill effects. Some illnesses can be either caused by small amounts of LLE or large amounts, but feel the same from the outside. So if two people with apparently the 'same' illness go to see a healer and one walks out all healed after just a few sessions but the other doesn't – it does not mean that one client is less loved and looked after by Ultimate Good. More time may be required, that's all.

Then there is the matter of LLE external support. Any reprieve after a healing session may be of short duration. Of course a good healing session comes with an increased buildup of your spiritual defenses and protections, but it depends how lucrative a suffering is for the relevant LLEs. For example if a disease is widely believed to be incurable, it could be likely that those energies will invest heavily in defending that incurability illusion. Some illnesses might be linked to greater collective subconscious energy structures. So unless one manages to somehow disengage from them, the structure might have to be healed for the recipient to make sufficient healing progress. I believe that everything is energy, ergo I also believe that diseases/sufferings/confusions of whole countries, cultures or religions have energetic roots. This can sound overwhelming, but in turn it also means that such ailments can yield to spiritual healing and there is enough Spirit out there to tackle any suffering, however large!

If for example a nation is in the midst of civil war, where that civil unrest is fuelled by widespread fiery temperaments amongst the population, as well as e.g. racism against a part of the population, then healing such unrest will require healing the collective subconscious of that nation. Obviously, if you are one of the oppressed, you could just leave, but that might be easier said than done. There might be financial restrictions, emigration issues and/or strong emotional bonds. I believe that even healing on such large scale, such as a collective subconscious, is possible. It would be naïve though to believe that just one prayer will solve such problems within a short period of time. I believe it healthier to keep yourself free of expectations and prepare for the worst. If the healings end up being more effortless and speedier than the worst-case scenario, it is a nice bonus.

I love my home country of Germany and I pray for it too. Every time I go back I feel continuous improvements. On average people appear more flexible and friendly than when I left years ago. But every time I do go back, I can still get hit by an overall feeling of lethargy, which I believe comes out of the collective subconscious belief in 'science' over spirit – a very left-brained devotion. There are obviously spiritual people in Germany, but they may encounter more spiritual resistances than in other countries. They might be hit by more doubts than a Lightworker in another country.

When I used to walk into a hospital in Germany, all those years ago, and think about spiritual healing, I would automatically feel like a lunatic or charlatan. When I walk into a hospital in London today, thinking about spiritual healing, the resistance is less severe. I might feel like an eccentric, but not shaken to my core and like a candidate for the psychiatric ward. Of course one could interpret this in such a way that in Germany I was still studying medicine and under the (Peter created) illusion that I was responsible for harmonizing the whole medical apparatus. Whereas in the UK I am just a patient. Perhaps it is a mix between that and the national collective subconscious attitudes towards spiritual healing in the two different countries? In Germany spiritual healing was still illegal when I lived there, whereas in the United Kingdom is has been legal for some time.

Some collective subconscious ills might go beyond national borders, but may not be interlinked. If asking for Ultimate Good healings against e.g. religious sexism or homophobia, the healings may or may not have worldwide spiritual repercussions, depending on how the relevant LLE structures are set up. For example if you are a citizen of country A and pray against sexism in A, and the sexism LLEs of country B do not support the negativities in country A, the sexism in country B will likely remain untouched. That is until someone prays or meditates against sexism inside country B – or these sexism LLEs attack a Lightworker in another country, the rule of self-defense!

I have a healer colleague who becomes frustrated by and has tiffs with her husband – an 'unbelieving' GP. Even after years of her involvement with healing, he still thinks little of it. I feel that here too there might be a greater battle taking place than just between two people (and their personal negativities). I suspect that the husband's conservative medical and spiritual skepticism is backed up by outside conservative medical and spiritual skepticism LLEs. Those LLEs still get a lot of fodder from plenty of people, who think the same way, so they can invest extensively in keeping her husband skeptical. However strong and real some collective illusions/negativities are, their funds are not unlimited and they can be healed, even if it takes armies of Ultimate Good helpers. I believe that if one prays for perfect cleansings and healing for something, i.e. that these cleansings and healings are as powerful as necessary, possible, available and sensible, and as far-reaching and complex as necessary, possible, available and sensible – these prayers can move spiritual mountains.

I feel it is never too late to set out on the path of self-healing, but I still support Western medicine and would never recommend forsaking medical advice. Western medicine may in areas 'only' produce temporary plasters, but from what I know and have seen, a lot of energy, time and love goes into creating those plasters so they can be pretty good and effective. Sometimes they might even be all your body needs to heal effectively, by itself, under the protection of such a plaster. Plus who says that doctors, medical researchers (even pharmaceutical ones) are all atheists and that some might not have prayed for e.g. medicines available to us today. Even if some medical treatments are just plasters, sometimes they might very well hold things together and give one extra time to spiritually heal the roots of one's illness.

There still seems to be accelerated healing if I get involved personally. For example if my mum would tell me that her knee hurts, it usually has a greater helping effect if I send her healing rather than if I 'just' pray for her. I am not 100% sure why that is. Perhaps (subconsciously) my mum puts a bit more effort into her healing (if that is possible) if she feels that I have spent 20–30 minutes in healing channel mode to help her than if I sent a 20-second prayer? Could it be that to heal another physical incarnated being it is easier and more effective if the healing comes through another physical incarnated being? Does the healing get somewhat amplified and/or anchored (in the physical) if it comes through a healer? Is it because we might be closer than an angel in some other dimension? Or do Ultimate Good helpers try to support Lightworkers' self-confidence?

Even though the healing workload is sometimes crushing, it does make me feel needed and satisfied that I can be a channel and not 'just' fire off quick prayers. Obviously there is a lot that requires healing on Earth; if physical bodies are required, I am not sure if there are enough healers. I trust there is no need to fear though. Compared to the body mass of all beings on the Earth's surface (which might require healing), there is a whole lot more body mass of the Earth's mantle and core. I am pretty confident that Ultimate Good helpers can utilize the Earth's mantle and core for their healings too. And the Sun and Moon have physical bodies too… Identifying and understanding the bigger picture required to effect a healing has not brought me down, but rather empowered me. It has helped me to ask for sufficient help, and exercise greater patience.

Should you seek healing and fear that my above observations might just 'create' more suffering (which has not been there before) do what I do – simply pray for perfect protections for yourself, your bodies and your life, including against any 'confused' ideas (still) inside you or coming through you. And again, not all healing processes are necessarily long-term; it is always wise to hold onto the hope that your completed healing might be just around the next corner! That could be through self-healing, medical advances, finding a great healer or that particular herbal mix or food supplement which is just perfect for your condition. Also, maybe I stirred up too many hornets nests at once in the past to have had chronic fatigue; so if possible at all, I recommend to just start with your own stuff first, be solid in your health and strength before you try to save the world.

So far we have looked mostly at negative energetic structures outside of ourselves and our control. Obviously that does not mean that 'normal' human self-healing blockages and problems, which might hold up a healing, should not be considered. These considerations are more along the lines of what most literature on the matter of energy healing cover. You might live with guilt energies for things done in the past. It is easy to fear that you are not worthy of being freed from the burden of such guilt, especially if you cannot unconditionally love yourself enough to forgive yourself (yet). Other people might fear that they get hit by God's wrath initially for stuff done in the past, so they rather keep that door shut and not pray for divine help! I recommend leaving the decision up to Ultimate Good (whose love and help, in my experience, is unconditional).

It takes guts to believe in Higher Powers, which are pretty

much invisible and often initially impalpable. I too used to be a skeptic. The main argument usually was, "If there is an all-loving, all-powerful God, why is there so much suffering?" Spiritual healing seemed to produce measurable results, so I gave it a shot (and got hooked). Then again I was young and in the beginning of my education. I can understand that if you seek healing at a later stage in life – admitting then that good spiritual help exists comes attached with the problem that, directly or indirectly, you have to also admit that your life might have been more effective, happy, had you started to 'believe' earlier. Also to embrace the belief that everything is pre-chosen, you have to concede that ultimately all the suffering you have experienced was up to you.

Still all such psychological problems, I believe, don't have to take too long to heal. As soon as you allow Ultimate Good to help, they will also start helping to clear your 'Higher Heart' (Thymus) Chakra, which helps us love ourselves unconditionally (and hence forgive ourselves unconditionally). After all such unconditional self-loving blockages are nothing but energy too. I believe you can either dissolve them by understanding their source or by just sending healing and cleansing into your Higher Heart Chakra.

Now we come to 'Passion'. Passion has the potential to serve us in healing matters, but it can also add fuel to the fire. Passion can be a powerful, resilient engine driving you forward in your quest for success, happiness and healing, if coupled with wisdom (love + intelligence). Blind passion though, without the strong reins of a sound, grounded mind, can be like a bull in a china shop. This kind of 'Hollywood' passion is, in my experience, often short-sighted, not long-sighted. Mostly I think that passion goes down the fiery, blind path if people are not well informed.

I sympathize with everyone on a journey of conscious self-discovery. Our bodies are quite resilient and have the capacity of enduring and building up astonishing amounts of negativities and blockages without completely breaking down. When I was still brimming with chronic fatigue LLEs, meditation made me just more aware of the large amounts of blockages and negativities I had in my being. Most such negativities came with a fair amount of desperation attached too. I really just wanted to cleanse them all out in one go, there and then.

As mentioned before though, trying to blast too much Light through a clogged system can create further problems. Going too fast may trigger booby traps etc. A healer has to try to remain calm, just like a surgeon. For example if a soldier gets delivered to a surgeon with an arrow stuck in his torso, the soldier's first instinct was probably to rip out the painful missile. The surgeon though has to remain calm; he has to consider if there might be major blood vessels or other vital structures that could be damaged when the arrow comes out. The surgeon knows that, even if it takes more time to carefully excise the projectile, the long-term healing will be easier, less painful and more effortless. Also the scar may heal better. From the soldier's viewpoint the surgeon may appear dispassionate, even uncaring. The surgeon will have invested large amounts of time and energy, and potentially great forbearance, to learn their healing skills in the first place though. Is that not passion too, just the wiser kind?

Sometimes the feelings of desperation can be overwhelming. If you intuitively discover that a client is severely ill and has little time left, the urge to 'give it your all' can be great. This may not only damage the client, but also the healer, if they give too much of their own life force, in addition to the energy they channel for the client. If the healer gets sick he/she will potentially not be much use to themselves and their other clients anymore. That is why, as healers, we have to ask for perfect protections against ourselves as well, to protect ourselves from overzealous healing help. Overall as healers we have to trust the expertise of our divine helpers and that they move at maximum speed already. Likened to the previous example they are the expert surgeons.

For larger scale healings I feel that it is important to stay grounded and patient too. I understand that people can get very passionate about injustice etc. Passionately pushing too fast, too quickly against too great a confused collective subconscious opposition will probably just get one arrested or worse though. On larger scales it could trigger civil unrest or even war. Besides education and the general furthering of rational thought I would say that spiritual work is key. Once restrictive LLE structures are weakened enough the general mood and attitude of the collective should change automatically.

A parable might look like this... *Imagine you have a house (your body) built on the edge of a sandy desert. You cannot move somewhere else, nor move the house (at least initially). The house might be your dream home or maybe it needs work to be perfect – it can be altered. The desert represents life, emotions, stresses etc. Over the years the desert starts to encroach on the house, filling up the front garden and getting closer to the front door. By conventional means you might be able to use the backdoor as your entrance, so the house is livable for a good while longer, but the desert will eventually go over the roof and render the house uninhabitable.*

Now spiritual healing is like getting a shovel and, depending on what point in your life you use this shovel, you have to remove either more or less sand from the property. Unfortunately the wind does not necessarily stop blowing and you might have to keep shoveling. You might be able to upgrade, over time, to a bigger shovel (having built up more muscle already) and perhaps even to a little motorized digger. For a while it may appear though as if every time you upgrade your shoveling equipment the winds pick up too. You start to recover your front garden, but it may be a laborious process.

However, the great thing about working with spiritual healing is that you discover you can ask for help – you do not necessarily have to do all the shoveling yourself. And yes, you can ask for even more help... and over time, the desert could be pushed back. Through irrigation and planting projects it can be vegetated. And the more the plants grow the more their roots hold down the desert. Or you might get the equipment and resources to move the whole house. One might get the skill to command the winds to blow away from the house, towards the desert!

So if life's adversities were the desert, how long you can live in your house in peace, without much shoveling, would depend on how close you live to the desert and the strength of the winds blowing. Some illnesses might just be annoying gusts of wind, others incessant breezes, others veritable sandstorms, where most us might not have much of a reliable weather forecast available though. It would also depend on how much time and/or help you have to 'plant' the desert – most people still have a job and cannot devote all their time to just their house (body). Prevention would be the sensible way to go. So even if all appears quiet, learning how to shovel and ask for help is useful. The lucky person will have initiated and completed the cultivation of wide enough stretches of peripheral desert, so that even if the winds change they won't be able to wreak much havoc anymore. At times it may feel as if there is no hope at all, and the desert will never be tamed, but one day it will happen.

Chapter 13

Going to Ground

I am a big fan of 'grounding' as it has done, and continues to do, a great deal for me. It helps me to be in my center and helps to strengthen all my chakras. Furthermore it has helped me to be more of a 'grounded' and rounded spiritual person, with a sensible head on my shoulders and good common sense, rather than wishful thinking or blind belief running through my veins. If I am well-grounded I feel stronger, more resilient and better protected. Unfortunately I did not learn about proper grounding until a few years after I came to the United Kingdom, as it might have saved me some suffering in earlier spiritual years.

If you do not know what grounding means, spiritually I understand it as the conscious effort to establish and maintain a good connection with the Divine/Ultimate Good core of the Earth. Regardless of the terms – 'to be grounded', 'to be a well-grounded person' which are commonly used – until someone actually explained to me what grounding work is I had no clue really. I might have had a general idea what someone might have meant when saying – "Oh yes, he/she is well-grounded." I would have understood a person with a level head, who does not get carried away with fantasies, but acknowledges potential physical limitations.

The purpose of establishing an energetic connection with Ultimate Good Earth energies is to connect to a large body of divine, good and healthy energy. Large amounts of divine energy, all-loving and all-capable, as well as willing to help. If you connect to Ultimate Good Earth energies with a healing intent, you will primarily help by pulling negative and stale energies from our bodies and giving us fresh, healthy energies back (up from the ground) in return. I see Ultimate Good Earth energies as some of the most attainable, pure divine energies that we can access and ask for help. Being so close I am fairly sure too that Ultimate Good Earth energies are well informed about our needs and have the perfect tools to help us.

As with most spiritual tools I have discovered over the years – it took patience, some tweaking of general teachings and the abolishing of many a fear before I became comfortable with using grounding work. Today it is second nature, but just in case you do not know about it already or might be stuck in similar traps, as I was, the following may help.

Believing that everything is alive and has consciousness to varying degrees, I obviously considered Earth to be a living being already, before I was told I should utilize Earth energy to help myself and my healings. I knew that martial arts practitioners used Earth energy to give them strength and stability – but initially I was wary, because I was not sure if Earth was trustworthy! If she is part of Ultimate Good or just another being on a suffering experience journey, i.e. a being having forgotten about her actual divine, ultimate good nature and, at least in part, confused.

I was also not free yet of fears that humankind is hurting and potentially destroying Earth. If we did hurt her and she were part confused, she might hate or at least dislike us and be rather reluctant to help us, if not lash out at us when we connect. Furthermore when one grounds one supposedly dumps one's stale and negative energies into her, and had she not suffered enough already? Did we really have to give her our crap-energies too? Would she take them? Finally a healer colleague told me that passing one's energetic rubbish to Earth is not hurting her, she transmutes it – it is like putting fertilizer on a field, it actually helps new things to grow! That felt right! During some meditations I think to have seen powerful connections between the Earth and the Sun and Ultimate Good (heavens) as well. So she gets healings and cleansings too. The chance of hurting her with our stress, fear, guilt energies is, at worst, minimal.

I had decided that an all-out, back to nature approach was unrealistic and hence would just give me grief. I pray for the harmonization of humanity and humanity's relationship with nature, but do not get all desperate about it anymore. Initially I feared that connecting to Earth she might potentially try to force me to become an eco-warrior (again)? If I opened such a connection, surely Earth would have more power than me!

I used to see drilling for oil as a major intrusion into Earth. But then I realized that if we compared Earth to our bodies, the size and depth of an oil drill would be tiny. I imagine the drill would be so thin we would not even feel the prick. I have given healing to people working in the oil industry (and other geological explorations), and when grounding them I didn't sense Earth being upset either. I once even had the intuition that removing oil from the crust is a bit like draining pus from under the skin. Who knows, maybe she actually wants us to?

It also helped to see other healers, during my training with The Healing Trust – NFSH, who did not seem to have any worries about connecting down. Even after having done so for years, these healers were not fanatic eco-warriors. So I started to connect down, asking Ultimate Good to monitor and guide that connection. If it was unwise to connect to Earth energies, they should please detour the connection to wherever else I could get the required energies on a similar frequency. Another tool I used was to set my intention to connect to the purest source of divine energy inside myself (the soul star – about two fingers wide above the belly button) and to Earth's soul star. When connecting from mine to Earth's soul star, it felt reassuringly large and accessible!

Another impediment is the widespread belief (especially in religious circles) that good is 'above' and bad is 'below'. Would grounding possibly connect me to some kind of Hell? I did not believe in the existence of a Hell, but negative forces have to reside somewhere. I was hoping that Earth is an enlightened being, not ignorant or naïve about what humankind gets up to, but aware that she provides the stage for living and experiencing suffering incarnations. As long as we do not try to blow her up, she would therefore not interfere. I was hoping, but I was not confident. I did what I usually do; I used Ultimate Good as an agent, a go-between. I prayed to them. I asked my Ultimate Good helpers to either heal Earth and/or our relationship with her; or in case she is enlightened already, to please extend my apologies about doubting her and to ask her to help cleanse away all the energies that are still trying to create mistrust against her.

I now feel the 'what is good is *above* and bad is *below* subject' is confused. Again, what would be 'up' in Australia would be 'down' in the UK and vice versa. I am confident that there is plenty of Good below our feet. I do not know where my other (heavenly) Ultimate Good helpers live. Are they indeed 'up'? Some healers attune to the center of the galaxy. I do not even know where that is. Above, right, left, front or behind me? Plus the Earth rotates! Would I possibly hit some planet or sun if I tried to connect to it in a straight line? I usually ask Ultimate Good energies to connect to me; I am not even going to attempt to follow instructions such as, *After 4.2 light years keep right. Turn right. Use the gravitational pull of the Sun there and travel in a right hand curved line for the next 10.6 light months.*

What of hell? I do not believe in it. If everything is pre-chosen, there is no need for eternal damnation or a demon in exile. I imagine being sucked into the Ultimate Good Earth core is not like going to a 'hell'; it will be more like a cleansing, purifying fire. Either that or these LLEs are beamed onwards by the Earth – somewhere where they can be rehabilitated or recycled effortlessly. From a conspiratorial viewpoint, perhaps LLEs have actually helped create the image of hell, to make humans afraid about grounding?

When I was taught how to ground the common visualization I was given was the widespread roots of a tree. I can see the reasoning behind this – a tree requires roots to anchor itself and create a large amount of surface area, through which it can exchange water and nutrients. As humans we would want roots to exchange energies with Earth. I believe that most people have rudimentary roots, and our spiritual bodies physiologically push some negativities towards our feet, heels and ultimately roots and some might even be excreted through these. Humans with rudimentary roots might manage to get rid of some negativities through them, but depending where they are they might just suck them or others right back up again – as roots work both ways.

Maybe I am just trying to be difficult – the image seems to be working fine for many of my colleagues, but I had a few problems with the root image. Classic tree roots would be wide and relatively flat. It is a good image for a stationary object, such as a tree, but we humans move about. To imagine schlepping a whole large root system about feels cumbersome. Maybe it works in the countryside, but in a city or town? What if there are loads of other people around? Must take a lot of planning and possibly energy, so that everyone's roots do not get all tangled up, ripped off etc. Or what if you live or work in a high-rise?

Initially I therefore changed the root system visualization to just visualizing one deep root, connecting my heels to divine Earth energies. That or just a few steep angled, rooting beams of Light, in case this makes it more likely for enough good energies to come through, should one root be 'attacked'. It/they won't tangle with other roots and has/have other benefits too. Living in a big city, and visited other cities, it feels like there can be a lot of energetic muck below my feet; a whole lot of energetic rubbish people have dumped, released in cities and which has accumulated over the centuries. I.e. a deep root can poke through all the rubbish energies, extend far down and connect with pure, healthy, abundant Ultimate Good Earth energies further down. There might be another reason why poking through the Earth crust or at least upper crust might be advisable. I have often thought about where LLEs outside of human bodies live. It seems feasible that they might hide in the Earth's crust. A bit like vampires, it may be healthier for them to stay away from sunlight?

I cannot say exactly how deep my connection goes. Initially I pushed the roots down from my heels, and asked the Earth energies to come up and connect to me. I plead with Earth: to help me connect, come towards me and protect the connection. Earth energies will have a lot more power behind them to get through potential energetic muck or LLEs actively trying to impede our connection. And while they were at it, they can also (at least) disable such attackers from striking again. Another benefit in asking Earth energies to come up towards me was that that way Earth could adjust how deeply I ground. I think one has to ground deep, but I did not want to go too deep either and/or hit any energetic structures that Earth needs herself and which are not there to support us.

There is a saying about putting one's roots down in a place or country. There might be more to this than just a colloquial expression. For a while I thought I could feel some of a country's collective subconscious, culture, beliefs when working a client's roots (i.e. the collective subconscious energies from their native country). I do not as much today though. It stands to reason that when a person moves countries and 'leaves some roots behind' in the old country, it might be harder to feel completely at home in the new one. It might also mean, as mentioned before, that by leaving some energetic roots behind the collective subconscious confusions of the old country might keep a stronger hold on them, compared to someone taking all their roots with them. I feel that if we leave a chunk of our soul or energetic bodies behind somewhere, it is stolen or given away – this piece of soul will (unless completely disconnected) maintain a connection with us. So if that (left behind/stolen/given away) piece of us suffers, it could have a direct effect on our well-being. Like a mother suffering if her offspring is hurt on the other side of the planet. Obviously when moving from one place to another, you may leave family, friends or property behind too. Any connection we make in our lives is a potential entry point for positive and negative energies. If a connection is burdened or unhealthy, it probably conducts negative energies more likely though.

No need to become all paranoid and never leave the house or meet (new) people again though. Some connections may have self-healing abilities and you can always 'ask' that all your connections are regularly healed, cleansed and protected. I feel that a perfectly healthy connection/cord to anyone/anything will only conduct positive energies. And we can obviously endeavor to never create or leave behind any burdened connections by resolving any conflict before moving on. That is if time permits this; some might have to be left to Ultimate Good to clear and heal.

Connections are not only established by you, but by everyone else too. So even if you only create healthy connections and are well protected, if some negative person or energy is out to harm you they might succeed in connecting to you from their side – for a while at least. Until their resentment can be healed or they find another target. I would ask Ultimate Good that in such cases any negativity flowing towards me is diverted and simply grounded until such beings cease to trouble me.

If you have left bits of yourself behind somewhere or have given a part of your heart to an ex-lover for example, I'd recommend grounding yourself and asking for perfect healing regarding scattered soul bits. When it comes to matters of the heart you may also want to 'return' any parts of your ex-lover's heart that they have lost to you. As applicable you should then either be reunited with lost soul parts (after they have been cleansed) or receive replacement soul parts for the ones lost (from which you will be disconnected and which will be freed and consequently cleansed) – whatever option is quicker and more effortless.

With regard to one's roots, I wonder if humans who connect to Ultimate Good Earth energies, rather than superficial confusion (including cultural and regional collective subconscious confusions), might not only be healthier and happier but feel more like citizens of the whole Earth – not just of a particular country? Feuds between countries or cultures might just melt away, once enough humans do this…

There is one more thing I have changed and which works better for me. Initially I learned to ground to the Earth through the root/base chakra, between my legs, and that hence grounding energy is red in color. Later I learned to ground through the heels of my feet, but some confusion remained – were the heel chakras just an extension of the root chakra? Today I feel that my root chakra and my grounding are two different energy systems. They are connected in parts, but not one and the same. I now see a solid 'white' energy connecting me to Ultimate Good Earth energies, from the heels of my feet. It makes sense to me that an advanced being such as a planet would not just be red, i.e. just a part of the spectrum of energies, but white, containing all the colors – like us. It is a great upgrade to previously believing there is only red/physical energy available from below. Earth, I feel now, can help with all color energies – she can strengthen me on all levels. She can also then remove all kinds of energies too.

Today I feel that even the 'one root' visualization might not be ideal, and I feel that my connection is actually 'wireless'. Healthy Earth energies just beam energies in and out of my heel chakras. If the connection is indeed wireless then LLEs sitting in the Earth's crust might actually not be able to interfere with the connection. I mention the root scenarios anyway, in case you still feel more comfortable with a 'root' visualization. I have used it successfully for years. Perhaps it is a natural development to have roots first, before going wireless?

Recently I was at a healing where the facilitator had supposedly trained with Peruvian shamans. She warned me that I was open to receiving Earth energies, not just having my rubbish sucked out. In her opinion the Earth holds a lot of pain and you can potentially suffer from pulling up those energies. But I believe, and see, that there are plenty of the purest, happiest and healthiest Ultimate Good Earth energies down below. As mentioned, I have also seen strong connections between Earth and other 'large' Ultimate Good beings (many times her size), which help her cleanse and heal, if necessary.

The healer also said we have to 'bring in' Light and Healing for Mother Earth. But I regard it as rather a romantic notion to imagine healers channeling cosmic energies through themselves and into the Earth to help her. I am sure she is grateful for it. Not to disregard the strength of such cosmic energies, but it does sound impractical. If there really is suffering and pain accumulated from millions if not billions of years stored inside Earth, if she hadn't blown up already, having to rely on humans to channel enough healthy energy into her to heal seems impossible and too herculean a task for humankind. We are so small – the amount of energy we can channel through ourselves, to help a being of her size, would be an exasperating bottleneck! Also if you believed that the Earth is in pain, why would you still consider it a good idea to ask her to suck out more suffering for you?

And if Mother Earth were in such pain, how would she release that energy? Would all humans have to channel energy out back into the Cosmos for her too, including all those supposed millions of years of pain? Again, I cannot say that this is definitely not what is needed. It seems too paranoid a belief though. Such paranoia would potentially keep a Lightworker in thralls of guilt and create fear and angers inside them against all other humans who do not channel cosmic energy for Earth's benefit. It could be a lifelong obsession. If Earth needs healing, it would be much more effective to ask large beings, like the Sun, for help. If I can give distant healing to someone on the other side of the planet, the Sun could initiate distant healing for Earth as well.

I could write another chapter about the Sun, however, my experiences are quite similar to what has already been discussed. Initially I was afraid to work with Sun energies. What if the Sun wasn't trustworthy? Could her energy be too strong, could I burn myself? As with Earth energies I used (heavenly) Ultimate Good energies as a go-between for a few years, but am confident today that Sun energies are Ultimate Good and not confused. Today when attuning to Ultimate Good forces I usually invite Sun energies to help as well. At times it feels like the Earth deals with LLEs residing inside her crust and the Sun helps with those above ground. I also feel strengthened in my belief that the Sun is a force of 'good' having discovered that vitamin D3 improved my health markedly. But I don't advocate people letting themselves get burnt basking in it either!

I spent two weeks in Australia, where the sunshine is intense, and lathered myself up to the hilt. Fear of the Sun's rays was very palpable there. Any other place, I just put some sun protection on and then forget about it. In Australia, even with sunblock, the fear was always there. However, on the last day I spent over 30 minutes in the Sun, without any protection. I meditated with the Sun and asked it for its help to keep me safe (a friend of mine burned within five minutes unprotected, and he is dark skinned). I didn't burn. I admit my skin had been somewhat prepared and tanned, thanks to the two weeks already there, so the risk was lower. It got me wondering though, is it the Sun that gives us skin cancer or our fears of it? Still I had to actively meditate and, especially if on holiday, I would rather put on sunscreen, relax and not think about my sun exposure anymore.

These days I recommend grounding exercises like the following...

Grounding Exercise

This 'Grounding' can just be done for a few seconds or for longer. Totally up to you. Grounding work can be performed standing, sitting, lying down or on the move. (Just don't run into things please!)

Concentrate on your heels. Imagine a beam of light coming out of each heel and going deep into the Earth to connect with healthy, divine Earth energies. (Ultimately the beams of light connecting you to Ultimate Good Earth energies should be white, but go with what you can. At times (especially initially) white might not be possible. Translucent usually is possible or try specific colors.) Now ask the Earth energies to help you connect, to come towards you and protect the connection. You might feel connected straight away or it may take a few attempts; just go with the flow, don't force it. When I do it with my feet flat on the floor it usually feels like my feet are being sucked firmly in place. With growing confidence just ask for Earth energies to connect to you, be that with beams or wireless.

Once connected the Earth energies will pull out negative and stale energies and replenish you with fresh energies. Like most chakras grounding can work bidirectional, i.e. pulling out energies as well as pumping in energies at the same time. I feel that grounding energies mainly work on the skeletal system. If you follow the grounding energies into the body, it will flow through the bones and interact with the rest of the body from there. Once the whole skeleton is cleared and cleansed, the bones should be all bright, white and shiny if looking at them with the mind's eye.

When you feel ready, thank all the energies who have helped in Ultimate Good for their assistance, end the exercise and go about your day.

Chapter 14

Purpose of Protection

Feeling sick and spiritually attacked for years, I delved into the matter of 'protection' frequently and intensely. Initially, to protect myself, I used one of Peter's prayers, "My energies are perfectly protected, I send all disharmonious energies back to their origin. Amen," but I was not all happy with it. If I create the belief that my energies are perfectly protected already, then consequently it would not make any sense for me to pray and ask for more. Sending back negative energies is probably not the wisest course of action either. I would stoop down to the same level as the attacker, it might actually feed their LLEs, or I might send such energies back to the wrong person. If I remember correctly, after becoming unhappy with Peter's tool, I just started to ask the Divine for perfect protections.

I was a fan of visualizations back then as well, and the easiest protection visualization I learned was to just put myself in a white bubble of light. I might feel a slight cessation of attacks when praying for or visualizing such, but then the attacks would usually return full force. I still felt attacked, regardless how often I prayed for perfect protections, visualized a white protecting bubble or indeed asked for a perfect white protecting bubble. I hence spent years thinking about potential loopholes that – at least my visualization – might still include. Every time I found a potential loophole I tried to plug it, but it seemed a never-ending process.

For example the white bubble might only last a limited amount of time. So I prayed for a self-healing and self-replenishing white bubble. That should have fixed it, but it didn't. Maybe some negative energies, already present in my body, were acting as portals for more negative energies to enter? I asked for perfect inside protections too. Any negativities should be capsuled off until they could be removed. I prayed to make it impossible for negative energies to beam/teleport into my bodies, still there were more negativities attacking and apparently getting through.

Perhaps I replenished them by breathing or eating? I asked for a perfect spiritual filter on my nose and mouth to block any negativity from entering with my breath and reaffirmed my prayer to please bless and cleanse all food and drink I take in. Just in case, I asked for my lungs and whole digestive system to get spiritual protections, so that no negativities could enter through them. No good. Had I forgotten to ask for all these new protections to be self-healing and self-replenishing? Okay from now on all new discovered protections should be self-healing and self-replenishing. I begged too that my protections should be perfect and all-considering, not allowing for any loopholes.

If it wasn't food, drink and air then maybe the energies I took in through my chakras weren't 'clean'? I always asked for the best, cleanest and purest Ultimate Good energies available. But if some Ultimate Good forces, helping us, reside light years away, they travel a long distance. They must be using hyperspace, wormholes or such, but maybe the energies still got tainted by negativities in transit and arrived 'infected'? Consequently I asked for perfect protections for all transiting healing energies and, just to be sure, to check and upgrade my chakras, to make sure they filter out any pollution.

When that did not help, I rechecked my grounding and asked for sufficient transit protections for these Earth healing energies helping me. Maybe I had only thought about my main chakras and neglected any side-chakras, sub-chakras or even acupuncture points? I kept on having to decide if I was forsaken and all my protection prayers were not answered, or if I got what I asked for and the negativities still managed to get through?

Then finally, after years of the above, I understood how LLE systems worked, that they can be powerful and extensive and that a breach of my perfect protections can be unavoidable. I feel better since understanding this. I try my best not to resist and most 'attacks' wash over/through me within minutes or, if heavier, hours to days. They do not manage to terrorize me for months or years anymore though. As mentioned before, I hence have started to ask for more and more e.g. pillars of white light, light pyramids or etheric crystal pyramids around my house and part of town – worldwide if necessary. Pillars of white light that can be used for LLEs who want, consciously or subconsciously, out! A bit like flypaper just more loving. I do ask for these pillars to be created and installed by Ultimate Good, where they think they are best placed and in such a way they cannot, if ever possible, be traced back to my prayer. No need to create unnecessary backlash.

I have asked for a large etheric crystal pyramid to surround my house, with a pillar of light on top too. Since I do not fancy unnecessarily increasing the amount of LLEs (and with it LLE backlash/resistance) attracted to my house, I have asked for perfect camouflage – camouflage that tints all healing structures, so that if you look at my house (from a spiritual perspective) it just blends in with the 'normal' surroundings. It is a consideration not only for my own well-being, but also for my clients'. I ask for perfect protections for them and am confident that during our healing sessions their spiritual protections will usually be improved. And if necessary, I ask for perfect camouflage for them too.

The next consideration is the reach of protection. If I had a pillar of light on top of me, a mile in diameter, it might filter out all attacks and protect me completely. The problem is that I live in the middle of London. Just next door is my neighbor and yards across the street in the other direction a block of flats. I would include these and many, many more neighbors in a pillar of light one mile wide. Now I might be hit by LLE retaliation attacks if I inadvertently started to heal and cleanse everyone around me in a mile-wide circle.

The backlash from healing so many people might require that I increase the light pillar protection say tenfold. That would result in exponentially more backlash and even larger required protection. There is only so much I can take, so I leave it up to Ultimate Good to judge how many LLEs I should piss off at any given time. It is not only my well-being I need to consider; others affected by my protection pillar of light might suffer in their ignorance, getting e.g. healing crises. A healing crisis is bad enough if you know they might be coming, but if you don't know what is happening, you might panic.

I try not to feel negatively about others. I ask for perfect protections for all beings against any negativity inside me, coming through me or associated with my life and work. I make double sure that my clients are protected against any confusion inside me, associated with me and/or coming through me too. Any time I get a client who seems to be somewhat more spiritually aware, perhaps meditates or prays, and he asks for others to be protected against negativities associated with him, it's a pleasant change. Obviously such clients will usually have less LLEs in the first place. Those healing sessions are usually much more peaceful. I would think if all humans would ask for others to be protected against their own negativities, the world would be a good deal more peaceful.

I described to another healer how I sense so many energies from my clients, mostly the negative ones. He advised me that I was taking on too much. Supposedly I could ask my Ultimate Good helpers to adjust the amount of negativities I feel from my clients; it is like a contractual agreement which can be renegotiated. This did confuse me. I already asked for as many protections as necessary, possible, available and sensible, and for my life to be as effortless as possible. Should that not cover it? For a while there I feared I might have Ultimate Good helpers who were negligent or worse, and I was being treated unfairly. I asked to take on less, but had no immediate change. Then after a few days I calmed down again and understood that Ultimate Good was doing whatever possible already, and that I would just have to bear with them.

For years I spent loads of energy trying to ensure that I only got connected to Ultimate Good energies and stayed connected to Ultimate Good only. Furthermore, that my protections remained impeccable even more so when I was channeling healing for others. During a healing session I would 'squeeze' with my entire body and mind – trying to force only the very best of connections. As energy follows thought, I tried to control everything and anything during my healing session, the connections to all chakras, sub-chakras, the protections and my thoughts. I soon discovered that there are limits to how many things I can concentrate on at once though, beside the fact that it was exhausting.

After some time I relaxed. I decided that my intentions were clear – I only wanted the best for the client. If the negativities creeping in were that considerable that they could bypass awesome Ultimate Good help (including prayed-for protections), then putting my puny body into the firing line would not stop much anyway. Better I relax and hope and pray for the best – expecting the impossible only leads to feelings of guilt and failure.

In my understanding, I am the most protected when I am fully attuned to Ultimate Good. If one imagines Ultimate Good energies attaching to my chakras, like a fuel hose at a petrol station to a car – then my chakra is actually fully covered and protected by the connecting Ultimate Good energies. Even if Ultimate Good connects 'wirelessly' to my chakras too, it will fill my chakras with its presence and protect them fully. I also assume and sense that Ultimate Good will keep somewhat of a protective light mantle around all aura bodies when I am in healing mode. I.e. if I get attacked while in healing mode, any attacking energy will be like the moths flying into the flame. I actually ask for 24/7 attunement and protections, as much as necessary, possible, available and sensible... well at least as long as Ultimate Good can see that I am being attacked or even just about to be attacked.

Today the theory behind all this does not occupy my mind much. I had some run-ins with other healers about the 24/7 bit though. I too had initially read that when giving healing, or going into meditation, you consciously 'open' your chakras to channel more energy and/or become more receptive. After a healing or meditation, you are advised to 'close down' your chakras. Keeping my chakras open would be like leaving a door open for all sorts to wander in. I soon found though that consciously visualizing opening and closing my chakras took a lot of time. Luckily I then came to understand that when I go into healing mode, and Ultimate Good connects to me, I am actually more protected against intrusion of negativities, not less. Furthermore I handed the controls to my chakras over to Ultimate Good. If they connected to me from the outside, they should be able to open and close my chakras as required, which also took care of the 'risk' of falling asleep during meditation! Negativities attacking did not give a damn if my chakras were closed; they found ways to get in and pester me. (And chakras are never 100% closed; we would energetically suffocate!) LLEs did not really care if I was at work or otherwise occupied and did not really have the time to battle them either; they attacked whenever they wanted.

Today I am in healing mode as much as I feel I need to be, wherever I am and whenever. And whereas some years ago just going to the local shops had me exhausted, this has markedly improved over the last years (still without me closing down my chakras consciously), which I feel supports my beliefs! Perhaps if one does not pray for Ultimate Good protections for one's meditations etc. because one might be agnostic or atheist, and opens the chakras consciously, one should close them consciously again at the end? Could be! The following affirmation is useful…

Protection Affirmation

Thank you, Ultimate Good, that the protections you provide are as strong and perfect as necessary, possible, available and sensible. Thank you that you protect me and those dear to me against suffering from the inside and outside as applicable. Thank you for protecting the outside against negativities associated with me, my body, my life, whether I am aware of them or not. Please protect yourselves as necessary and don't overexert yourselves on my behalf.

Now when looking at the bigger 'protection picture', investing in long-term protective effects we have to take 'spiritual cleansing' into account. It can have some significant long-term protective effects, in addition to aiding and maintaining general well-being. Because any kind of 'energetic muck' can potentially make you feel uncomfortable, and at worst be used as a point of entry for other negative energies. I find that cleansing and healing our energy and light bodies regularly is good practice – basic spiritual hygiene if you like!

I believe that loving and happy thoughts, emotions and beliefs will increase or sustain our well-being; whereas stress, fears, guilt, frustrations, sadness, jealousy, anger offer no such benefits. Our bodies do have a certain capacity to 'digest' and/or excrete negative and stale energies, but most people's bodies seem to struggle to get rid of all of them. So they accumulate over time and muck up the system. From my work with clients – and I have seen a few hundred different individuals – I have sensed that no client ever has 100% clean, bright and happy energies. I always find some resistances or blocked/slow chakras for example, despite many of my clients leading reasonably healthy lifestyles, eating decent food and exercising.

Perhaps humans today are overloading their systems with stress, or our lives are otherwise too disharmonious? Maybe so, but then again some clients only need a little work on them and then their energies feel happy and strong enough. When I ask such clients if they do any spiritual work, they most always say – yes. So with a reasonably healthy lifestyle and a bit of spiritual cleansing, a relatively happy and healthy life seems achievable. And just as people usually do not complain about having to wash regularly, one day we might not complain about having to clean our 'Lightbodies' regularly either.

Of the 'big four' in energy work – healing, cleansing, protection and recharging – cleansing seems the most important for most clients. Initially when I learned about Spiritual healing it was mostly explained as giving energy/life force to a client, to help their body heal itself. This explanation places the emphasis on putting energy in. I feel though that most clients need (negative and stale) energies taken out. Else it is like giving food to a constipated patient. Yes one might have to put something in to help such a client, but that would be a laxative, not more food. Similarly before changing into clean clothes you usually take a shower. The same applies to most healings. You might have to give a client a bit of energy to help them cleanse out negativities; once they have unburdened themselves, you can give them more healing energies, helping them heal any damage the old accumulated stale energies might have caused.

I would now like to share with you a few cleansing methods I have gleaned. I often hear about 'just brushing off' energies. You sweep down energies by holding your hands over your head and then sweep down along the body. To do the legs you would have to bend then finish the sweeping motion with your hands flat on the floor – to ground the energies that have been swept off. It is obviously about the intent. If taken literally you would have to sweep down all aura bodies individually (could be hard, some aura bodies may be so wide they are out of reach and you might not know where the individual bodies really end either). Also you would have to make sure to cover every inch (hard with the back). Since it is mainly about the intent, I prefer to just visualize a spiritual shower hosing/sweeping down my bodies. It's easier too and less conspicuous in public.

But what about 'within'? For a good inside cleanse of energies you need to practice a cleansing meditation. Intense prayer might work too. These mechanisms will utilize the natural openings and exits of the spiritual bodies, mainly the chakras, but also the lungs and breath, as well as all the energies that get cleansed through our heels with our grounding. I frequently get clients who 'just' watch their breath or say a Mantra for their meditations, and think that is enough. They do not consciously ask for or visualize a connection to Ultimate Good forces before their work, nor do they ask for energy cleansings. Not every meditating client of mine has relatively clear energies; maybe that is why? Many of my meditating clients seem to think or believe that meditation is simply relaxing, but do not seem to have much of an idea why.

When I was ill my bodies were swamped with muck. I would get quite desperate and zealous about cleansing myself. I did not understand back then that this is a continuous process though. I believed that once I had cleansed out all negativities (and was perfectly protected) I would never have to meditate again. I did not see it as a necessary exercise like my daily shower. I'd ask all negative energies to leave as soon as possible. Usually every-thing would grind to a halt quickly though. With all these energies mobilizing at once, they'd pile up and clog up avenues out.

I then added to my prayer – to please leave in an orderly fashion and without causing any further harm to my bodies. I'd also ask my bodies, organs, cells to try their best not to react to the negative energies passing through. It still took years to heal though. (I did tell a friend, who complained about heavy side effects during a detox she held, to ask the leaving energies to do so as harmlessly and effortlessly as possible and her bodies to react as little as possible – and after that supposedly her detox was much easier.)

And there are 'tools' that can help cleanse; you may know most of these already. (Sea-) Salt is said to be good for binding negative energies, especially if dissolved in water (you bathe in it, do not drink it). Again, in my opinion, this works mainly for energies that might be sitting outside the body. To help with inside stuff, you would need to 'intend' to release negative stuff inside, either through the chakras and/or hands and feet, into the salted water to be bound or neutralized. One can just visualize being in a saltwater bath too.

Then there is smudging, most commonly cleansing your energies with herbal smoke. One of the most popular is sage. Supposedly such smoke is inter-dimensional, binds negativities and carries them forth into healthier dimensions, where they are taken care of. I am not sure if smudge smoke mainly just deals with energies sitting in top of/outside the body, as it can be inhaled in the process and might therefore cleanse from within too? Sometimes I just visualize cleansing sage smoke and others just use a (non-burning) sage stick, which they wave around or tap on their body, from top to toe. Just visualizing sage smoke is cheaper, burning bits do not fall from the stick (and burn holes in your carpet), plus I do not like when the smoke gets cold. If burnt inside the house, cold sage smoke is almost as unpleasant as cold cigarette smoke. Not to forget all the different types of incense one can burn – which can smell great too. Supposedly Dragon's Blood is especially good to smoke out negative energies. I love Nitiraj Original incense sticks, they are very wholesome and calming. Smudging can also be done using sound to disrupt negative energetic vibrations. Most commonly used are rattles, bells, gongs and sometimes drums. But you can also visualize violet flames cleansing a space, or silver light works well too.

Furthermore there are several crystals which can help one (especially during meditation, when connecting with and/or through them) to take up negative energies (and channel them out). The main ones are clear quartz, amethyst and white selenite. There are so many, but personally I especially love zeolites, shungite, hematite, black spinel, amber and black tourmaline. Or there are aromatherapy oils, crystal, plant, animal and flower essences too.

For internal cleanses I sometimes take charcoal capsules or zeolite powder. Also I take milk thistle as an antioxidant for the liver, assisting in its detoxifying function, and vitamin C as a general antioxidant. Furthermore garlic is supposed to help kick out negative energies (as well as being a great cleanser of the blood). I take one or two odorless capsules before bedtime. I found black pepper has qualities that can exorcise LLEs too. Then there is the wide range of herbal teas that might help. Nettle tea is said to be especially good, and not to forget plain water!

You can ask special angels, elementals, and totem animals, the Ultimate Good beings inside the elements (earth, fire, water, air and ether) for cleansing help too.

Being barefoot on the beach or spending time in the Sun usually has some healing effects anyway, but I find that communicating with the elements, planets, Sun, saltwater and so forth intensifies the process. I assume that without our asking for help there is only so much they are allowed to do for us, as not to violate our right to 'free will'.

Whichever methods you use always give thanks. In so doing we communicate and acknowledge that our cleansing helpers are alive and conscious. They might be more enlightened, but would you, in their shoes, not rather help someone who sees you as another divine being rather than an e.g. inanimate piece of rock and completely in their service? (I admit it is hard to think about communicating with beings that society keeps on telling us are inanimate. I forget too. When I remember I send a blanket thanks out, plus I'll especially thank all the helping beings, crystals and so on in my house. I used to feel guilty when I forgot, but then realized that I had assumed that without me communicating with them, my crystals would just sit there and not have anyone to talk to. Then I realized that they have all the other crystals to talk to. Who knows, they might have more fun than me in my human interactions!)

Besides the chakra systems and aura layers I also cleanse all other energetic systems – mainly Hara, Kundalini and the Soul Star. Some claim that especially our Kundalini energies and the Soul Star are particularly divine. This used to make me think that they probably do not require any cleansings. Over the years I have dropped those assumptions and conducted cleansing and healing meditations for all of them. I also tend to at least check them with my clients, and it often feels as if healing happens on those levels too.

I have read and heard several warnings about raising one's Kundalini prematurely. Apparently Kundalini rising if your chakras are not all cleared can be problematic. I am still careful, but am not so sure that is all true anymore. I have had quite a few clients with more free-flowing Kundalini energies. I am not sure if that is because I attract such clients or if generally Kundalini energies are starting to rise across the population (or have always, on average, been more flowing than some gurus might tell us they are)? It is noteworthy that not all such clients actually do any spiritual work or even yoga. I had more than one client where the Kundalini seemed active in areas where chakras had blockages, so 'cleared (back-) chakras' do not seem to be a prerequisite for Kundalini to flow either. It feels more like Kundalini energies will become more active if we lead reasonably happy, content, inspired and/or creative lives – are more the individualized divine beings we are. Whenever I have clients whose energies feel particularly psychopathic (and self-aware), these energies seem to usually reside in their Kundalini. I.e. to assist the healing of psychopathic tendencies in humans (especially criminal ones), more and more healers might have to become competent in working with such.

And just as a reminder, for all my cleansing work I have a standing plea with Ultimate Good to mop up and please safely dispose of any negative energy being set free from my bodies, my clients' or anywhere else associated with my healing work.

So how long does it take to cleanse a chakra? Honestly I would not be able to say for sure. To cleanse a chakra one does not only cleanse that chakra, but also the associated aura body. When working on a massage client, my (main) chakra healing scan usually takes between 5–25 minutes, front and back each. For a healing client in the healing center (where I used to volunteer for a few years), where a walk-in healing should last 20–30 minutes, the chakra scan, front and back, will usually take up about 60% of the time. The same applies to private healing clients, who I see for an hour (of which about 45 minutes is healing work). There does seem to be some adjusting to circum-stances and time restraints by Spirit. And obviously just because I or any healer feels that they should move onto the next chakra does not mean that the last chakra and aura body are all clean already!

Usually I sense when I should move on to the next chakra. Often there is a deep breath, which can be a sign. A healer friend of mine counts in her head and moves on when she gets to a certain number. I used to be paranoid that I might stay too long or not long enough on a chakra, but I have learned to just go with the flow. Obviously if I feel a lot of resistance, blockage or sucking of energy and it seems quite obvious that a particular chakra needs plenty of TLC, I'll stay longer.

All this is client work though. Working on myself is different. Ultimate Good does seem to pay some consideration to how much time I might have for a meditation. There used to be plenty of times though where healing meditations could last for hours (if I'd have the time). I might work for one hour or so on just one chakra. Again I would move on to the next chakra when it would feel 'right'. I would have the benefit to be able to feel more accurately if a chakra was free. A dissolved blockage usually gives me a great sense of relief; and as mentioned when I send energy into a chakra, and it is free and connected, my breathing will be deep and slow. When I hit blockages, my breath will be shallower and labored – as if the air breathed is thicker.

When all my energies are in a good state, I can feel the Hara in the midline of my body, my chakras, my Kundalini – all flowing. It feels right! Thankfully that is usually the case today. During my chronic fatigue years I would not be able to feel my 'middle'. I generally just felt like one big blockage, nothing was flowing at all. It was a horrible feeling and it lasted for years. It was hard to imagine that it could be different. I started doubting that the flowing state existed at all; maybe blocked was 'normal'?

And even now I can still find improvements to implement. I just discovered that the Kundalini seems to be an open system, just like our chakras (i.e. energies flowing in and out constantly). I used to have this image that the Kundalini system is mostly closed; considering that it is our most divine essence and is often described like a snake, I might have feared that if it flowed out I'd flow out of my body. That fear feels unfounded now, and with my Kundalini system open and flowing my energies feel even stronger and more stable.

Possessing such 'ideal' energies does not mean that I feel ecstatic and happy all the time. There can still be plenty of grumpiness, anger, depression, pain etc. I also read so many reports that once the Kundalini is fully awakened you will be able to perform superhuman feats. I'd e.g. be able to access Akashic records, be fully clairaudient, clairsentient or clairvoyant and be able to get so hot that I could melt myself free, if buried under snow. Well I sometimes get visions – fleeting and not always accurate. I am rather more clairsentient. No Akashic records though or out of body experiences. And I have not been buried under an avalanche recently, so no way to know if I could melt snow.

Back in the day I could not wait for all those superpowers to materialize. Today I do not really care too much; if they do materialize and/or improve – great, but I refuse to be unhappy because they have not. My most desired ability is to be a good channel for healing energies and I believe that has materialized. I am very grateful for it. It might not be an ability that is too hard to achieve; basically if one wants to channel divine energies for healing purposes you just ask for it and those energies will come and help. Pretty much everyone should be able to do it. But I think it is one of the most useful abilities if you want to free yourself from suffering. What use is being able to levitate in deep meditation when you are still a slave of all your emotional negativities? You might be able to attain outside recognition for levitating, but that does not buy you the love inside.

Chapter 15

Method in Meditation

I have not read tons of books on meditation or travelled to faraway lands to meet spiritual masters to initiate me; I have spent thousands of hours in what I would consider meditation though. To me meditation is any activity which is dedicated to being/becoming more connected to (benign) higher powers; an activity directed towards strengthening, focusing, enlightening and calming one's mind. It is an activity devoted to healing, cleansing, protecting and recharging our being.

There are plenty of forms of meditation – the classic sitting down and connecting to some Ultimate Good power, exercises (like Tai Chi or Yoga), automatic writing or improvising a dance or piece of music and so the list goes on. At some point one's life might even become nothing but meditation. As soon as I started to understand that I wanted to become a healer, it seemed unavoidable that I needed to 'learn' to meditate, but how? My first attempt was to purchase two books on meditation (cannot remember the titles to save my life). Sadly they just confused the issue for me. They claimed that the aim of meditation is to be empty – one should empty one's mind, and relax and rejoice into a 'nirvanic' void. I should not think about anything, not even about my not thinking about anything. I was given the anecdote of the 'pink elephant', i.e. if one tells someone to sit and think of anything but a pink elephant, one will probably think about a pink elephant. The biggest challenge was supposedly to become proficient at not thinking about anything, regardless of being told that. I tried to sit and think of nothing. I failed miserably.

Even using 'tools' like imagining a big iron cauldron (inside my head), into which I placed all my thoughts, fears and worries and then closed it with a heavy lid, left me with plenty of thoughts and emotions – did the cauldron have a hole, and some stuff could escape? Thinking of nothing seemed impossible. I do not think I was overambitious, but I did have certain expectations on myself. I expected to be able to learn things and over time excel at them. Sitting down and doing nothing sounded too easy, and I really could not comprehend why it would be good for me in the first place.

What helped was meeting Peter. He said that meditation is a process. The main thing is to just do it, sit down (morning and night) and dedicate 20 minutes to meditating. He propagated that a mantra meditation is the best and gave us each a supposedly individual mantra word, which we were supposed to repeat in our minds. If we 'dropped' our mantra and got lost in our thoughts, we were to return to our mantra as soon as we realized. This seemed achievable. I religiously meditated (with my mantra word) first thing after getting up and last thing before going to sleep. I had some profound meditations with this technique. My mantra was a bit of a mental broom too – sweeping away superfluous thoughts and emotions.

After dropping out of the cult, I dropped my mantra too. It might just have been a spoof word Peter had invented, but I did not want to take any chances. As mentioned before many gurus seem to instruct their devotees to use mantra meditations to drum out their supposed 'useless mind-chatter', but might actually try to cut their followers off true divine ideas and intuitions coming through in meditation. I don't mean to say that there might not be non-destructive ways to use mantra meditations, but for me my mantra was too connected to Peter, so I did not use it anymore.

But I am still an avid fan of a 'working' meditation. My goal is to get to a point where my life is continuously happy, joyous and effortless. There still seems a lot to do and I am not sure if I could just sit there and 'be empty'. I'd rather use the time to actively heal or cleanse something. There is this implication too that 'thinking' is wrong, non-divine or at least a lower, less developed form of being. But I still enjoy thinking, as long as it is not destructive or otherwise mood dampening. I ask, is it not 'being' if you see a beautiful vista, are at peace and happy, and reflect on it in awe? In that moment you know 'this is beautiful', you just don't verbalize it. I feel that in ideal (carefree) being there might be less thinking with words, more thinking without words: being, feeling, enjoying and knowing. That would still be much more than just being empty!

As long as I have problems in my life, my mind usually is a powerful tool to find solutions with too, either by finding different ways of looking at a problem or finding ways to get out of these problematic situations. I guess one could discuss endlessly if the actual aim of meditation is being empty or not. I am sure there are many supposedly enlightened old masters who think or thought and teach or taught that emptiness is the ultimate goal. I do notice that the more content, happy and connected I feel, the fewer thoughts I generate. Perhaps one day I will hardly need to think at all – be that with this body or zillions of years from now…

I find that meditation is a great tool to help our bodies get rid of negative or stale energies, such as stresses, angers, fears, doubts etc. Besides that, Ultimate Good might use the time we meditate to help us rediscover spiritual abilities, heal energy systems and/or enforce/protect them.

Many a guided meditation suggests you look at the events of the day – as if from a distance. That you should let go of all your troubles and relax (on cue). But is that a realistic or practical way of approaching meditation? I would think that most people concentrate on what they are doing when working i.e. they will have 'meditated' for a whole day – just that what they meditated on will have been their profession (OK, many people might not consciously stay attuned to higher powers when working, but usually there will be focus, trying to understand, problem solving, goal achieving). After which most people will be filled with some amount of stress. They are brimming with residual adrenaline in addition to all their other everyday worries now kicking in like – What shall I have for dinner? Damn… I need to pay those bills. I need to do the ironing; I promised to call him… To be told they can only relax and recover by now sitting or lying down and becoming empty is almost grotesque.

Meditation should be a tool to cleanse and heal. A quieting of the mind will then follow naturally. Therefore I prefer to meditate in such a way that every meditation becomes a (working) healing and cleansing meditation. I will usually ask Ultimate Good Earth energies, Ultimate Good Sun energies and Ultimate Good (heavenly) energies to connect to me and help me heal, cleanse, protect and recharge my energies – as much as necessary, possible, available and sensible. I will also ask Ultimate Good to connect to all relevant energy systems as necessary. Besides asking for perfect protections, I would also recommend to ask to only be connected to Ultimate Good energies. To just ask someone to sit down, close their eyes, become quiet and open up seems almost criminal to me today. There are just too many forces out there which are not all benign and who love to take advantage.

Okay, at times I get skeptical clients and asking them to meditate/pray feels like a step too far. In such cases I agree that it might be necessary to water down one's meditation instructions. I may e.g. tell such skeptical clients to work with Earth energy or Qi (like some martial arts practitioners) – and I'll omit to call them divine. I'll tell them to just concentrate on their heels to activate their grounding chakras and to visualize a (white) beam of light connecting them down. I will then in addition (silently) pray for them and ask Ultimate Good to please look over them. Should they attempt to use my watered down instructions on grounding – I ask Ultimate Good to always connect, help and protect them as well as possible and dispose of any cleansed out LLEs safely. All this for them and anyone else my clients might advise in turn.

For my own meditations I'll usually ask to be a tool and channel for my own healings (or the healing of others). Usually I will just lie on my bed and put my right hand up (sometimes the left too, unless I am holding a crystal with it) and intend to send healing into whatever situations, beings which negatively attack or influence me, my bodies and my life. Today, during such meditations, I will pretty quickly feel connected. I will feel stronger, calmer and more centered. I will feel satisfied that by having been a healing channel during my meditations, I will have helped to bring more healing energies into our physical plane and will have helped to kick some LLE's butt. Becoming more relaxed, breathing deeper can be a nice natural side effect of this. To feel Ultimate Good helping is one of the greatest feelings of all – even if one might doubt it again shortly after.

A 'watched-over' by Ultimate Good meditation should be safer than just sitting down, relaxing and becoming empty. Not asking for protection and grounding is a bit like driving drunk without a seatbelt – very risky. Sure, even meditating protected can get one attacked by negative forces, usually the resistance of whatever LLEs I am going against with my healing – but at least when connected the Spirit Police are right there to grab the LLEs trying to intrude, or at least prevent them digging in as deeply as they might when not opposed.

I like to think of this kind of meditation as an active healing meditation. I would not be surprised if some people might feel that after a hard working day they just want to relax though and not have to do anything 'active' anymore But this kind of active meditation is, in the long run, much more effective and beneficial than just plonking oneself in front of the TV. It is like a quick workout in the gym after work. Even if you are tired after a day's work and exercise, and the additional energy required for this seems nonsensical – you will actually 'burn-off' some stress energies. After proper (regular) exercise the additional energy investment will actually result in endorphin release and feeling better and stronger. Now you can enjoy watching TV even more.

Admittedly in my worst years I often did not feel much benefit from regular exercise and/or meditation; sometimes I felt worse for it after. I also believed that my 'unwellness' was energetic though and that whichever energies made me unwell would feel less comfortable if I exercised and/or meditated. So that gave me some indirect satisfaction at least. Today I am pretty confident that I was dealing with healing crises and I am glad that I stuck to my exercise and meditation routines!

Initially I learned that to meditate I should sit in the lotus position, on a chair or lie down in a quiet room. Later I heard about walking meditations, but that sounded relatively advanced and surely required an idyllic natural setting? To combine meditation with exercise felt blasphemous back then. Today I experience some of my most powerful meditations while on the cross trainer, rowing machine or exercise bike with two major benefits. In my chronic fatigue days many a meditation lying or sitting down simply resulted in me falling asleep. Strong LLEs seem to have some kind of spiritual valium in their arsenal of self-defense tools. As you might have guessed, I have never fallen asleep on the cross trainer though.

Additionally, deeper and more vigorous breathing during exercise feels like it helps to pump more negative energies out of my bodies. As aforementioned when engaging some negative energies my breathing will feel more labored or blocked. The stronger the energetic resistance I am working against the more difficult it will be to breathe deeply, as if the air is becoming more viscous. When undergoing a power-healing meditation in the gym it is easier to 'breathe' through these thick patches of negative/stale energies. Breathing is a great thing, especially during active healing work. During most healing work on clients I breathe a lot. Funnily if clients already meditate or do some spiritual work themselves, they seem to breathe deeper during their massages than those who don't. In turn I often feel less of a need to breathe so much and so deeply myself.

Some people put too much emphasis on breathing. They can get so passionate about it – just breathing deeply and calmly seems to be 'the' panacea to achieve all sorts of healing and enlightenment. Sure, a few deep and calm conscious breaths might give you extra energy in a crisis, possibly help defuse an edgy situation, but I would think if one has a e.g. short-fused temper this is a short-term fix and will only be able to do so much. In my experience one problem is that, unless combined with exercise and/or spiritual work, there is a limit to how much one can breathe deeply, as without it there is heightened risk you will just hyperventilate.

Initially when Peter told us that one can just hand-over one's negative thoughts and/or emotions and then breathe them off, I used to sit down and keep breathing deeply and heavily – beyond the point of it feeling natural and intuitive. I did get tingly hands and once or twice started to convulse and cramp, arching my back etc. I therefore now don't like to 'force' my breathing – and get somewhat antsy if people (especially other therapists) try to tell me that I have to breathe in this or that way. If their healing work is any good, and manages to make me feel comfortable and safe, deeper and calmer breathing will be a natural intuitive side effect.

I am also quite proud of my body (and very thankful) that it breathes, whether I think about it or not. It is a wonderful thing; just ask someone who has to breathe more consciously, like a person suffering from emphysema. It is a lot of work. And who knows, there might be some higher, intelligent reason why my body's breathing is shallow at times too. Some say that Westerners do not breathe into the stomach. However, stomach breathing usually implies neglecting most supporting muscles in the chest and shoulders. I guess what I mean to say is that breathing correctly is important and plenty of people potentially could do with learning this, but I would advocate that this comes as a side effect from other things undertaken, be that exercise or spiritual work. If people cleansed their energies properly and regularly, they would flow better and with it their breathing would be generally deeper and calmer.

Is it essential to actually sit still or lie down during meditation? If it were essential would my gym meditation be wrong or ineffective? I think some more sedentary meditation is a nice gesture – plus it relaxes my muscles. Also being able to close my eyes, forgetting about my body and only solely concentrating on Ultimate Good and my healing goal focuses my attention and can really help to calm anxiety. Still meditations may include some more healing and fine-tuning work. So yes, I appreciate both sedentary and exercise meditation. Obviously for some people, who are always on the go and exercise already, adding meditation to their cardio routine might initially be easier than 'finding' the time to sit in meditation regularly. Those who do not exercise might prefer the sitting kind to start with. Do not worry how much you do of which, it is better to do just one kind than nothing. As you progress you should find the time to sit or get the energy, time and motivation to exercise respectively.

This leads nicely into the importance of posture. I have encountered many a spiritual person who seems very determined to only meditate with a straight back – best with sitting in lotus position. A more lenient version would be to sit on a chair with a straight back. Personally, as mentioned, most of my meditations I perform lying flat on my bed, or exercising. I am in healing mode most of my waking hours though and don't tend to walk about as if having swallowed a broomstick. I have no qualms to channel energy half lying, half sitting on my sofa and watching TV or when going to sleep curled up on my side. I cannot say it feels as if such bent-spine positions create any problems. One of the more sensible things Peter said was, "Enlightenment does not depend on body posture" – I agree. This does not mean that I did not get attacked by feelings of guilt when first starting to meditate lying down. During my cult years, and a bit after, I religiously meditated on a meditation cushion, seated on the floor. But that was just it – guilt feelings because I went against the mainstream. Germans can be so eager to follow rules to the letter. Once these posture-guilt LLEs found they could not engage me anymore they soon stopped.

Even though I don't really consider myself to have chronic fatigue anymore, I still do most of my meditation lying down. And do not think it is because I am lazy. Lying down I can fully concentrate on my meditation and spiritual, mental work. I don't have to worry about starting to be uncomfortable, falling off a chair or my legs falling asleep. Furthermore it feels easier to ground through my feet if my legs are not in lotus. I believe Spirit is practical. Some energies might have come from light years away; I doubt they care if they have to work with a bend of my spine or if my head is slightly off center.

Also from my experience as a healer and masseur, it is impossible to conduct, give a full healing session (unless maybe performed from a distance and not on the body) and especially a massage with a straight spine. As a therapist working on the body, one will bend over the client, kneel and I don't get the feeling that the healing effect diminishes because of this. At times the energy seems to stretch my back when possible. I interpret this more as a stretching out of my back muscles though – which feels good after just having been bent over a client for some time.

My advice would be to meditate in whatever position is most comfortable for you. Feeling guilty about not sitting with a straight back brings guilt energies into your meditation – and guilt, in my opinion, is one of those feelings which has nothing to do with unconditional, divine love. It might be alright to tell healthy, fit people to meditate sitting straight-backed (it does have the benefit of slightly helping to keep one awake if meditating when tired), but I feel sorry for anyone tied to a sickbed or with a deformity somewhere, trying to help themselves, considering meditation and then being rebutted by silly rules. Some teachers might even insinuate that meditating in any other posture is harmful. I really don't understand why they believe that energies, especially Ultimate Good ones, all-powerful and all-capable as they are, should be incompetent to work with and around a curved spine or the like.

Another point involves crossing legs. Whereas some traditions might suggest that sitting in lotus position is near imperative for effective meditation, on the other side of the spectrum I have heard plenty of individuals claiming that you should not cross your legs when meditating or receiving healing. The main argument here seems to be that you should have your feet flat on the ground (to maximize grounding?) and that crossing limbs can result in a sort of short-circuiting effect. What I can say is that, even lying flat on my bed, grounding is not an issue (especially through my heel-chakra). It is comforting to feel the ground under my feet at times, but I have learned that it is not imperative.

I have meditated with legs crossed and cannot say it felt wrong. When watching TV and in semi-meditative healing mode, I still frequently cross my legs. It feels fine! Sometimes it helps keep warmer and feeling warm and comfortable will probably have more of a beneficial effect on 'relaxed' meditation than feeling cold and uncomfortable. Again I cannot believe that Spirit cannot work 'around' crossed legs! Also when considering that we might extend beyond the physical body, with our aura – if one would seriously follow the route of 'un-impeded', 'short-circuit-free' meditation, one would potentially have to insist on having one's legs wide apart, feet on the ground, arms out (like the da Vinci *Vitruvian Man* drawing) – and I have never heard such. Not to mention some religions having spiritually worked in 'lotus' position for millennia and still having achieved spiritual advancements and healings!

If you start falling for rules like, "You must have your feet planted flat on the floor!" where does it stop? Next thing grounding is only effective if one lives and works on the ground floor? What if there is a cellar underneath? Or even worse one has to ground only on greenbelt land? That would make meditation and spiritual work very hard for most city dwellers. Even if one had a garden or went to the park – what about potential sewers below one's feet? I think 'rules' such as these just invite unnecessary paranoia.

Today I also meditate when I want or feel like it. I have found that meditations can feel differently according to the time of day. In grumpy morning hours I'll feel less connected and calm, whereas later in the day meditations feel more powerful and serene, so I prefer to meditate then.

We ought to now look at 'mindfulness'. During mindfulness meditations you might focus on sounds, how your body feels, or observe the breath. The aim is to widen your awareness, become more self-aware, but also somewhat detached – to become more of a spectator in one's life (at suitable times) rather than solely the protagonist. Mindfulness can be great. One learns to see and follow one's thoughts, but also to just let them pass – be detached. Being aware of thoughts may help prevent you falling into negative spirals. You discover that most thoughts are just thoughts and often just speculation. For example if I am in the shit and my thoughts tell me, "You are in the shit and hence your whole future life is going to be shit," who says that thought is truthful? Most likely it is just some grumpy and paranoid energy talking.

'Just' being mindful might be enough for some. I am not sure though if it is always powerful enough. Does it actually change anything? If one is laden with negativities, becomes more calm and lets them drift by, if one does not get annoyed by them, not feed them, they might get bored and leave – ergo one experiences healing. It is often likened to children playing and one trying to annoy another. As soon as the annoyed child stops letting itself be annoyed the perpetrator usually loses interest.

Mindfulness may help with 'normal' amounts of stress – but when it comes to really hefty energies, I have my doubts. Our own mind, our own divine essence is strong and capable, but some energies can be totally overwhelming. They might be fed by the collective subconscious of hundreds if not thousands of humans, maybe for decades or centuries. One needs outside help – Ultimate Good help – to tackle such energies. A fitting analogy would be to say that our divine self could be seen like a bucket of water; impeccable, crystal clear, delicious spring water. If we sweat a bit and get some dust from the daily road on us, it will be perfect to refresh us and clean us up. If we have been trekking through a smelly swamp though (and many people's lives are probably more of a swamp expedition than a dry-land trek) a bucket of water won't be enough. We need a veritable waterfall (and some soap!). That is why I would always recommend some form of meditation that is connected to Ultimate Good help. That way you always have a cleansing waterfall at your disposal!

Mindfulness may help to monitor thoughts and emotions. It is good too, because instead of suppressing the mind one gives it a task! Furthermore it might be useful initially if people are atheists and you do not want to scare them off with talk of divine help. Some people in my experience have problems asking for divine help, even if they believe in it. Mindfulness here is still better than nothing – and I have heard too that even 'just' mindfulness meditation causes positive changes to the brain. Any kind of meditation will probably help you become more aware, observant, detached (where necessary) etc. If anything I believe that such lessons will be learned quicker with Ultimate-Good-connected meditative work though!

Generally I think one cannot do too much spiritual work. Of

course if you have small kids and they start going hungry, because you'd rather meditate than cook for them, then you have a problem – but that is common sense. You see, a few years ago I saw a TV program about addiction and addictive behavior. I got scared that I might be addicted to meditation. Maybe I was craving its calming effect, but I needed hours of meditation, because a 10–20 minute meditation just could not give me enough tranquility. If we look at the neurotransmitter model in addiction, a drug triggers the release of neurotransmitters, like serotonin which cause a high. The neurotransmitters get used up by the body and you end up with a comedown. One needs more and more of the same drug to get the same effect.

Now with meditation I am working with Ultimate Good energies; besides a potential healing crisis, there should not be any side effects and/or addiction. But esoterics often say that healing is 'totally' side effect free as well, so maybe they are wrong about the potential of addiction too? The whole question did unnerve me a bit. One solution would have been to not meditate for a while, see what happens. To me that was like being in a battle though and not shooting at the aggressor enemy, believing that the aggressor is only shooting at me because I am defending myself. I felt I really had no choice but to meditate or feel shitty. Again if I were drug addicted and stopped taking drugs, I would feel shitty for a while as well...

Still I was stubborn and kept doing my stuff, including meditation. Besides, I had a massage and healing business, so had to give healing for 15+ hours a week as it was if I wanted to pay the rent. I was convinced that I meditated out of self-defense not because I was addicted. It would be another 1–2 years though until I got so much better that on some days I do not take any special time out to meditate anymore at all. I.e. the average amount of time I spent doing active spiritual work, especially for myself, has gone down, which pretty much disproves the addiction theory!

I would like to share three meditations (basic, intermediate and advanced). Feel free to 'tweak' them as you see fit. They are tools designed to help you rid yourself of negative/stale energies as well as healing, protecting, and recharging your energies. If you do not have a standing order with Ultimate Good already, first ask Ultimate Good for perfect healings, cleansings, protections and recharges.

The Bubble of Light (basic meditation)

Imagine a healing bubble of white or translucent light around you and your aura. Intend for this bubble to be self-generating, self-cleansing, self-protecting and self-healing. Then breathe in the light and breathe out whatever your bodies want to expel. The Light will take away any negative or stale energies and put them on the big cosmic recycling heap. If you feel like another color to white, feel free to change it. White includes all colors, but might initially be too strong – translucent should definitely always work though.

Chakra Meditation (intermediate meditation)

It is best to look at a picture of the main Chakras before commencing. It will help to visualize whereabouts specific Chakras are. Begin the meditation with Grounding and if you want a Light-bubble as well. Then ask Ultimate Good to connect to all your Chakras, with the respective color(s). Once you feel that all connections have been established work through your main Chakras one by one, top down or bottom up. Keep your attention on each respective Chakra, with a healing intent. You are guiding your own healing energies and some of the Ultimate Good healing energies you have connected to, to that area.

Now let the healing energies do whatever they need to do to help that Chakra: cleanse it, improve it, heal it and/or protect it. If you can feel or see blockages already, stay on the Chakra until they have been resolved; or alternatively, once you feel like moving on to the next Chakra, do so. Initially completely resolving accrued blockages might take too long, so this will have to be done in more than one session.

No worries if your attention wavers. Once you have 'guided' the healing energies to a Chakra and are generally in healing/meditation mode, the energies can work without you keeping your attention on the process. The healing might be slightly stronger or speedier, if you stay focused, but it is not essential. No need to feel guilty about thoughts 'wandering off'. The concentration should improve with time. Especially as energies become clearer and LLE resistances lessen.

Hara Meditation (advanced meditation)

Hara is the energy harmonizing and connecting our Chakras; it also supports our grounding. I see it as silvery-white light coming in at the bottom through the heels, through the Base Chakra and from the top through the Crown Chakra. The Hara energy flows through the vertical midline of the body and connects all Chakra centers. It also has three main power-centers (Dan Tien) – at the height of the 2nd Sacral Chakra, the Higher Heart Chakra and the 5th Eye Chakra. To me Hara energy is a bit of a turbo boost to the Chakra system and the grounding energies.

To meditate on the Hara energies, I usually focus on the entry points: Heels, Base, Crown, then visualize it in the midline of my body and go on to meditate on the Dan Tiens. If I find any blockages or grey/black areas, I'll rest my attention on that area until I feel them dissolve or feel like it is enough for that session. At times I will concentrate on how Hara energies benefit, help my whole bodies, including arms and legs! Or I'll concentrate on the interaction between the Hara energies and my Chakras. I usually see Hara energies as silver (white). I started off though with seeing Hara energies as translucent.

The Dan Tiens are said to be energy reservoirs, but I find they are somewhat access to intuitive knowledge as well. Also I used to think that it would be up to my bodies to use the energy from a Dan Tien, but realized I can actively pull energy out of Dan Tiens, especially the first/lowest.

Chapter 16

Sight, Intent and Attunement

To attune to a respectable energy source, to intend to help heal and to visualize for your own, or a client's benefit, are essential tools for Lightworkers. Furthermore it took me a while to find methods of attuning which I felt comfortable with.

Visualizations vary from depressing and nightmarish, lightly entertaining and titillating, to powerful healing tools. And to just simply put your mind in a healing space, to just set your intentions on healing is always said to be so simple, yet I have battled in the past to achieve this with any real conviction too.

So what is visualization, this special sight? It is a tool to change your subconscious and ultimately your life. How do you visualize? You just close your eyes and picture something with your 'inner eye'. What is the inner eye though? I guess it is the mind's little cinema of your imagination and memories. I have met people whose inner visions seem to be just as powerful and colorful as their 'real' vision, but with me (and I guesstimate most people) my inner vision is more like quick flashes and a heavy reliance on memory recall. If I am supposed to visualize a cube, it is more the knowing of what a cube looks like than actually seeing a cube. It seems that as soon as my mind has received all that information and knows it, it is happy and moves on.

My real interest in visualization was triggered when I read *Urban Shaman* by Serge King. It was suggested that by entering inner worlds and vision quests, you could learn more about your subconscious, your beliefs and strengths, as well as your fears and weaknesses. You could change things in your inner world and affect the outside world with this. By visualizing/imagining a problematic situation in a more ideal way, that process can supposedly change your outside life. By e.g. visualizing how you stand up to an old foe, you might be more confident the next time you encounter that person.

Visualization is said to be an incredibly flexible and multi-functional tool. Supposedly if you have money problems in the outside world, you just have to visualize your ideal shopping trip (on inexhaustible funds) and more money will flow into your life. Or you could visualize opening your bank statement and see a 6-figure sum in the black! Apparently our inner world can influence our outside world. So if there are visions of poverty inside us, we attract it. If we then visualize the life of a billionaire (for ourselves) will we really attract that though? In my experience it is not that simple.

I have found that there are several factors that complicate the process. Whenever I heard any esoteric lecturers talk about visualizations, and dared to ask critical questions, I mostly got stung by at least an annoyed look or even a snappy remark though. I have been accused several times of over-thinking every-thing, including visualizations. But I feel that argument is a cop-out because whoever says it does not have a proper answer to my questions. It is always okay to ask questions, because you should be able to feel comfortable with the spiritual tools you use!

In *Urban Shaman*, Serge King describes the vision quest of a student. He tells the reader several times beforehand that their inner worlds are theirs – they have the power there and can do as they please! On the vision quest they enter a lower dimension world, and the student encounters a wild bear, roaring at him. First he is stunned and fearful, but then he grabs a sleeping pill from his pocket and throws it into the bear's mouth. The bear drops over and falls asleep – danger averted. The student realizes that he has to work more on his inner fears, and his creativity in facing and taming them. I was really impressed by that story. I felt I was creative and if by manipulating my inner worlds/visions I could change my outside (for the better), then bring it on!

Initially my visualizations seemed effortless, but over time I had more and more complications. Every time I got all hyped up and ready to do a creative visualization (battle) inside myself, I'd encounter some kind of snag. In the previous example of the wild roaring bear I would wonder – what if I did not bring any sleeping pills with me? I usually do not tend to carry any barbiturates or the like with me, so why would I in my inner worlds? But wait, if I can do as I please in my inner worlds, I can just materialize some sleeping pills! When trying that, it turned out harder than expected though. Do I have to know the name of the sleeping pills? Do I need to know their molecular structure? Do I need to be able to visualize that structure? Chemistry was always one of the subjects in school and during my medical studies which I did not excel at. Could I just visualize any structure and it would work? How would that translate into the real world? If quizzed in a medical exam, I could not just go up to the board and make up some molecular structure! But let us just assume that as long as I name the pill I materialize in my vision Creation would do the rest.

This made me realize though that even in my dreams and visions I am not all-powerful, and dependent on other forces to assist me in my creations! The next problem was that any sleeping pill I know about does need a few minutes, at least, to come to full effect! Now a roaring, angry bear can rip me to shreds in a few minutes! Would I need something stronger? Would something stronger be potentially poisonous? Why not shoot the bear straight then? Well, I was a vegetarian back then – and refused to kill a bear, even in my imagination! Especially knowing that what I imagine in inner worlds can have an effect on outside events!

Not helping was a constant nagging telling me that I am in a real crisis situation here, just as in real life. I cannot just think about it for ages before I come to a decision about what to do; by then the bear would have eaten me. Luckily I have found over the years that I can take all the time that is required. I just press the imaginary 'pause' button. Any energy trying to rush me into decision making is mostly a negative one. As with everything, the more you practice the more proficient you become at visualizing combat/crisis resolutions and the quicker you will be able to act too. The best insurance is to always act under perfect Ultimate Good supervision and protection.

Okay, let's just trust that I have a sleeping pill that works in milliseconds! I am cross-eyed though (in real life), which in real life means I cannot see three-dimensionally, and makes me one of the worst shots (and catchers) around. Surely I could just imagine that I could aim and hit my target (the bear's open mouth) effort-lessly in my imagination? Yep – I can do that! Still just that little detail gave me the first cracks in my beliefs that simply imagining something could change my outside world effortlessly. I am confident that I would have to visualize throwing a lot of hoops perfectly before my ball playing skills in the real world would improve at all! Believe me I have tried! A shaman might say that it is my doubts – that it will take a lot of visualizations to change my eyes and ball playing skills – which limit me. Well I did visualize that it only takes the one visualization, visualized it and – oops, still did not catch that ball!

The next problem is that visualizations can have a life of their own. Okay, I have thrown the millisecond-effective sleeping pill successfully into the bear's mouth. Then I suddenly realize that I stand on a steep mountainside foot path. To my left is the mountain, to my right the abyss, and the bear is falling towards me. I better realize there and then that I can stop time, for I only have a second or so before that sleepy bear crushes me under-neath him. I can move backwards, but there is so much loose gravel on the path I stumble. In that millisecond I have to learn to either fly or teleport. Teleportation sounds good, but where to? I suddenly realize that I do not really know where I am. So I need to visualize where I land, potentially visualize a whole new country. By now I am exhausted. A 'simple' vision, supposedly empowering, has given me a plethora of problems in a few seconds… Don't get me wrong, I like a challenge; I have learned a few things, but a little warning that things might get tough would have been nice.

And I have to wonder – are the inner worlds real? Why do I care? Well, if they are just a figment of my imagination, then they are all me – the bear attacking me is part of me! Which makes me wonder, why are parts of me attacking me? If the worlds I travel to – especially during guided shamanic journeys, and potentially in the company of others (like I did in Peter's cult days) are real worlds, then I cannot act like a tyrant and/or an all-powerful being without potentially affecting others too. If in such a world, I suddenly got attacked by a horde of Orcs, I cannot just bomb them. If I were to use a bomb, it would have to be a smart bomb, which only neutralizes foes and considers that there might be allies amongst them, fighting them in their midst.

Over time I found that a lot of 'inner' visions seem to be more than just imagination. If I visualize an angel in the room with me, chances are that an actual angel will appear (spiritually). If I visualize a specific chakra, I will see it free flowing or blocked, depending on its 'actual' state etc. Initially such e.g. chakra visualizations annoyed and confused me. I would try to visualize my ideal and perfect bodies, trying to affirm them and give the ideal state more power, but started seeing all these things that were wrong with my bodies. My visualization turned into an actual vision of the state of my light bodies. Or I would try to visualize how a blockage of a chakra would dissolve, but the blockage would just not budge – which taught me that some blocks need either special tools to dissolve them or more patience.

A common practice in visualization is 'cord cutting'. Cords symbolize our connection to someone. If we have unhealthy relationships, problems with an ex-lover, for example, the cords get sick and might be more conductive to negative emotions. What we want is light, bright cords, that only conduct love and happiness, and protect against receiving negative emotions from someone else. You imagine cutting the (sick) cord to release and heal the relationship (let's just assume you always carry a cord-cutting sword with you). Now this can have a direct effect on another human being. I have had to realize that I need to cut selectively i.e. I cut through the sick, darker elements of the connection, leaving the actual light-cord intact. Furthermore some darker cords I cut would immediately reattach to each other. I would need a flaming sword to cut them, to cauterize the ends and prevent them from reattaching. These loose ends would possibly start to rot and release toxins, which could affect me or my ex-lover negatively. I'd have to ask for a blessing and perfect healings for the stumps

Really scary would be though if I just went and cut a cord and that would trigger some booby trap reaction inside myself or (even scarier) whoever I de-corded from. I cut the cord to heal a relationship, not cause problems – even if they are healing crises. I'll feel especially bad if they might have been avoidable. I'd therefore have to scan all cords for booby traps and ask for them to be deactivated before attempting to cut anything. With all this there is always the potential risk that what I visualize is wrong, my visions are somehow blocked or distorted. I might not find any booby traps, but there actually are some. Or I might think that I am negatively affected by my ex's emotions, but the cord is actually healthy, i.e. I'd be fighting imaginary foes, wasting time and energy.

One particularly scary occasion was when I tried to visualize one of my angels next to me in the gym. I saw them, but the negative energies in the gym attacked them. Had I not cut off that vision there and then, they could have exploded. I am not an angel killer. I am not sure if an angel can be killed, but I am not willing to find out. I think to understand though that my angels would not have come down into the gym if they knew it was dangerous for them; I could visualize them there as much as I wanted. What I saw was what would happen if I insisted and they obliged. It was a visionary/hypothetic vision…

I also found that when I enter into any visualization I do not necessarily just see my own inner worlds! My inner worlds are not independent of the outer world and others' inner worlds. If I go and face a particular fear inside myself, and that fear energy is connected to and supported by outside LLEs, they may strengthen whatever I encounter within my inner worlds. For example during one healing I encountered a menacing, pitch-black statue. I tried shining healing light onto it, without any joy. I asked for the healing light to be turned into powerful lasers – not a scratch. I tried to blow it up – nothing. I asked for it to be carried off, but it seemed deeply rooted into the ground. Only when I asked for all LLEs in the outside, who must be visualizing that black entity into my inner world, to be engaged and removed was it possible to dissolve and remove the statue safely.

The main thing with such visions is to stay calm. Try to stay open for inspiration – the solution usually comes. I do feel that if working with Ultimate Good they will always try not to overwhelm one with visions that one does not have the time, skill or energy to master. Battles cannot always be prevented though, especially perhaps in the beginning stages of one's spiritual path, if one starts off with e.g. a lot of accumulated heavy energy inside one's bodies, or one is thrown into the deep and cold end by spiritually 'waking up' to a foe like cancer. After a while things should become more manageable.

Again I recommend to not force a visualization, like insisting on dissolving some blockage there and then – Ultimate Good might still be busy defusing booby traps connected. I do not mean that one should resign and admit defeat; we just have to give in to the fact that it will take some more time to clear or heal something. It also does not mean that I feel it is wrong to fight something spiritually. Staying in healing or meditation mode is not forcing something; one has a right to stay assertive in that. When staying in healing mode and 'holding' a frequency, my whole body might tense. But I feel that that is initiated by Spirit; I am holding that frequency (the Energy does the actual manipulations of e.g. the client's energies), not forcing a specific outcome of a healing!

The time it takes for a visualization to 'translate' into the material world can be frustrating. I have visualized many riches for the last 17 years. My financial situation is alright. I still pay off credit cards and do not have any savings or major assets to my name, but it has been much worse! So even if you can visualize that perfect shopping spree in your mind, you see the millions clearly (in front of your inner eye) when opening that visionary bank statement, I'd be cautious about spending that money in the real world just yet.

During my chronic fatigue years visualization was near impossible. Anyone telling me I should just visualize feeling healthy, fit and energetic – I could have shot on the spot. I nearly always had aches and pains in my muscles and joints. Even during meditation I would be aware of them, so trying to 'feel free' of them was futile. After feeling terrible for years on end I could no longer even remember what feeling good and healthy was like. I would have had to take heavy drugs to make me forget and feel different. I did try some recreational drugs. They can have amazing effects – they did make me remember happiness, I felt happy and pain free for a few hours at least. The comedown afterwards was usually horrendous though; I felt even worse than normal. I would not really recommend them as a regular or standard therapy.

Yet without being able to visualize well-being back then (all I could do was pray for good health and perfect healings), my health improved! So much for those who claim that we create everything ourselves – i.e. I could not visualize good health, ergo it should have been impossible to come to pass, but it did…

For all visualizations I recommend a general disclaimer:

May this visualization only come into effect if it is good for me, my bodies, my life, my long-term well-being as well as the Universe.

I already mentioned that I am very careful about any visualizations in my healing work, but that especially extends to visualization work regarding my or a client's bodies. It might stem from my medical studies, and again it might be part-paranoia, but I do have a healthy respect for the complexity of all our bodies and how they function. Just because e.g. my white blood cells are a crucial part of my immune system – and fight off pathogens and potentially cancerous, mutated cells – does not mean I visualize how they multiply when feeling off. Because I also know that if I have too many white blood cells it can be detrimental too. As I would not know what level my white blood cells are, and where they should be, I would not just give a command to my body to double the number of all white blood cells. I find it is much better for my well-being and healer's peace-of-mind if I just pray for perfect blood health, white blood cell numbers and then just offer myself as a channel for extra energy that might have to come through to help adjust any deficiencies or surpluses.

Initially, when learning about chakras, I was more brazen when it came to healing my light bodies. I would visualize my chakras opening or closing, pumping more energy etc. When I would feel a blockage, I might pour spiritual acid onto it to dissolve it. I am not sure if Ultimate Good kept on telling me off in such circumstances or if it was paranoia, but as soon as I would visualize something I often got some intuition that it might actually cause more harm than good. I realized over the years that our light bodies probably are likely just as complex as our physical ones (if not more), and that I really did not have a clue what I was doing.

I do believe that any spiritual work we do can be incredibly powerful. Visualizations can be a part of that. The more we begin to not just visualize/imagine, but actually see real spiritual things, events and work with them, the more effective and accurate our spiritual work should become. I recommend keeping an open mind. At times visualizations might just be a form of occupational therapy, designed to keep our minds busy and give us a sense of empowerment, a sense that we are doing something for our own healing (or that of others). That might not sound like much, almost defamatory against visualizations, but from my own experience – when in the depths of despair, when the mind does not seem to be able to come up with any kind of encouraging or positive thoughts – it is very comforting to have tools that keep the mind occupied.

Some people might initially have problems visualizing anything. Sometimes it helps to just call it imagination instead of visualization. If one has problems visualizing one can just verbalize, for example for 'Grounding' say:

I affirm a perfect beam of light connecting me to healthy, divine Earth energies and thank them for perfect cleansing, healing, protection and recharge of my energies. Thank you! Amen.

Or any other way one wants to verbalize it. Amen is supposed to be a power word (meaning 'so be it'), but you can leave it if it has too many religious connotations for you.

Overall, after years of working with visualizations, I try to not let myself be goaded into the visualization arena anymore. I am not free of 'visions'; when working on a client I might have a picture of a blocked chakra or a swollen aura layer, but I try my best not to 'react' to such, other than facilitating the relevant healing. Sure, 'seeing' things during a healing session can be exciting, and my medically interested, inquisitive spirit is eager to learn and understand. It also makes a healing session more interesting. If I encounter a blocked chakra, I will only make 'visualization suggestions' like the use of a spiritual, intelligent laser beam removing any stuck gunk. I will only visualize this 'speculatively', not practically. I'll leave the actual work to my Ultimate Good helpers. If they want me to see or learn anything, great, but I'll keep my know-it-all healer ego out of their way.

I am cautious about what I visualize, but I have stopped being paranoid. I do not take any unnecessary chances, but feel there are some safety mechanisms built in (definitely if one asks for divine protections and guidance), especially in their translation into the physical world. After all Earth is still round, even if millions of humans believed it flat for centuries. Still I try to not create any unnecessary work for Ultimate Good, having to block my visualizations or repair possible damaging effects. I feel that what is even more important, than the actual visualization, is the 'intention' with which we do it – intention is the true driving force behind the effectiveness of our visualizations.

We are often told to 'set your intention' or 'intend for it to be healing and it will be healing' and so on. Initially that call for the right kind of intention baffled me. If I intend to go to the cinema tonight, I am planning to go to the cinema tonight. I will have checked what's on, what time and where. I might think about meeting friends. Still, to my feeling the use of 'intention' here is describing something somewhat vague and immaterial. If I intend to go to the movies it is less certain than if I say I 'will' go to the movies. In the intention phase I can still withdraw, change my mind.

So why is intention so important in healing? Or is it? Especially during the initial years of my spiritual awakening, I ended up constantly testing my intentions. Were they all good? Was I acting for the highest possible good? I do not regret spending that time; it's healthy to take an audit of our beliefs and behaviors at some point, if not regularly. I did find some things that merited improvement and weeding out. In retrospect though, I spent far too much time worrying about my intentions. During my time with Peter and for years after – I worried and looked for evil where there was none. When healings did not materialize for me in the past, I started to question everything – including my 'intent'.

Maybe I wanted to destroy myself? That must be why I had McDonald's the other week? And a chocolate bar after lunch? Was I practicing healing, wanting to channel healing to satisfy some ego desire or because of an unconditionally loving heart and due to my divine intrinsic nature? It did not help that I felt sick with all my chronic fatigue problems. The voices had a ball, trying to convince me that it was some karmic punishment due to past evils. If I could not heal myself there and then, it must be because something was seriously wrong – how could I dare to then channel healing for others. Was I channeling evil energies? I did not think I intended to do so, but then I might be blinded by the evil inside myself...

As a result I prayed quite vehemently for everyone's protection against any potential evil inside me, especially when channeling energy. Even to take me out of my bodies in case I became a serious danger to anyone's well-being. I would think that kind of prayer shows well enough that I cared about doing Lightwork and not serving shadier masters. It still took me years to really regain self-confidence. I generally trusted that when I asked Ultimate Good to perfectly protect a client against any confusions or evil inside me they would. My emotional body was so riddled with guilt and doubt though, and these fears frequently felt much stronger than any comfort or wisdom I could get from my heart or rationale.

I knew that Ultimate Good is bigger than any evil that could fit into my body. The screwed-up emotions I felt though were mostly all I could feel – the unfathomable vastness of Ultimate Good might have just as well not existed. Funnily enough you still get 'spiritual' people telling you that your intentions must have not been clear if what you prayed for did not come to fruition. Today, if someone comes to me with that one – I politely 'intend' to wring their neck – just kidding. I try to be understanding; after all I fell for some esoteric propaganda slogans in the past too. One single truth does not make the whole book true though.

So if you ask me how to be sure of your intentions – just verbalize them. You could say:

Ultimate Good, I always want to work in your Light. Should I stray out of the Light, please guide me back. Help me see and understand what I need to live harmoniously. Please help me to be and live my true individualized divine nature. Protect all beings (including myself) against my errors. Any harm I might still inflict please help to heal perfectly. Thank you for helping me to lead a happier and ever more loving life, free of suffering. Thank you. Amen!

Or when asking for something specifically, "Dear Ultimate Good, I want to be more self-confident. Please help me in any way you can to rediscover my full self-confidence potential (without becoming a pompous ass). Thank you. Amen." Or, "Dear Ultimate Good, please help me be a good healing channel and make sure that all healings only happen for the Good. Thank you! Amen." And just as a reminder if you were to e.g. fight self-consciousness LLEs, they might not want to go without a fight, so it might take some time to be free of such. So even though you have prayed for perfect self-confidence, you might still be attacked by doubts and feelings of self-consciousness. Now that won't be because your intentions to become self-confident weren't clear enough, but because your self-consciousness LLEs will try their best to dissuade you from believing that there is any self-confidence inside you, or that Ultimate Good will do everything in its power to help you dig it out!

Finally we come to 'attunements' – the process of connecting to a spiritual energy source – whatever size, shape or form that source might be. As a spiritual healer, to attune I initially learned to visualize a white beam of light rising up from my crown chakra, and connecting to 'Source' in the depth of the Universe. That energy would then go through the vertical midline of my body. From my heels I'd send down a beam of light to connect with Earth energies. The two energies would meet in my heart chakra and from there flow through my arms into my hands, to be passed on to the client. It sounds so simple, yet I came up with problems here too. Because I do not just attune to Ultimate Good energies to heal myself, but also to channel energies for my client's benefit.

I am quite keen not to attune to some dodgy, halfhearted, semi-divine source, or even worse. I am willing to experiment with my own well-being, to a certain extent, but not with that of others. I do very much hope that if a healer just really wants to help and channel (all-good) healing energies, that that will happen. I have met healers who seem to worry much less about the technicalities of attunement – they follow the above method and seem to have healing successes. With all the negative stuff I have encountered, I rather play it doubly safe when I attune though. After trying the above-mentioned method of attunement for a while, I started to get too many doubts. What I was doing did not seem ideal. So I came to ask Ultimate Good healing energies to attune, connect to me, rather than the other way around. I do believe that Ultimate Good does hear our prayers instantly and that help arrives pretty instantaneously too, even if some Ultimate Good energies are eons away. Distance seems no hindrance.

It feels good to believe to know a bit about the heavens and the different Ultimate Good helpers, but I am careful not to give my clients the impression that they might have to know names or e.g. angel hierarchies to receive help, as some 'angel experts' claim. If you have no medical training whatsoever, do not even know where which organ is, and feeling unwell go to the accident and emergency unit, the nurses and doctors are not going to send you away again because you do not know which specialist is supposed to deal with your complaint... I thoroughly believe that the heavens are no different there; we will be hooked up to the right energy source if we ask for help.

When attuning I was told to pull in white light through my crown chakra. But we are also taught that the color for the crown chakra is violet/purple. I have had healings where I ended up seeing white light coming through my chakras, and not their individual colors, but I am not sure if that is the norm. Might I have fallen for a delusion? I would be careful to recommend to a novice to channel white through any chakra – it feels as if it would be stronger, more advanced, and I would not want to judge if someone is ready for it or not. I was told to just use the crown and the base chakras (plus heels) to get energy for healing. The base is more of an anchor, helping to ground; the main energy for healings comes through the crown. After a while I questioned, why just the crown and the base, what about the other main chakras? Could I only use crown energy to effect highest possible good healings?

I felt thrown back into the cult delusions of feeling guilty for being human. Actually Peter does not seem to be the only one who made his followers feel guilty about having a physical body. I have heard slightly different versions explaining why we have physical bodies: "We need physical bodies because they are more inert – if we had more subtle bodies every thought we think could potentially kill us," "We keep on reincarnating into physical bodies until we escape some karmic wheel by doing sufficient 'good'." All seem to assume that it is some form of punishment to have a physical body, or Earth is a kindergarten for the soul. I do not believe any of it! It would be a rather poor education if everyone forgot everything each time they incarnated. And what happens between lives; how come such loose cannons, such as ourselves, have not blown up the heavens yet with all our unruly thoughts and emotions? I choose to believe that the physical body is just another form in which we experience individuality, on our eternal soul journey – on this planet with the added twist of suffering.

When going through these thought patterns I realized that if my physical existence was not a punishment, then there is no 'sin' to having physical, emotional and mental 'bodies' and hence there should be an ideal, Ultimate Good frequency for all my chakras – an ideal red, vermillion, orange, yellow, green, aquamarine, blue, indigo and violet. Therefore I attune through all my chakras, and ask to be hooked up through all of them since.

There is another consideration for some chakras. Traditionally one might learn or assume that one only needs limited amounts of energy on e.g. the lower chakras. I.e. for e.g. with the heart chakra we ideally have the capacity to love everyone and everything unconditionally. Whereas with e.g. the naval chakra we only emotionally bond to our family and close friends, on the sacral to an intimate partner (or a few partners), and the base chakra we need for just our own physical body. As healers and Lightworkers, I find we often channel energy for more than just ourselves and a handful of people though. Not just via the upper, but also the lower chakras. If you want to be a healer, you might want to ask for upgrades on relevant chakras to be able to handle sufficient energy flow for greater healing.

Different people might use different methods of attunement, which is perfectly alright if they work for them. There is the use of words/names of the Divine, symbols (such as religious symbols or e.g. the Reiki symbols), attuning via a holy figure/master (alive or departed), nature spirits or totem animals. They are all but doors one can open to gain access to divine energies. Some symbols open blanket connections to the Divine, like e.g. the Christian cross symbol connects to the divine in general, whereas connecting via a totem bear might mainly connect you to divine qualities of strength and self-confidence.

Or the pentagram, for example, can have especially protective qualities. If I experiment with any other forms of attunement, I generally first attune to Ultimate Good and then ask to connect to the Ultimate Good version of e.g. my wolf guide and protector. That way, if I do not have an Ultimate Good wolf guide yet, I might get one, and if there is a 'confused' wolf spirit that wants to connect to me, I won't connect to it and will be protected against its efforts as good as possible.

As a healer/Lightworker we attune to Higher Powers as to not use our own energies for a healing (and deplete ourselves, as well as not to potentially use energies inside us, which might still be confused). Our intention is the power inside us and given to us to 'hold' healing energies in our being and to stay attuned to them as long as necessary. Intention is our love-, wisdom- and desire-to-help-energy, the link between pure divine energies and the recipient. It is obviously the shifter as well which decides if we want to attune to divine or confused energy sources in the first place. Visualizations help to gently guide (not force) these healing energies onto a certain target, like a specific chakra. If we attune to Ultimate Good energies, which have their own intelligence and know where they have to go and what they have to do, the visualization part of a healer's work is optional. It can just help make a healing more interesting, further our understanding about healing processes or e.g. understand more about the causes of a client's ill health. Over time I have learned to shift most of the energy I initially used for visualizations in my spiritual work into the intention element of my channeling. I use it to help me hold the connection to divine energies which become most needed if hitting LLE resistances.

Chapter 17

Intuition and Divination

When I first read about spiritual healing I was fascinated by 'experienced' healers' claims that everything can be diagnosed accurately and healed without negative side effects. This sounded heavenly. My medical studies were much harder than I expected. The amount of knowledge and research available for study was mind-boggling. Yet you still hear of patients being misdiagnosed or it taking years to reach a diagnosis. And there is no guarantee of help – many a disease is still seen as something you will have to live with as a chronic condition. If treatment is available, it might come with uncomfortable side effects. I dared to dream that one day I might be one of those spiritual healers who could help diagnose and access powerful healing energies, all this side effect free.

I felt assured that everyone could rediscover their intuitive abilities to heal. As there was mention of potentially painful confrontation of 'inner demons' to do this, I was full of youthful optimism. I would not want to go back to before I embarked on my spiritual quest, yet many of the promises made by the esoteric books I read remain unfulfilled. Today I am not so confident that 100% clear intuition and psychic abilities are even possible on this planet, yet. If I get any extrasensory information about my life or my clients, it leaves plenty of room for all sorts of interpretations at best, or is wrong or even damaging at worst. I don't regret not finishing my medical degree years ago, but at times I almost long for what feels like the simplicity of looking at an MRI picture, reading an EKG or getting black on white blood parameters from a lab report. There are plenty of uncertainties in Western medicine and basically many a diagnosis and treatment is based on statistical likelihoods – but on the other hand plenty of those statistics are backed up by large amounts of 'comforting' data.

The biggest stumbling block with trusting psychic abilities is that intuition can be wrong or misleading. Today there are hundreds of gurus on the planet who claim to have been Jesus or Buddha in a previous incarnation and most of their devotees will believe this. I once talked to a cult advisor, and she told me that one day she had five people from a specific cult in her office. They all had performed regressions, but were not allowed to talk about their regressive experiences to each other. She managed to get them to a point where they 'came out' with their previous lives though. It turned out she had three Cleopatras in the room.

Aside from the improbable pre-incarnation of myself as Mengele, I had three psychics tell me what they saw about my 'previous' lives. They all came up with very different incarnations – just in the twentieth century I was supposedly a famous American novelist, a Jewish-American female primary school teacher and a Manchester fishmonger. No mention of me having died early in any of those incarnations. Obviously I could have died in my twenties in each and every life; still that would not have left me much time in between lives to digest my previous incarnation and prepare for the next one.

During my chronic fatigue years I experienced what felt like definite attacks on my emotional, mental and spiritual health. The whole symptom complex had started somewhat during my time with Peter and more and more after leaving his cult – I had the strong suspicion that perhaps Peter was attacking me with 'black magic'. Experiences and sensations that, according to what I read about other ex-cult followers, are not uncommon after leaving a cult environment. From what I had observed Peter had strong psychic abilities, a manipulative and evil character and last but not least access to a lot of energy he could 'suck' from his devotees.

I tried to protect myself as well as I could, by praying for such and constantly requesting plenty of Ultimate Good healing for him and the cult, but the intensity of my symptoms did not abate, even after years. Sure psychopaths might have a tendency for revenge, but how feasible was it that he was still acting out against me years after me leaving? For example, I'd get hit by severe melancholy when smoking during the daytime (not at nighttime), but knowing that Peter used to treat three to four patients at once all the time – would he really have the spiritual capacity to monitor me 24/7 too, so he'd know when I was having a cigarette? Over the years I figured that he must have some strong 'negative' spiritual support behind him, helping him. But was I important enough on which to expend so much effort? I figured that I was probably grossly overestimating his actual abilities.

I was confident I had plenty of angels on my side too – should they not be stronger than whatever he could come up with? In the scheme of things, even if his circle had increased to say 200 hundred devotees, what was that against potential armies of angels helping me? The most frightening thought was that he actually was Jesus in a previous life and had some 'confused' Christian heaven backing him – and through this access to the life force of 2+ billion Christians. Closer inspection of all my experiences with him pointed to the diagnosis he was just a charismatic sociopath. But the voice of reason inside me did not help much – especially considering that my well-being did not improve, and I did not have too many other viable explanations for my un-wellness yet.

I kept on giving healing to myself, analyzing myself and seeing healers – some specialized in removing black magic, curses etc. Whenever I saw such healers or psychics there was a common pattern. At the beginning of the session I was asked to tell them of my troubles. Why I had come to see them, and why I thought I was feeling the way I did? It was nice to have a sympathetic ear, so I'd usually tell my story. After the healing the healer would then tell me that, yes, I had been attacked by my ex-guru. They had to fight him, but managed to banish him. I should not be bothered by him anymore. Or alternatively, if I returned for six sessions I'd be completely cleared of all negative energies.

Cause for celebration? One time I walked out of a healing session with supposedly 'the' healer in London for black magic problems, and I actually felt it all dissolve away. I felt free and un-pestered again. What a relief after years of attack! Unfortunately it only lasted about ten minutes, and then it all swamped back again. I did give this healer two more attempts – maybe she had overlooked something? After each session, she announced, "You are completely healed! It has all been taken care of," but unfortunately I felt just as bad as before each session, not even ten minutes of respite this time. After the third time I was fed up with it – either she was an unreliable psychic, a charlatan or perhaps even in cahoots with dark force?

Why should another's healings be more effective than those I initiated anyway? It's Ultimate Good doing the healings, regardless of who they use as a channel. Other healers might be clearer channels than me, but then I only saw that healer for a total of three hours, compared to hundreds of hours I had spent in potentially less-clear-channel self-healings. When I remarked after the third session that I still felt the same way, i.e. crap, she told me that if the angels wanted me completely healed they could do it in the blink of an eye. There must be something I still had to learn. That remark really pissed me off. Why then tell me beforehand everything was clear?

In more lenient moments I think that maybe some healers are too scared to question their intuitions – it takes guts to admit that there might be forces out there which can warp psychic input. Perhaps by telling their clients that they are all-healed they believe that, if the client just believes strongly enough in their all-clear diagnosis, they will 'attract' such an all-healing (as per Law of Attraction)? In my experience that is ignorant and opens doors to feelings of guilt and doubt, plus some patients might stop taking lifesaving medications etc. Sometimes I am not all sure if some healers and psychics are actually aware of the damage they can potentially inflict.

It is bad enough if a regular therapist or doctor says something wrong; they might claim they are definitely right, but one can still believe that they are human and hence might make mistakes. If a healer or psychic claims something to be divine and 'absolute' truth, it could be seen as having eternal implications. Who is eager to spend eternity with sadistic or careless angels? Fortunately I had had experiences before where healers or gurus were wrong, so I knew about it and did not let her remarks bother me too much. Still it had been a waste of money and time (taken off work).

I found another healer and, now wiser, refused to tell him what was troubling me. I wanted to find out how far he might be able to 'see' what was attacking me, without being 'led' by my suspicions. He saw some things that did not make any sense at all – I had supposedly encountered some evil energy in a cave? Except for a brief visit with Peter and the group to a tiny cave on Maui, Hawaii, where I only stood at the entrance, I cannot recall any cave visits – and these five minutes did not feel any more evil than the rest of my two years in the cult.

After years I just got fed up with the whole Peter-attacking-me construct. It was giving him far too much power and was becoming more and more unreasonable. I had now read that plenty of cult leavers show similar symptoms to mine (so Peter's cult was likely no more special than any other). As mentioned, after I talked to the cult psychotherapist and he told me that he had been threatened multiple times by cult devotees and gurus against talking out, but his health had improved over the years, I refused to listen to any more voices trying to tell me it was Peter attacking me.

I had other 'outside' attacker theories in those years. At the time I was praying for anti-ageing and rejuvenation – if I was ever successful with this kind of healing, I might make a lot of plastic surgeons unhappy and unemployed. I had a very hard time though picturing some Association of Plastic Surgeons sitting down and holding black magic ceremonies – invoking evil spirits to destroy all beings which might pose a threat to their enterprises. The same applied to all other kinds of doctors who might one day have less to no work, if spiritual healing gained full momentum and fulfilled all the promises many a healer made.

I tried to either find a healer that might be able to help me or a psychic who might just be able to tell me what exactly was going on with me. Was the cause of my troubles inside or outside or both? But none of them ever introduced their divination by telling me beforehand that what they were doing was not an exact science, that they might be interpreting impressions they got (potentially wrongly) or even got confused input. (There are experimental psychologists, parapsychologists, and the like, who do publish percentages as to their experiments into extrasensory perception et al, but I am talking one-on-one sessions with psychics here, outside a scientific setup.) I got some assessments about my character which I could agree with – but nothing too accurate either. Usually when asking about my health I'd get answers such as, *Your energies are strong, all is well*, or when making clear that I was actually feeling sick, *You have all the tools and help necessary to solve all your problems.* Not one psychic suggested I might be caught up in a battle between Light and Dark, that many of my troubles I picked up empathically from people around me and that the solutions to my problems were to go bigger, to ask for more help in fighting negative energies on the outside, to cleanse my energies regularly or even to take vitamin D3 and get more sunshine!

All this should not be interpreted that I believe all psychics are incompetent or frauds. I just suspect that it is virtually impossible to guarantee any reading as accurate, especially to guarantee that one is 100% connected to Ultimate Good and Truth only, and that nothing else can interfere! Like man-made pollution we also have to contend with 'spiritual smog'. Even if we manage to establish a bit of a clearer, more protected spiritual bubble (where we live or work) most of the spiritual input will have to 'travel' through the smog and may well arrive tainted. Still, if you receive a reading and say 70% of the given information is correct, that could be helpful and healing, as long as you are aware and grounded enough to discard the 30% of tainted or rubbish info.

I also suspect that there are different categories of resistance. If a person who is somewhat interested in the supernatural keeps an open mind and visits a psychic – telling them something accurate is less of a threat to LLEs then if a healer or a person with a strong spiritual practice seeks help. These individuals are generally a much bigger threat to LLEs and hence LLEs have a greater vested interest in hurting or trying to weaken them with misinformation.

I have talked to friends that have seen psychics and who have been told astoundingly accurate future predictions. About 20 years ago a psychic told me that I would write a lot one day; back then I assumed it would be composing or some medical publications – maybe she saw me writing this book? I have not lost hope yet either that, as predicted, one day I will be fabulously rich (well I would not want to be greedy, but financial independence would be most appreciated and I believe it is confirming creation's abundance too).

During my chronic fatigue years, my intuition in general was often very negative, 'Spiritual Tourette's' I called it. I could just walk along a road and, in my mind's eye, see cars flipping in accidents. I'd send a quick prayer for their protections, in case I was picking up premonitions – but it was still stressful. What if my thoughts helped create such events? Before just about any flight, I'd see the plane crash. It took a lot of prayers, blessing the plane and meditations to get onto planes, and it wasn't a very relaxing experience. I saw people being blown up too. In retrospect might some of it have been LLE resistances? They sent me visions of planes crashing so I would not travel to their countries? Or might I have been picking up others' flying fears? Today it rarely happens, and even then I can remain calm. I feel I am stronger as well, so directing Light and Healing to wherever the problem may originate from seems to dissolve it somewhat faster these days.

Not only were my intuitions mainly negative, but contradictory. I would not only get the negative version of something, but also the comforting message that the negative input is untrue. Both felt like genuine intuitions though. I might be barraged with heavy energies trying to convince me I was crazy – and then at some other point I'd feel a more loving energy telling me all would be well and I was not crazy. Since the negative input was so frequent and intense though – the 'nice' voices were almost just a cruel joke. I think I could tell right from wrong (before joining the cult) – it is mostly common sense – but my feelings were at times very confused! People say just listen to your gut – it is always right! But what if one suffers from an overactive conscience, gets hit by confusing LLE resistance, or is on the receiving end of a sociopath and access to gut feelings is totally blocked or the gut all messed up?

Today I go more with the flow and follow my gut instinct, which appears right more often. I might go as far as disqualifying a subtenant applicant who does not feel right. Maybe not see a client again who felt too creepy. I might take a detour one day, to see what's on offer in one of the more-out-of-the-way secondhand shops and find that red sweater I had visualized. I would not rely on my gut though if I were called up for jury duty, and send someone to prison because my gut did not like the defendant.

When I first tried to communicate with the Divine, I followed the guidance I found in books. To just go into a meditative state, pray for perfect connection to the Divine and perfect protections and that is it. It sounded easy enough; trouble is, even 17 years later, and much better protected and connected than as a novice, I still get plenty of 'interference'. Over the years I have added to the above formula about intuitions from Ultimate Good beings. I ask for 24/7 protections, as much as necessary, possible, available and sensible. I also ask that, should I fall for any mis-intuitions, I should please be brought back to my senses, the real truth, as soon as possible.

During a healing/massage session (often before or after) I get plenty of input (about my clients), most of it thoughts, emotions and sensations (inside myself). Most intuitions are vague, ambivalent and generally harder to read than say a medical lab report. All I have to interpret my sensations are my past experiences. Having regular clients is a great help. I can monitor how I feel before, during and after our sessions. With this information and the few pieces of knowledge about my clients (and their lives) I get – such as ethnic origin, country of origin, professions, age, outside appearance, mannerisms, spiritual/religious beliefs – I can guesstimate how viable an intuition I have about a client is likely to be.

Even then I rarely share my intuitions, it has to feel right and it has to make sense to me that sharing my impressions will be of some benefit (and not just scare the client or be damaging in some other way). Plus, it is not always definite that what I am feeling might not be cross over, i.e. energies from my previous client or the one after or perhaps the friend I am supposed to meet that night. So am I just cold reading after all? I am definitely switched on, connected to Ultimate Good while I massage and channel healing – this in turn causes things to just 'pop into my head'; in that sense I do not just use my intellect to come up with stuff. Some input is completely unexpected.

Usually I will try to keep interpretations (in my head) quite general. When working through the client's chakras, for example, I'll just be aware of what chakra I am working on, and if it is the front or back of the chakra. (The front chakra being more current affairs, the back chakras being more past events.) When giving healing to the navel chakra for example and it is blocked, I'll infer that it is likely that there exists some relationship issue on a family or close friends level. I had clients where it felt like they took their employees into this chakra (instead of just being connected to them through the solar plexus chakra – where most professional connections are found). As most people have some family issues – if I voiced my concern I'd probably be right in most cases.

The next thing to consider is that a chakra block can be due to actual events, a person's fear that something might happen (without it actually having taken place – yet); plus it can be caused by inside or outside LLEs. They all pretty much feel the same (to me) though. E.g. a person fearing that they are cursed can feel the same as a person with an actual curse. A person fearing cancer might feel the same as a person with cancer.

I cannot guarantee it, because I do not always check many intuitions regarding their likely correctness – but I have a suspicion that according to the 'self-fulfilling prophecies rule' I get more humbug intuitions with clients who probably believe that psychic abilities are all mumbo jumbo. Disbelief is a belief as well and hence an energy that creates something – in this case the client would expect that I do not have accurate psychic abilities and I would affirm these beliefs if I voiced some mis-intuition.

I can understand that some psychics or healers might feel particularly blocked in a skeptical environment, like a demon-stration in front of doctors, and potentially perform less success-fully than usual. I feel it is a question of numbers too. If in a one-on-one with a client the skeptic energy will be less strong as the cumulative skeptic energy if in a room with several skeptical people. In contrast when attending healing seminars with exercises in psychic intuition, my intuitions often feel easier, more comforting and certain. I am then usually in a room with a bunch of other healers though, all being at least open to the potential of correct Ultimate Good communication, having asked for Ultimate Good protections etc. I often feel more serene and confident about my intuitions too when my clients are more spiritual and have energies with less resistance.

What saddens me though is that usually the lecturers, of such healing or psychic seminars, do not mention such beneficial group effects. Plenty of people might go home after such seminars – all enthusiastic about their newly discovered psychic abilities – only to find that at home, or the next time with a bunch of skeptical friends in the pub, they get it all totally wrong. Relating this to my client work – I'll usually be careful about my intuitions. I usually wait until I have given healing to a client's crown, 3rd and 5th eye chakras. Especially if their crown is strong and feels well connected – this usually is a good indication that the client has higher beliefs and is connected to Higher Powers. This in turn will often make them more truthful (about their own energies and emotions too), more intuitive and open to concepts of divine intuition, psychic abilities and so on. There might be a higher chance that things I pick up may be relatively accurate as well then.

It is not all that easy though. I have had clients that had a strong crown and strong higher belief with it, but also some very conservative religious belief that in turn would have demonized psychic abilities. Their 'fear' of psychic abilities and intuitions might create mis-intuitions for a healer or psychic as well. In the book *The Celestine Prophecy*, a non-believer finds the Divine and his extrasensory powers somewhere in a rainforest. He sees vivid colors and feels energies. Then militia show up and he only survives because he is following higher guidance/intuition. Admittedly it is a novel, but I am sure that there are gurus who also imply that following your intuition is so important, you are in mortal danger if you don't. Peter implied that if we (his followers) did not find our perfect intuition and follow it, we would be guilty of causing the apocalypse in 2012 (well that didn't happen). Such teachings can create panic and paranoia. I simply pray to Ultimate Good that I won't ever be in a situation that is so dangerous that I have to rely on my intuition to survive – I am not much of a thrill seeker.

There is another facet to intuitions – being emotionally involved or not when receiving an intuition. Some say that intuitions will have a greater chance of being accurate and truthful if one is emotionally detached. There is certainly a lesser chance of me going into a state of panic if I feel a bad and threatening energy with a client, rather than a member of my family, but to be emotionally detached is almost impossible either way. I have become more serene with the years; it helps to be more confident that life does not end with our physical bodies and that suffering is pre-chosen and a finite illusion, but going down the spiritual path has made me more empathic and sensitive too. And even if I believe that even the worst suffering will come to an end sometime, to feel that a client might have some nasty illness that is pretty definitely going to serve him up a good deal of suffering, even if I do not know that client very well yet, it is going to trigger an emotional response in me. I would think that true divine intuition has to be strong enough not to be warped by possible emotional responses of the receiver. Negative predictions are going to be   worse than positive ones, but even these could do damage. If I predicted some great event to come to pass and, it didn't, there would probably be at least disappointment.

Maybe one day I will be able to rely on my intuition, and I will be so serene in my disposition that even in a life-threatening situation (and maybe even being surrounded by a bunch of skeptics), where I require full capacity to use my intuition to survive, really won't faze me. But until then I am confident that

Ultimate Good will do all in its power to avert any such situations, before I even get into them – or make me act intuitively right, even if in a confused state. I feel strongly that Ultimate Good does not mind me asking for this. I don't think that my Ultimate Good helpers are gamblers and eager to gamble with my life and well-being either. And in my experience intuition flows best if there is no pressure involved.

The Celestine Prophecy example is quite drastic for portraying someone who has just discovered his intuition and very soon after has to fully rely on it. Since it occurs in the jungle it might be slightly more feasible – considering that the trees and plants around might be more enlightened, might help to strengthen his intuition and keep him attuned. If the same scenario would have been set in a large city, I would have judged the author's imagination totally far-fetched and unrealistic.

Then there are those intuitions, even when right, that feel inappropriate to discuss. I gave healing to a healer colleague once and her back-base chakra was blocked. She knew about this already and told me that she suspected it was because, as a youth, she had been sexually abused several times. Now as a healer and spiritual person (and knowing me for a few years already), she did not have any qualms talking about this. Once during another client's massage and healing I encountered a particularly blocked back-base chakra. Her story popped back into my head; perhaps the client had been sexually abused or had had some other severe childhood trauma too? I saw him for the first time though and our connection was not particularly strong, nor did he seem a very open-minded or spiritual person. I therefore just prayed that he might receive all the healings necessary, available and sensible for whatever blocked his back-base chakra and that if he needed to talk about it that he may get the strength and trust to do so.

I try to remember that I might get a high on accomplishing a feat of sixth sense. I would love to be able to accurately see what is wrong with my clients – hoping that this in turn will help me help and advise them perfectly. I have to watch out that I do not build up too many frustrations as long as perfect sixth sense has not materialized yet though. If frustrations do come up, I make sure I cleanse them out regularly. I mention this because in my experience, if I build up frustrations about something, if it then feels as if my actual wish might be coming true, this can cause ecstasy and a sense of a high, which in turn threaten to make me act rashly.

I also must not forget that even if my help and advice might be perfect, it might not be sensible to 'force' it on a client that has not asked for it. Clients might not be comfortable if their masseur/healer sees their deepest secrets the first time round. If a client would not have the strength or wisdom yet to confront such memories, bringing them up might actually be more damaging than to let them slumber. LLEs can pass on truthful intuitions, as well, if with them they can cause damage…

I had intuitions about clients not making it much longer; their energies seemed in such a bad state, the only thing I could think about was their demise. This is scary though if the client is still young. Two clients come to mind, both workaholics. Both have come to see me on and off for five years now and both are still with us. Call me a coward, but I do not believe it would have helped if I would have told them five years ago, "By the way it feels like you might not make it much longer. I could be wrong, but you might want to get your things in order, just in case." Both clients are quite wealthy too, so I really try to avoid meeting such clients and creating a situation where it looks like I might just want to sell them multiple healing sessions in one go.

Some esoteric authors claim that to distinguish a real from a false intuition (i.e. interference from one's mind) you have to look at and judge how expected the input is – true intuitions will supposedly be unexpected. Sure, intuitions can be useful in giving 'outside the box' hints (if they are truthful), but I am not sure why that should be true in general. Everyone is individual, but then again many people share common traits and experiences. Let's take a common complaint – backaches. When a client complains about back problems, finding the culprit might just take some common sense. A probable cause is that they never had a workplace assessment, sit crooked in front of their PC at work and/or they do not get enough back strengthening exercise and stretching. If I 'felt' any of those causes, they would be more credible than that the client fell into a ditch on Mars, in a previous incarnation, as a Venus spaceman.

Furthermore I have encountered plenty of LLEs which were quite creative and came up with intuitions and explanations to some problem which were very surprising. These explanations often had a certain logic built in, but upon further testing they still turned out to be wrong. For example never did I expect it when I was told that I was Josef Mengele in my last life. It made sense at first, because it seemed to explain why my life seemed to be so hard and burdensome. On further investigation it was impossible (as he died after I was born in this life).

I believe one should always keep two feet on the ground when trying to diagnose the cause of illness. Everything is spiritual, but that does not mean that the laws of the physical body do not apply, that decades of medical research have all been totally confused and in vain, or that common sense should be kicked out the door. I try to find the middle ground and not forget about spiritual elements influencing me, my bodies and my life, without going crazy and trying to theorize every little thing that happens to me.

Sometimes I get the impression that there are other factors too. The really helpful intuitions, which will potentially enable the quickest and least painful healings, are potentially most protected by LLEs. Therefore it may be easier to get spiritual, psychic information that is perhaps interesting, but won't crack the case and if anything will just cause peripheral healings. I am not saying that one actually always has to find the exact cause of the disease in the first place!

I used to follow the often propagated rule that to heal perfectly you need to find the root of your evil. Only by identifying the exact causes will you be able to eradicate and heal perfectly. I spent hours upon hours of meditation trying to go deeper and deeper, to find some truth about myself or my past. I knew that my intuitions were not always reliable, so even if I found something I was never sure if it was a truth or an illusion. It used to drive me mad. Even if I forgave myself for whatever truth I had found, and let it go, I still felt crap again within minutes after coming out of such a meditation. I would definitely feel crap again when waking up the next morning. I am very glad that today I can trust that as long as Ultimate Good knows what needs healing, where and when – I am covered.

I have also learned that if I have a question or need some insight to heal something or help me grow, there often is no use trying to force finding the answer or that insight. At times I might find such an answer or insight during a meditation or healing I actually dedicated to finding it – often enough I won't though. Some of the most valuable intuitions I get are actually kind of 'slipped in' while doing the dishes or the like, and when I least expect them. I suspect this is because at such times the LLEs might be more negligent in protecting such insights or the insights are ripe for the picking.

Sometimes I will be highly certain that something I experience/feel about a client is correct, but when probing the client they will disagree. For example I sometimes feel a marked drop in my energies an hour or two before a client arrives. I might start to feel like in the darkest days of my chronic fatigue. Usually this appears to be the case though because my client is running on almost empty with his energies. My suspicion is frequently confirmed by the fact that when I start to touch them, and I open up to Ultimate Good healing energies to come through for them, their energies/bodies will 'suck' very hard.

They really seem to be energy starved.

Generally I recommend vitamin D3 supplementation. Most clients are grateful, as they have not heard enough about the benefits of vitamin D3 or sufficient sun exposure before. I tell them that it is supposed to be important for bone health, immunity, energy, mood, cardiovascular health and may help protect against several forms of cancer, as well as preventing diabetes. I have had especially exhausted-feeling clients who got upset when I told them about vitamin D3 saying, "But I feel fine and I am a very happy person!" Does that mean that my intuition about the client's energies being depleted was all wrong?

I do not feel exhausted before every client, and with new clients I have no way of knowing that they might have a particularly demanding job until they actually arrive and tell me so. Have I possibly fallen for LLEs' influence? Or are those clients too scared to admit exhaustion? Some clients might be scared because they do not have the skills, knowledge or tools to help themselves out of their exhausting patterns. Admitting exhaustion, and with it finding themselves helpless, might exhaust them even more.

I have had clients whose energies felt atrocious, all blocked up, low, quite aggressive and who, when telling them about vitamin D3, claimed happiness. I kind of believed them too. It felt as if part of their 'illness' was due to the fact that they actually could not feel the state of their energies and bodies. As opposed to above scenario, where the client might feel his exhaustion but live in denial. So there actually might be those people who genuinely believe and feel as if all is well, happy and healthy and then one day just drop dead with e.g. a massive heart attack.

Sometimes it's maddening the discrepancy between what I feel and what the client might tell me when probing a subject. At those times I have two very real and strong realities about the person, and they can be quite contradicting. There is no reason to actually go mad about this though. Again the healing energies will just work on fixing whatever is really true and needs fixing. I rather not insist on my version of what I am feeling and suspecting than insist and fully project it back to the client, just in case it is a delusion. And especially with negative intuitions, I rather not make up my mind until my intuitions are proven true beyond reasonable doubt (by that time they might have been completely cleared away anyway). If I am not fairly certain I don't even comment on good or peaceful energies. If someone were a tyrannical manager or family member I would not want them to start believing that their character flaws are sanctioned by the Divine and could not do with a little work on them on their part.

As long as I work with Ultimate Good help, the important thing is that they know what to do – where and when, during, before and after the healing, and I trust they do. It helped a lot that during my spiritual healer training I was reassured that healing energies are intelligent and will go where most needed, regardless of the healer being clued in or not. I have found this assumption in turn verified by clients quite regularly reporting that, during a Spiritual Healing session, they might feel warmth or pressure on a particular body part; when they then peek though, to see where the healer's hands are, they are on or above a totally different part of their body. I also assume that Ultimate will know where outside LLE support resides and go there to clear them, as applicable.

Furthermore I trust that they protect my clients against any mis-intuitions or misinterpretations landing in my lap and potentially being strengthened by me thinking about them and having emotional responses to them. I would think that on this planet it is not uncommon to have encounters where the outside picture and one's internal responses/interpretations/intuitions do not match. It is good to act as a channel, for your life to slowly and steadily heal such discrepancies but, as long as they still happen, there is no use getting upset about them either. Such discrepancies might be felt more in a healing environment. For example an untruth might be felt more intensely during a healing session. I feel that most of my clients are not attempting to deceive or disrespect me though. It can happen that clients lie to me, but then they might have their reasons for doing so – and nowhere does it say that they owe me truthfulness as their masseur or healer.

Most clients won't have much control of their energies, so they are not directly at fault for having LLEs in their bodies. Even with potential psychopathic liars, they are coming for a healing massage, so some part inside them appears to be seeking help. Their LLEs might be strong and uncomfortable to work with, but as long as I do not feel my physical safety is in jeopardy, any spiritual, mental or emotional hits my bodies may receive are usually healed again.

I have noticed too that just because I am more energy sensitive does not totally protect me against people screwing me over. Sometimes I get a warning feeling in a situation, but at other times I do not. Last year a cabbie in Rome defrauded me by switching notes on me when I paid him. I ended up paying him twice of what I owed him, and the meter showed too much in the first place. I only realized what had happened three hours later. Had I had more of an intuitive warning, I might have been more attentive during the payment process. Or last year I had a client who defrauded me on payment. I went to his house, massaged him and then he said he had no cash in the house, but offered to pay via bank transfer. I agreed, but six months on there was still no money. I had just massaged him for two hours, including healing work. His energies were not the best, but I got no intuition that he might be out to defraud me. Both cases were obviously just monetary losses, but I feel that some LLEs might just be protected well, so well that only hours or days of healing will actually reveal the true state of affairs. I recently found out too that the above client has now gone to drugging, raping and not paying escorts, so I was actually quite lucky (or well protected) that my damage was just monetary.

I think Peter was similar. His disciples were 'protected' from feeling that there was something wrong. One cannot simply point fingers and say that a person was just too stupid to see what was happening or that they must have known or felt something was wrong and chose to ignore their intuition. Then there is the complete opposite: people following their intuition too much. I spoke to a fellow masseur the other day. He said that his client 'block' list was about 800 strong. He said he blocks everyone that books and then does not show. I understand that and mostly do the same. He also blocks anyone where he does not feel 100% okay with the client's energies or behavior. Not sure if I would still be working and able to support myself with my massage work if I too blocked everyone where I felt uncertain of their energies, or they might be uncomfortable to work with.

If Lightworkers were to avoid all 'uncomfortable' situations, there would be far less healing taking place on this planet. If I feel discouraged, listless or annoyed by a client's energies attacking me, I tell myself, "What I can help heal today will help make my future more effortless and happier sooner!" Not to mention that letting myself be bullied by LLEs into staying away and avoiding situations or encounters will possibly only make me more isolated and restrict me in my life choices.

As for End of World/Apocalyptic intuitions and predictions – I was sold on them when I was with Peter, but with time I found that most of his fear mongering was just that – fear mongering. Once I understood that suffering is pre-chosen, there is no real need for divine 'punishment' like a worldwide Sodom and Gomorrah. Sure Ultimate Good might intervene if enough beings pray for help, but I doubt that would be in such a way that they destroy our entire infrastructure and send us back to sticks and stones! Plus if LLEs caused the apocalypse, they'd lose all their 'hosts' at once.

Psychic abilities and intuitions can be empowering. I still dream that one day I will be able to diagnose my clients' ills 100% correctly and help to heal their suffering as quickly and effortlessly as possible. But being psychic can feed the ego in a way that it makes you feel as if you are more important/special than others. It can be a fine line between being happy about a healing-channel job well done and getting smug about it. It is important to learn to distinguish which intuitions are of use to the client and which aren't. If a person is not ready or strong enough to confront some reality, pressing it upon them can do more harm than be healing. Some believe that everything should be shared with their clients. I'd say, the truth shall set you free, but only if the time is right and people have the tools they need to deal with their troubles and the strength to do so.

I don't want to insinuate that all psychics are evil or bad at what they do; I obviously have not met all of them yet either. From the ones I have met, I am not convinced that they all (even if well meaning) fully vetted their spiritual sources. Perhaps some psychics are tempted to just trust their guides because they sound enlightened and feel powerful, but in the end could these sources have ulterior, unholy motives? Perhaps some people still enjoy the sense of power that comes with psychic abilities too much, even if they cannot be certain that their intuitions are accurate? It is not just some psychics who might be careless, but other spiritual people too. For the time being, I feel, we still have to be very careful (and ask Ultimate Good for constant protections, cleansings and healings), else we might fall for entities or ideas that in the long run will cost us.

Chapter 18

Relationships: Good, Bad and Spiritual

Up till the age of 25 I was a 'Hollywood devotee' with regard to relationships – a good chick flick can stir some powerful emotions. I was convinced that finding 'the one' was a most pressing endeavor in my life – if not the most pressing. It seemed essential to finding true happiness. I could not become 'whole', unless I found my other 'half'. I was a hopeless romantic, believing if I managed to find 'the one' I'd be with him till death do us part – monogamous and faithful. Since I started on my spiritual journey quite a few of my relationship dogmas have changed. The main factor in the 'eternal love and romance' ideal was the introduction of actual eternity. I am not so sure that I would not get bored with the same spouse for all eternity… And if we add reincarnation into the equation, what happens if in my next incarnation my eternal lover is unreachable – incarnated as my mother, father, sibling, the wrong sex or got mistakenly married to someone else already?

Not to doubt the awesomeness of the Divine, but I did used to get worried too that if I needed to find the one amongst billions of humans – was that achievable? What if I did not listen to my intuition that one time that Ultimate Good set us up to meet again, and I went to the wrong bar that night? Surely Ultimate Good would try again, maybe the supermarket. But what if I did not listen to my intuition again and went to the wrong super-market too? What if I had met the one already and let him go because I did not recognize him? 'The One' theory does come with a big bag of potential headaches and potential pitfalls.

So I was on the lookout. I managed to 'pull', but somehow the perfect relationship never developed. There were a number that lasted a few months, but most only lasted a couple of weeks. I fell in love many times, but for the initial few years usually the subject of my infatuation would quickly fall out of love again. After a few years I started to experience the same, i.e. I'd have a stormy first week of a relationship and then suddenly my feelings would cool down. My unhappy, unfulfilled relationship status was one of the main reasons why I was so fascinated by the newly discovered spiritual concepts. Could it really be that I could master my destiny? If I called out (spiritually) to my perfect mate perhaps that would attract him sooner?

With all the guilt and saving the world pressure at Peter's, I was pretty much celibate during my years in the cult. With all the work we had to do, to save the planet, it felt too selfish to worry about meeting guys and having sex. And as mentioned before, there were the fears too that celibacy might be necessary to reach enlightenment, at least to speed up the process. I couldn't really go to a disco anymore; I was feeling far too guilty about all the electricity used there. There were parks where gay guys cruised and had sex at night. Before embarking on the spiritual path – places like that were out of the question, surely no true love could come out of such places of promiscuity? These cruising grounds had their benefits though; you didn't have to talk before engaging in sex. Small talk was very optional! The giving and receiving of pleasure was usually mutual and theoretically no one got hurt because of it. (If the other guy had a partner at home they were cheating on – that was out of my control.)

I also discovered that there were many beautiful men out there. It was fun to discover new bodies. At times I was attacked by feelings of guilt or emptiness after some encounters, but I was less certain that they were a natural response; they felt more like confused emotions. I could see that most of these encounters had no lasting substance, but it was still two humans coming together to give each other pleasure and maybe even some happiness – why should that be wrong? I started to compare sex to eating.

Obviously you won't starve without sex, but then again it has health benefits. It is great to have a lovely three-course meal, but that won't always be possible; sometimes you have less time and will grab fast food. The same applies to sex: some encounters are like a gourmet dinner, others are more like fast food – tying you over, till you can get another really nice meal. Over time my philosophical concepts/discoveries developed further and aided my notion that free sex was perhaps more creational too – than society had tried to make me believe until now.

At some point, way back, I believe we were 'one'. In this state of oneness, we were so close to each other – there was no separation. We were flowing through and around each other. At some point we decided to try something different. We went through the 'Big Bang' and were free to try many a different, separate body – in our quest to experience and create! I believe too that one day we will come back to a true state of oneness. We will be as one, flowing through and around each other, but we will be enriched through the individual experiences we had. We will also be in an eternal state of ecstasy, love and happiness.

I have no proof that I am right. But since believing such, monogamy has become even less logical to me. Eternally being bonded to just one other being? When we are 'one' again, flowing through and around each other, there cannot be any separation. Couples holding hands and screaming, "Don't touch us, we are promised to each other only, eternally!" would be nonsensical. In Oneness isn't everyone, everything connected in true, unconditional love? One of the closest things to this state of Oneness, I can think of on this planet, would be an orgy. Truly sexual encounters (especially with an additional closeness of spirit) are some of the closest encounters we can have on this planet.

Believing the above (and that my right soul-half is male and the left female) has also started to make me see that in my heart of hearts my true divine being is, if anything, bisexual! I still haven't had intimate relations with a woman, but I am not categorically excluding it for the future. Please! I advise to have sex where attractions lead though; forcing anything usually is not conducive to happiness. And happiness and love is what it is about. I do not believe in having to heal homosexuality, same as I would not ask a purely heterosexual human to go to therapy to become bisexual! In the past I have had fleeting pangs of guilt that I might not assist in enabling more human incarnations, i.e. have kids, but when thinking them through I always found them to have no merit. Besides having had a very hard time to financially and health wise look after a family (until just recently), if anything this planet is getting too crowded. To tell the gay 5% of the population that they should lead 'normal' lives and procreate too is almost ironic. Even if they do try to e.g. adopt and raise children, that usually is no good for conventionalists either. I have heard plenty of people argue wisely against homophobia and the usually unfounded arguments of the homophobes though, so I do not feel I need to add more to this topic here.

I do not intend to deny any couples the happiness they might have found with each other. I do admit that just finding (more) true happiness and love with one person, on this planet, can be quite a feat. Still, I am, in my heart, promiscuous today. I think it is likely that I might just have this one human incarnation and then I will take other forms. Since sex is one of the most pleasurable experiences I can have with this body, I hope I will not have to restrict my freedoms in this regard. To me beautiful bodies are more like pieces of great art (and beauty is in the eye of the beholder)! And shouldn't great art be shared, for all to see, in a museum or such – rather than being locked away in some collector's vault, only for them to see?

I know that some people might interpret my writings as the scribbling of a sex addict. That is fine by me. Not that I have to justify myself – but these days, even with the job I do as a tantric masseur, I rarely have sex. Like any other human encounter, usually there is some resistance when I engage sexually with someone. How much usually seems to depend on how much lighter I am than my counterpart. I rather stay at home and watch TV though, than have a quick, flat sexual encounter and potentially have to meditate for hours after to cleanse and heal my energies. If I were to even consider a longer term relationship today – I would need to be physically attracted to such a guy, but even more importantly he would probably have to have some spiritual substance too, meditate etc. There are not too many of those around yet. I have found several times that if I try to get closer to a skeptic or even atheist it is virtually impossible, as it seems to trigger the worst resistances.

During my chronic fatigue years I was less choosey. But then I felt so unwell and unhappy most of the time, I thought sex might give me a bit of happiness and joie de vivre. Today I am much more content and happy, and with it more patient. I haven't given up on the dream of plenty of good sex (or even great relationships) yet, but I can wait for it. What helps me the most here too is that since learning that I am individualized divine spirit, I have come to understand and feel, more and more, that I am 'whole' – I do not need a second half to be happy!

Monogamy might be the ultimate prize to many, but in all relationships past (especially since becoming spiritual) it always felt like a cage to me. Some cages were more comfortable and valuable than others, but they were still cages. In my worldview jealousy just isn't a part of (divine) love anymore. I feel jealousy is more a fear of loss and potentially worse an endeavor to own another person. I would wish my 'mate' to be a best friend first and foremost; if the sex is great – even better. I have found too that often people develop at very different speeds and in different directions. If my mate would find that spending more time with another person gives him more happiness, than being with me, it might sting a bit, but I would rather have him be happy somewhere else than less happy or unhappy with me. We would have grown in different directions or at different speeds; he would have outgrown me or I him. I feel life is too precious and short to spend it with upsets and regrets.

It is obviously easier to think and feel that way, not constantly fearing that someone might have been the only person one could have truly been happy with! Discovering that all humans are individualized divine beings, they are all potentially extra special and utterly lovable (even if many hide that side of them well). If what we truly are is 'all love' and 'as one', we love everybody and everything more than the perfect movie romance can even come close to. Again though – I am not propagating that everyone has to sleep with everyone; it definitely should be a thing of mutual, respective attraction and willingness!

I might have spoiled things for myself with a few potential suitors in the past by coming out early on about my 'open relationship' ideal. If we take the cage visualization above and one of these guys would have been truly stunning, I might have agreed to remain in a cage with him. Still I would prefer my cage door open – and funnily enough I can imagine that with an open cage door I would probably think about the other birds outside even less. It is funny how, at times, whatever isn't allowed just becomes so much more appealing.

Obviously I would allow the same freedoms to my mate. I would find it exciting and arousing. I'd see it more as a confirmation that I have chosen a sexy, attractive partner rather than risk the threat of a breakup if he strayed. But then these days I love myself unconditionally. Fifteen years ago when I asked myself if I would go out with myself, the answer was, 'probably not'. Back then if my partner would have had sex elsewhere, I would have been afraid I'd lose the one guy and his love for me. Today I love myself and am generally confident that Ultimate Good loves me – and what is one lover compared to 'all there is'?

Considering that I have asked Ultimate Good for 24/7

cleansing of negative or stale emotions or thoughts, I assume that if an emotion will make me suffer they'll take it away. If it won't make me suffer (but I might not like it) they won't; instead they'll take away whatever blocks my understanding of why it can make me happy. At times when going out I still see guys I fancy. If there is mutual interest, I am still not immune to emotions of infatuation stirring in my gut. Feelings of infatuation can be very convincing. They usually claim to be buds of 'true love', claiming him to be 'a one' at least, even if I know nothing about the guy. Any promise of a great amount of happiness should not be straight out disregarded on this planet; they don't happen every day. For me infatuation usually comes with a whole lot of fears and insecurities attached too though – will he come over, talk to me, have sex with me, call me, meet me again and so on?

In recent years, every time I handed the fears and insecurities, attached to infatuation, over to Ultimate Good the whole infatuation would usually disappear altogether. Now either that is because he wasn't a decent match or most romantic love (especially monogamous) is just one big LLE illusion? An illusion that does give happiness to some – true! I am just not all sure, if one added up all feelings of happiness and unhappiness generated by the concept of love and monogamy, the bottom line would sum up to more happiness or more suffering? For the avoidance of doubt, please note that I am talking about romantic love here, not unconditional, divine love. Unconditional divine love will obviously respect, but will not have any conditions attached to it.

There are obviously merits to couples sticking together – especially when looking after and raising children. I do not mean to sow evil thoughts of doubt amongst happy couples, nor would I advise that every couple in a crisis should just take the quick and easy route out and split up – there are many factors to consider. Every situation or circumstance where people come and potentially live together in happiness is a step towards what we really are – individualized divine beings and 'All Love'. I do admit to the possibility that just because I haven't found the right one, I may be rationalizing this chapter (or at least some of it).

Perhaps some people are freer in their capacity to love? I think I am. Who knows? Maybe if that boy or girl cheats, they are actually living more of their divine intrinsic desire to spread their as-One love? The problem is that society keeps telling us that only one-on-one, monogamous relationships are true. So even just thinking about open relationships opens doors to guilt and fears of being unholy or abnormal. I find the thought that we are capable of loving more than one individual (including sexual relations) comforting though. If a boyfriend of mine should stray, even if he should really enjoy and love having sex with that other guy or girl – I do not automatically have to start fearing that this means the definite end to our relationship! He has the capacity to love more than one person… So if a partner errs and is unfaithful, perhaps it is not the end of the world – like portrayed in so many movies?

This scenario is a very fitting one to describe emotions with – false memories. Whenever I felt 'betrayed' by a partner's behavior, pretty much 'everything' he ever did before – which previously was cute, adorable and romantic – suddenly just turned into a big ploy to make me hopelessly dependent on his company and then crush me like a bug! Feelings of jealousy, fears of deceit or betrayal, I have found, rarely came with cool minded, honest objectiveness. I can easily forgive myself today. Even without the knowledge that such emotions are sometimes near impossible to resist LLE illusions, I can see that, back in the day, my main hope for happiness was finding my second half. Crushing that dream was potentially a condemnation to life without any true happiness. Damn I was confused and insecure.

I am not saying that even in what I today would consider a more spiritually mature and free relationship there are guarantees that there will never be feelings of jealousy, or fears of loss or separation. I know from personal experience that jealousy energies can be very strong and uncomfortable, but so can the feelings of being locked into a relationship where one constantly gives more than one's counterpart, or is elsewise manipulated into agreeing to more compromises than feel fair and bearable.

I have several clients where I suspect they are coming for a tantric massage without their partners knowing. Initially I was not sure in how far I might enable (potential) suffering in their relationships. I decided though that it is not for me to judge. And if they come for an erotic massage with me, at least it is in conjunction with Ultimate Good healing. With healing work included, undesirable constellations and situations have a greater chance of finding harmonious solutions than if they saw a masseur who does not also work as a healer. I had a client, the sweetest, elderly gentleman, who told me after his massage that he had the first orgasm in thirty years that he did not reach through his own efforts. Supposedly he has been with his partner for 39 years, he still lovingly is, but they stopped having sex after about nine years into their relationship. I really cannot begrudge him going for an erotic massage after such a long time. And who knows if his partner is still faithful? I would recommend striving for as much honesty as possible, in any kind of relationship. It has taken me years to really find out what I am and what I want from life – i.e. being honest about my desires and dreams at 25 would have looked very different to being honest about them today. But then most straight, child-bearing relationships start in their twenties… I guess the best recipe is to try to keep loving and respecting one's partner. If one finds, over the course of time (no haste necessary), that certain promises one might have made to each other have become untenable, one can only forgive oneself for one's lack of insight when making such promise, and communicate with one's partner. I obviously understand that partners might have made promises to each other, such as promises of monogamy. It can be painful if one partner might even think or suggest at a later point that they might want to go back on such a promise. I feel that is why the Bible says, *'swear not, neither by the heaven, nor by the earth, nor by any other oath'*, i.e. we should not make promises which we cannot foresee we can keep (and our human perspective is usually quite limited). It is an easy mistake to make though, especially in conjunction with feelings of strong infatuation etc. But once we have had the experience that feelings of romantic love can be fickle and that we might overreach making eternal promises, we can still forgive ourselves and pray that our partners do the same.

If communication is not possible straight away, I would pray or meditate until communication becomes possible. Last but not least – I would try to never forget that, even if I feel manipulated or otherwise hurt or unfairly treated in a relationship, I have chosen that experience before I incarnated. I would do my best to not forget that even though some relationships seem hopeless entanglements of problems, resentments and so forth – there is nothing that cannot be healed. I'd forgive myself for these choices and pray and meditate until the suffering is resolved, be that with or without that partner. And I hope it is needless to say that obviously one is allowed to leave abusive relationships ASAP. If one feels the relationship does still deserve some attention and healing, it can just as well be performed from a safe distance!

Chapter 19

The Esoteric Market Laid Bare

I believe most esoteric followers: New Agers, spiritualists, religious people are simply seeking an understanding of life – trying to find out what we are, where we have come from, why we are here, and where we will go. Though there are plenty of books and other forms of information out there, such wealth of resources can be not only a blessing (if one does not agree with a belief system, one can find alternatives), but also confusing, as many books claim they (alone) have the answers, but they contradict each other too (at least in parts). Whereas I found some teachings made no sense at all, others had some merit, but seem to omit critical parts, which can leave a student confused, at best, or coming to destructive conclusions themselves, at worst.

I believe most spiritual seekers are looking for answers to Life! Answers that will help better themselves and give their lives more meaning. Since spiritual teachings are usually founded on personal experiences, this often leaves plenty of room for skeptics (be it the skeptic inside of us or on the outside) to argue the placebo or self-delusion case. I do have some sympathy for skeptics; I think it is healthy to keep our rational thinking intact. I am the last to recommend blind belief, be it spiritual or scientific. Honest critical thinking has advanced humanity. Most skeptics are not out to harm humanity with their statements; most seem to believe that by claiming that there is no proof of a Higher Intelligence they protect themselves and others against harmful delusions.

A lot of atrocities have been committed in the name of spirituality and religion. I too had problems in understanding how an All-loving God could allow so much suffering – until I understood that it is pre-chosen. Yet as objective as most skeptics claim to be, they often project nothing more than their materialistic scientific beliefs onto everyone else. For some it is easy to disregard thousands of years of spiritual or religious human experience as nothing more than superstition. Most modern science, as convincing as it appears, is but a hundred, two hundred years old, and who knows what humans in another thousand years are going to think about our contemporary scientific understandings.

It seems to be about finding a healthy dose of skepticism in this life, but it must be personally decided. Avoid becoming so skeptical that it closes off your mind, but still keep grounded. In the end often both factions accuse each other of being ignorant and/or deluded. I guess until humanity comes up with a machine that skeptics can accept as a viable method of measuring chi, prana, healing energy (in the greater scientific accepted context) and where they can see a dial moving, it is a dilemma we might be stuck with for a while longer. Though it can have incredible extension – I saw this medical professor on TV assessing alternative healing therapies and, even after having witnessed open heart surgery in China using acupuncture alone (for anesthesia), she still figured it might 'just' be a placebo effect.

With some people the assumption of a greater intelligence/power seems to engage the emergency brakes. The thought alone brings up so much aversion or fear that any further attempts to develop the required technology is ceased, or viable existing research is disregarded. There might be no technology yet which allows humanity to measure Ultimate Good powers, but that does not mean that there won't be in the future! Before humanity could see bacteria through a microscope – bacteria still existed. Supposedly mold was used for centuries prior to treat infections (where mold produces antibiotics, such as penicillin). These mold treatments worked, because the mold could produce antibacterial substances. Humans followed their observations. They could not measure or understand why it worked, until the invention of the microscope, but they had found something that made them feel better when they had infections, and they just went with it.

Spiritual people might be accused of wasting their time with prayer, meditation and so on. Worse they might 'infect' others with their delusions and waste their time and money too. Not to mention gurus and/or charlatans, who might not only waste their followers' time and money, but physically, emotionally, mentally or spiritually harm people. Yet there are 'skeptics' who invest endless hours and huge sums of money to investigate stars millions of light years away – are they not chasing dreams? There is no technology that could actually get us there yet. They are chasing after cosmic bodies they'll never reach and experience. They are happy to spend all this time, energy and money trying to understand where we come from (at least the atoms that make up our bodies), how the Cosmos was created, and where it is going. And considering how short and fragile our human lives are one could justifiably ask, "Why?" Is humanity that much more fulfilled in finding those answers, although they do not have any immediate effect on our existence and experience, to justify spending billions on such research? The answers don't feed hungry mouths, put kids through school or cure any disease – not for centuries to come and potentially ever.

Though I believe that spiritual people are often ostracized by the broader scientific establishment, this book is about esoteric/spiritual beliefs and since the aforementioned was mainly a 'heads-up' for esoteric people vs. non-believers, I'd like to swing back to observations I have made during my spiritual ventures, where some metaphysical beliefs and teachings could do with a bit of revision! I find no great pleasure in 'slagging off' fellow believers. But there is some comfort in the hope that the spiritual field may improve if more Lightworkers read this and some self-regulations and more (open) critical thinking come out of it. I do have to say that reading some books or hearing lectures by (often renowned) esoteric writers, I feel ashamed of my profession, and I worry how humanity is supposed to find the Light with such confusion. At other times, like talking to fellow healers and seeing their dedicated services to provide spiritual healing to the public (often for free!), my pride as a healer is restored. So let's hope that, as time goes on, there is less shame and more pride!

I am wary of books that base their theories or wisdoms on 'mystical' long extinct civilizations like e.g. Atlantis or Lemuria. Perhaps Atlantis and Lemuria did exist, but without anything archeologically or geographically 'concrete' yet people can pretty much claim anything they like. Usually both nations are described as spiritually highly advanced, which supposedly led to their downfall too. Why did the spiritually advanced nations perish and the 'confused' more 'primitive' ones persist? Perhaps it was just time for another era or maybe something more underhand came into the mix? Do Lightworkers believe that if humanity managed to evolve so highly before we can manage it again? I had to laugh though when esoteric writer Diana Cooper claimed online that the 2011 earthquakes in New Zealand and Japan were due the ancient continent of Lemuria starting to rise up in the Pacific Ocean. It did sound as if that was supposed to be a good thing – maybe we'd find ancient lost wisdom as a result. Have these people not thought this through? If a continent would rise up in any ocean, it would mean major coastal flooding. Furthermore we'd end up with a giant rather uninhabitable salty piece of rock (for a few decades at least).

Then there is the myth of the Lemurian Seed Crystals – laser shaped quartz crystals with line etchings on the side. Apparently, before Lemuria vanished, Lemurians travelled the world and etched their wisdom into these crystals for posterity. In my opinion a fun, romantic piece of esoteric folklore (good to increase the price of such crystals), but that's all. We are talking about normal quartz growth with the lines on the sides being similar to tree age rings, rather than artificial etching... Not to mention many of these crystals were found buried deep underground or within mountains – how would Lemurians have accessed them in the first place?

Even where archeological findings exist, like Egypt, a lot of spiritual abilities attributed to such people are still hard to prove. A lot of detailed, concrete knowledge has been lost over two thousand plus years! We might be able to say there were pharaohs, because we have found their tombs. We might be able to say that pharaohs were given divine status, because of hieroglyphs found, but whether that made them telepathic or telekinetic who knows? If in a thousand years an archeologist finds a lost copy of a Harry Potter book, perhaps they will believe that there were true magicians and witches in our time?

In 2007, at an unicorn lecture, a renowned esoteric author and speaker, let's call her 'Davina', proclaimed that the 'new' chakra system is pastel colored (I quite like the rich rainbow colors which are usually taught), and portrayed human sex as something rather animalistic, primitive and somewhat repulsive (such was her tone of voice). I saw Davina again in 2012, unveiling 'new' chakras just five years on, and the colors were different again! We did a group meditation, where we met our guardian unicorns and were taken up to the '5th dimension'. I seemed to experience that alright, but felt I went to some 11th dimension instead. I went up to Davina in the break to ask: was it possible to go to an 11th dimension? She was all smiles with all the other people in front of me, queuing to ask questions, but was short and flustered when I asked. And rather rudely and abruptly replied, "Yes that is possible, there are twelve dimensions." With that she turned around and walked off. I felt like scum. Was she jealous because she had only been to the 5th dimension? To be honest, I am not fazed by all that 'dimension' talk. My goal is to make my existence here on Earth as happy and joyful as possible – the heavens can wait.

Generally I reject any theory which even hints at hierarchies in the heavens, telling me that an angel has less worth than an archangel for example. If there are different dimensions, then I see it more as different skill sets, rather than stages of evolution, and I am certain that 5th dimension beings do not look down on e.g. 4th dimension beings. I see this as one of the main spiritual evolutions from polytheism to monotheism in our Western and Middle Eastern cultures. It is bad enough to suffer on Earth and have to pray for help – it would drive me potty if I had to constantly worry which deity to pray too. If the gods cannot manage to live in peace, how can one expect them to be able to help with human problems, help with peace, forgiveness, healing and so on. Also if Ultimate Good beings did not have a grip on themselves – my prayers and/or healing work might harm others; I would not want to end up channeling a god's angry energies! I still believe that there are countless beings we actually pray to and which help. The shift to 'One God' was more to help us understand that the heavens are 'as One' and in peace.

Whereas some lecturers seem too serious – perhaps believing themselves to be instrumental to the saving of humankind has stressed them out a bit – others I found too jovial. In 2008 I attended an esoteric lecture by someone with several books to her name. She started talking about 2012 – the world would then not end per se, just as we know it. Her face beaming she went on to declare that only 15% of the world's population is safe, another 20% have a fair chance and the rest are certain to perish. To my horror people around me smiled understandingly and seemed almost as ecstatic about the prospect of 65% of the world population perishing in 2012. That would be about 4.5 billion people. Not really sure what would be funny about that? She went on to say that we should learn to make choices and not stay in situations where we (as Lightworkers) did not feel comfortable. I took her word for it, got up and walked out!

Just recently I ordered a book about Hara energy – Dan-Tien:

Your Secret Energy Center. I had just discovered this energetic part of myself and wanted to see what others felt and understood about this energy. The author initially seemed clued up. Living in the Hara, kind of like living attuned to Ultimate Good energies, supposedly has improved his intuition and understanding. He does not get stuck in negative emotions anymore, but rather seeks to get 'back into the Hara' as soon as possible. What turned me off though, and eventually drove me to put down the book completely, was the author's insistence that in Far Eastern societies (especially Japan) kids are taught in schools to stay in their 'Dan Tien' (one of the main Hara energy centers). If the whole nation would have always resided in its Hara energies, being more connected to their divine essence and Ultimate Good, Japan's imperialist politics in the last century should not have happened though? I asked a Japanese client if it was true, that kids are already taught about the Dan Tien in school? He laughed and said that Japan is a highly secular society and that teachers would not dare mention anything so religious, parents would get them sacked straight away. My client had never much heard about the Dan Tien or Hara energies, his grandparents might have mentioned it once or twice, but that was it. A quick Internet search revealed, too, that supposedly religion is not taught in Japanese schools, as this would contravene with Japan's constitutional separation of state and religion. I am sure there are spiritual people and Lightworkers in Japan, but to portray Japan as a spiritual Shangri-La seems nonsensical.

Hara energy, when it is open and fully functioning and attuned, can be very powerful as well as comforting. Luckily I discovered and felt my Hara energy before I read the book, else I might have written off Hara work altogether, thinking that if the author is making things up (which are easily disproved) then what he says about Hara might all be pipe dreams too. Atlantis, Lemuria, Shangri-La – it makes me wonder if these authors are really connected to anything good or authentic, or are they just manipulative, sociopathic gurus like Peter, trying to confuse Lightworkers? Throwing them off the scent of things that really need healing? Suck their energies or confuse them so much that they get totally desperate and end up sectioned or suicidal? Or just out for a quick buck, without giving any thought to the possible consequences? If one believes that one is talking to the unadulterated Divine, it can be hard to object to what one hears. If I get questionable input, I ask for more information. If the input still does not make any sense, I disregard it. When I was in the middle of chronic fatigue and did not understand why I did not start to feel any better and contemplated that my Ultimate Good helpers were incompetent, I 'fired' (with the utmost respect) a few of them. (Well, I told Ultimate Good that if the apparent non-progressing healings were due to my current set of Spiritual Helpers and Healers to please replace them with a more competent bunch. Today I am sure they were actually competent – and that they have forgiven me.) I still do not verbalize or write down anything I might believe to have 'been told' which I cannot confidently stand behind. If I am uncertain of a claim, but it is the best answer I can give for the moment, I will say so.

Strangely some of the authors who claim the most outlandish things and/or create the most unrealistic expectations (along the lines of – just visualize that million bucks, smell it, feel it, imagine what you would buy and do with it – and the next lottery is as good as won!) sell books in the millions, hold worldwide seminars and so on. Take all those books on positive thinking, the Law of Attraction and cosmic ordering. These books claim that we humans are creators, i.e. our thoughts create and shape our existence, our bodies and our lives. If something in our lives is not the way we want it to be, we just need to change our thinking. Thoughts are supposed to function like spiritual magnets. If they are positive they attract positive events; if they are negative, they will attract negative things. To consciously consider that our thoughts influence our well-being seems self-evident to me these days, but I have to admit that for the first 25 years of my life I was totally ignorant of the concept myself too. Yet I have found that the Law of Attraction is but a facet of energetic influences shaping our lives, not the only one, like often claimed. To portray such life-shaping forces over simplistically though can lead to all sorts of confusions and even hurt. Of course positive thinking can make you feel better. Supportive, positive thoughts will feel better than destructive or negative thoughts, especially about ourselves. Even Western science agrees. Psychologists offer CBT (Cognitive Behavioral Therapy), where they help their clients to shift their thought patterns into more positive areas, and psychoneuroimmunology researches tell us now about the inter-action between the mind and the body. It is great when we first learn that we have a choice: to either simply just allow all thoughts, be they positive or negative, or to actively attempt to become the master of our own mind. Both the esoteric books I have read on the subject and probably most psychologists do not mention though that our thoughts, emotions and beliefs themselves are alive and (to varying degrees) self-aware beings. If our thoughts are alive though the question is, are we thinking our thoughts or are our thoughts making us aware of them? Perhaps both options are possible, where the latter will become more probable the more we think particular thoughts. For example if one thinks fearful thoughts and helps create ever stronger fear LLEs, these LLEs will want to live on and try to keep you thinking in the same way to sustain and feed themselves. Real food for thought!

There are different levels of negative thinking. If one is basically content and happy, but a little too critical of one's occasional failures, then to think more acceptingly, patiently and lovingly about oneself might be all that is needed for optimum contentedness, even happiness. But if one is stuck in the depth of a depression literally overwhelmed with negative thoughts and emotions, then changing a few thoughts will feel like a drop in the ocean. So I see 'positive thinking' as a mental/spiritual plaster that can vary in its effectiveness according to the 'wound' of negativity it is placed on. Alternatively staying positive might raise our energy and create an environment where weaker negativities just don't feel comfortable enough to stick around.

And what of the claims that our thoughts can manifest real events? Not like being positive and affable might make people stick around more, give us more friends, build more connections, which in turn might help on a professional level; I am talking indirect effects, like visualizing the perfect job and suddenly, the next day, you get a job offer from a totally unexpected source. Our thoughts and emotions are like radio waves, so if others are attuned they might pick them up and act upon them. Or would positive thoughts 'attract' Ultimate Good help? I am not so sure… I find Ultimate Good does respect free will and only helps if asked more directly. It might attract other more positive energies though.

The 'Law of Attraction' is portrayed as being quite binary. The Universe is painted as this huge computer program, where our good thoughts trigger good things and our bad thoughts bad things. As long as one is of a jolly disposition, half-intelligent and has reasonable capacities of concentration, the Law of Attraction is offered up as a cosmic money, success, love and happiness machine. You just have to switch it on. And if you don't then it's your own fault for being miserable, poor and so on. Perhaps 'just' positive thinking does work for some. Perhaps then these people just project their theories onto everyone else? Could they not be disregarding though that up to seven billion humans may keep creating negative stuff with their thoughts, which go where? Would people's creations not affect each other?

Funnily there is usually no mention of the Divine. Maybe the 'universal Law of Attraction' is supposed to be the Divine or replace it? The 'Law of Attraction' as this tool kit to live by without having to worry about the guilt and fear that can be associated with so many religions? I do not agree with many a rule or guilt propagated by the main religions, but I do love non-denominational Ultimate Good, and would not want to be without their help and the knowledge that they do help (if asked). During my chronic fatigue years, feeling miserable both physically and emotionally, I could use my mind to think positive thoughts, affirmations and prayers, but none of those would have enough short-term power to drag my emotional body out of dire straits. I very much hoped back then that the positive thinking books were wrong or incomplete by either denying or omitting the Divine. Today I think that the Law of Attraction is spirituality for beginners and those who reject higher, intelligent, divine powers, but want some spiritual tools nonetheless.

For those who still think that the Law of Attraction just does not work for me, because I allow for all those doubts – believe me, I have tried many a time! I'd set a goal (like perfect healing during my chronic fatigue), eliminate and disallow all doubts or fears to the contrary (including fears that a healing might take time!) and then concentrate on my healing goal, visualizing it as being real, now! The result would be a mix of being in healing mode and a 'whole body' squeeze to keep all the doubts and resistances, surfacing now, out. After a few hours or even days of this I'd be utterly exhausted and still not feel any better! If you want to sit down and change something (with a lot of resisting counterforce) by yourself and with positive thinking alone – you might be sitting there for a very long time!

As soon as one starts to allow for Ultimate Good help and prays to divine powers, the rules change. The Law of Attraction might still exist, but if we see it as the spiritual equivalent of gravity – praying for help will give you a set of wings and start to protect you and your life against any ill effects from the Law of Attraction. An intelligent being, like an angel, can distinguish between a true prayer for help and an LLE attack. The angel will not stop helping upon a prayer request because their charge has a bad day and doubts their existence or has other negative thoughts.

There is another side to the Law of Attraction, which I have not found a definitive answer to yet. As the Law of Attraction is not commonly taught in school, most people will not know about it. This in turn means that they will believe that their thoughts are just arguments they have inside their heads. They will definitely not believe that they create or attract anything in the outside world. Therefore would not all their thoughts be tagged with a *"Do not create in the outside"* label? Until one believes in the Law of Attraction, the creational value of one's thoughts (according to the Law of Attraction) should therefore be about zero. One could also argue that unpleasant and evil tyrants would just drop dead with so much animosity directed at them. Nor did our bodies fail when we had erroneous beliefs about their anatomy and physiology, in centuries past. Yet, I too admit that it often feels like I can sense my clients' emotions and beliefs. Is that because they have heard about the Law of Attraction or perhaps because there is some higher LLE intelligences/mechanisms involved?

If one lives in a country in the midst of a civil war, becoming more peaceful and starting to think more peaceful thoughts, forgiving one's enemies will do something, but as long as everyone else is filled with hate, their energy will keep going into the conflict too. I am not saying that the spiritual efforts of a single person (i.e. the person's work plus the countless number of Ultimate Good helpers potentially helping) might not be able to change the course of a war, but I would keep my expectations realistic as to the amount of time this might take! The positive thinking books I have read usually claim that the main (if not only) creational force in your life is you. So you might consciously or subconsciously start to take on responsibility (which can easily turn into guilt if things created are unfavorable) for things you have not created. I have been there and done that and it was no fun! I would not recommend it to anyone. If you manage to change your thinking, but things do not change, perhaps even get worse, you might fall victim to paranoia. I had paranoid fears such as: I might be 'crazy' without knowing it; I must have accumulated incredible amounts of negative karma in past lives; the Universe has forsaken me etc. And apparently being so laden with negativities, I feared I could become a real danger to myself or even others! The worst facet of the Law of Attraction, in my opinion, is obviously that one supposedly attracts more negatives if thinking or feeling negative thoughts or emotions. This is often somewhat appeased, as the books will tell you that the power of a positive thought is stronger than that of a negative thought. Still without telling their readers about benign intelligent higher powers with them and the option of asking/praying for protection (including protection for yourself against your own negative thoughts, beliefs and emotions), this can lead to quite substantial fears.

If you are clinically depressed or in chronic pain, as mentioned before, according to these self-help books you just have to imagine being happy and/or pain free and you'll attract more happiness and perfect health! To tell this to a depressed or chronically ill person though is grotesque! After a few years of chronic fatigue I could not even 'remember' what good health and happiness used to feel like! I am sure that most chronic, long-lasting ill people will have similar tales to tell. On top of having to fight their illnesses, having read about the Law of Attraction they'll now have to battle the fears that they will inadvertently attract more misery, as long as they feel ill!

What about genuine precognitions or intuitions? You might feel something is wrong with a situation and the situation then actually gets out of hand. If you follow the ABCs of the Law of Attraction, you would have to believe that having thought it before it happened, you are therefore responsible for creating it... I have experienced some healers advocate that if one even contemplates to look for any reasons to one's misfortunes or illness in the outside world, one is just avoiding responsibility and shifting blame! Ultimately, yes, I too believe that everything is pre-chosen, so one cannot really accuse life or the Divine of being treated unfairly, but that is not what these people seem to talk about. They say that everything we encounter has been thought up by ourselves (in this, or possibly a previous life). Following this train of thought, we might take on responsibility (and guilt) for things we did not affect directly in perpetuity.

Some positive thinking books recommend adding 'dates-of-fulfillment' to your dreams i.e. if you want a particular car you visualize it, cut out a picture and look at it every day. You imagine owning it, sitting in it, driving it. I do believe that doing so will help 'fill-out' that dream, but it depends on the amount of energy and/or resistance between oneself and the dream as to when the dream will become reality. A millionaire visualizing a Ferrari might realistically drive it sooner than a blue-collar worker (visualizing any car, especially a Ferrari). If the blue-collar worker gives himself a year to own a Ferrari, but after one year there is still little chance of owning one – what will he believe then? Will he blame himself for being incompetent or simply lose all faith in spiritual tools? Better to pray for Ultimate Good help, to achieve whatever you want to achieve, or visualize whatever you want to visualize, without a specific fruition date! You should then just get on with life as best as you can and leave the Universe to sort out the delivery venue.

Positive thinking books often teach the reader to use affirmations. Short concise messages to the self, affirming a quality for yourself – *I am confident and strong* – or something one wants – *I am successful and financially independent*. These affirmations are to be repeated, like a mantra, and are supposed to strengthen one's creative powers. The taught cardinal rule is that one has to use the present tense when affirming something. Using the future perfect will allegedly keep on creating that event in the continual future. However, if I would affirm, *"I am financially independent and rich"*, my rational mind would rightly so interject, *"But you are still in debt, you are lying to yourself."* I could use subliminal messaging techniques so that the affirmation would bypass my conscious mind, by e.g. subliminally being incorporated in a piece of music I listen to. Still I would deceive myself and I find it hard to lie to myself. (Well supposedly it is no lie, as I, by affirming abundance, would be affirming the divine abundance reality behind(!) the illusion of debt. Without reminding myself constantly about this greater truth, my rational mind still tends to interject though.)

When with Peter, and under more emotional pressure to perform perfectly, the financial independence desire took even more dangerous forms. I concluded that if I really believed, then I would still be allowing doubt if I watched my bank balance at all. And doubting the all-powerfulness of Creation was a sin. I spent beyond my means, trusting that creation would provide. It took me years to pay off. Therefore I believe that insisting on the present tense can be dangerous, besides being ridiculous, like a diabetic might affirm that she is perfectly healthy, stop taking her insulin and end up in A&E, or the morgue.

Even if one does not want to believe in more religious, divine powers, but 'just' in an all-providing Universe, which follows our thoughts to the letter, one could design affirmations which are not self-deceiving, but realistic e.g., *The Universe is working now and continuously on creating/unlocking financial independence for myself as soon as possible.* One will get the money one requires, for financial independence, as soon as it is available and accessible. Why would the Universe not understand that instruction? Or for a sick person: *My body is healing itself completely, as quickly as it can.* That clearly says that you are asking your body to start healing completely now and to do so in the quickest way possible. If one can believe in Ultimate Good powers and helpers

– it is even easier. One just has to ask, "Please help me to find financial independence as soon as possible," or "Please help my body heal completely as soon as possible."

Does anyone really believe that the Universe or divine helpers are so stupid to fail to understand such prayers? (I guess that is what affirmations really are, short concise prayers.) That they judge that if you did not say you wanted to be rich or healed completely right now, then you want to be rich or completely healed in the perpetual future? If something as relatively stupid as a human can understand that kind of instruction, why should divine powers not be able to? If they interpreted that as a request for something to be created in the perpetual future, they'd be sarcastic and cruel, not all-loving! Looking back now, I almost cannot believe that I ever fell for the 'You have to affirm in the present tense' scaremongering rule. Perhaps I was naïve, too trusting, desperate or not grounded enough. Writing this now, it all seems such common sense. It is almost embarrassing that I did fall for any fears associated with the topic. But then I am not the only one, and as with all spiritual topics, one cannot call a telephone number or research the answer on the Internet – reliably. One is reliant on one's own evaluation and judgment, and sometimes that is different to what others believe. I also believe there might be a possible (potentially dangerous) side to just thinking positive and more or less ignoring the negative. One example mentioned in a positive thinking book is a presidential election. Let's say there is a good candidate and a bad candidate running, and we want the good candidate to come into office. Supposedly if we keep fretting and bitching about the bad candidate, we actually feed the energies that want him to win, i.e. supposedly it is better not to think about the bad candidate at all and just think positively about the good candidate. I would both agree and disagree. Agree that thinking positively about the good candidate will strengthen them without feeding the bad candidate's LLEs, but disagree about simply just ignoring the bad candidate and their energies, as it does not necessarily dissipate these energies! If there is enough energy supporting the bad candidate they might still win! To just ignore a bad presidential candidate does not necessarily make them go away – one has to pray for the good candidate and ask Ultimate Good for all healing, cleansing, recharging and protection work necessary to banish and/or heal away the bad presidential threat and the associated energies! As a drastic example take Hitler's rise to power. Hitler's threat was ignored by the Allies in 1938 when he invaded Czechoslovakia. The rest of Europe was hoping all would be well if they just let Hitler have that one. Well, we all know how that shaped out – if anything Hitler was probably encouraged and saw the rest of Europe as weak and up for grabs.

The next step on the spiritual tools development ladder brings us to techniques such as EFT (Emotional Freedom Technique). It could be seen as more advanced than 'just' positive thinking, as it actually gets rid of negative emotions. For those who have never heard about EFT – as I understand it – one holds onto/brings up an emotion, which one does not want anymore, and then goes through a tapping process. One taps on certain acupressure points on the head, torso and arms and hands. By tapping on these acupressure points one supposedly activates the release of these uncomfortable energies/emotions. Some emotions are released swiftly; for others one has to go through the tapping procession several times.

EFT strives to release all negative emotions one engages. There are a few snags though. It is a cumbersome process. The tapping procedure can be quite extensive and not easy to memorize (and I am not too sure if the process works, if one might mess up the exact tapping sequence). It looks odd too. I would not do it in public or even in front of family or friends. To a non-initiated person it looks as if you are just randomly tapping the body. I tried it at home and I soon seemed to reach the limits of EFT. True, some emotions just vanish quickly and almost miraculously. Every (negative) emotion that 'pops up' needs a tapping sequence, and this quickly becomes monotonous. EFT takes more time than asking Ultimate Good to rid me of an emotion, which I can do in my head and in public. The only outside sign might be that I suddenly breathe a bit deeper and slower, as I breathe off an emotion.

When trying to release more complex and deeper rooted emotions, I went through the tapping sequence many times and still did not feel any improvement (but did feel very self-conscious). Last but not least, if one just releases these negative emotions, where do they go? One has just established that they must probably have some form of energetic body, how else could you release them; so if you dump your negative stuff, does it just float out the window and attach to the next passerby? I feel far more comfortable working with Ultimate Good help, as I am confident that they will always take away any negativity for safe recycling, rehabilitation and/or safekeeping.

Overall, for a spiritual novice it might be an enlightening and empowering experience to feel that you can actually rid yourself of negative emotions, actively and consciously. One is not dependent on time, which eventually heals all wounds (but can often take its time doing so). Advanced EFT followers supposedly realize that they can just visualize the tapping sequence and get the same benefits, but I still find it cumbersome.

I admit that using my handing-over tool, as taught by Peter, takes some time as well to verbalize, but, as said, these days I do not even say the words anymore, I just start releasing uncomfortable emotions and trust that Ultimate Good is there to take them off me. EFT might ultimately have the same potential, but I guess only if one adds higher powers into the mix here too.

Speaking of safe disposal of negative energies, at university I studied with a fellow medical student who also studied anthroposophy. One anthroposophical teaching, he told me about, did shock me and I still do not agree with it. They supposedly believe that there is always the same amount of positive and negative energy on our planet, i.e. if one effects something good – there will be negative consequences, because of this, somewhere else. If I heal a client, without Ultimate Good taking care of negative energies being released from the client – these negative energies might just wander off and inflict themselves on someone else. If I won a war and/or created peace in a conflict, without asking for the war creating energies to be removed by Ultimate Good – these warmongering energies could just move on and try to create conflict within or between other nations. He believed though that that is the rule! To believe that one's good deeds will have negative effects elsewhere sounds pretty debilitating! How could one justify helping anyone, even oneself, if that would just shift the problem elsewhere? The best thing one could do, under such a system, would be to take on as much suffering as possible, on oneself, in order to free others of it. I do not believe in masochism though or that Ultimate Good would want it for us. The worst case I can imagine would be that I remove a negative energy from myself or a client and that this energy gets taken away by Ultimate Good and 'recycled'. So if another being has pre-chosen to experience that suffering Ultimate Good might reuse that negative energy on them. Furthermore if one believed that good and bad are always equally strong one could possibly argue that both good and bad have always been and always will be. If we are a part of creation though then we would be both good and bad, and would never ever be able to rid ourselves of the evil part. So why even try? Not a philosophy I choose to believe in.

So on to the 'Here & Now' philosophy. As I understand it supposedly many a human does not live in the present, not in the place where their physical body is. Supposedly most are caught up in the endless chatter of their minds and instead of being where they are and when they are, they are floating about, thinking about other places, other things to do, events of the past or the future. As a result man squanders energy by not being fully present in his 'here and now'. Supposedly if man would be fully present, he would have more energy for what he is doing and more (if not all) of his divine potential and power. There seems to be this slightly romantic notion too that if one is fully present in the here and now one is in the presence of the Divine and should be much happier. Peter went as far as saying that being in the present means no need for planning, as all the answers and right things to do are always present. After learning all this, for a good while, every time I caught myself wandering off to thinking about past, future events or other places – I would feel very guilty. I wanted to be in the here and now and thought myself a failure if I wasn't. Today I am more relaxed. I have discovered that there can be good reasons why I think about past or future events. Usually when thinking about past events, I will look at them and analyze them. By looking at the past retrospectively, calmly and collectedly, with the added benefit of hindsight, I can learn from things I might have done well and things that I can attempt to do better next time. I do all this in the 'now', very consciously and actively, even though it is about the past. Furthermore after a particularly hard day or event, it is like a little holiday to look back at a nice memory or forward to an anticipated event. The joy generated in such manner relaxes and releases endorphins.

Of course one should avoid dwelling on past traumatic events, run in circles, just regurgitate them and get upset about them again and again. Being stuck in the past is not ideal. It's better to forgive oneself and anyone else involved, let go, and get on with one's life. (As quickly as possible. Some traumatic upset energies can be quite sticky.) Still when I heard about 'here and now' teachings, no one ever mentioned that there can be constructive ways to use the past. (I obviously did not read all the books; some authors might mention it!) Similar thinking applies to thoughts of the future. If I am going on holiday in a few weeks and have several errands to run beforehand, I am happy about every moment I get where I can think about the holiday. The more often I remember to buy sunscreen, the less likely it will be that I will actually forget on my next trip to the shops (even if not fully present then).

You could see it futile to worry about future events, they have not taken place yet and they might turn out to be less dramatic than anticipated, but I have found here too that thinking about the future can actually help! If I e.g. know I am going into a difficult situation or meeting a difficult person, I might, whenever I get a moment, picture that situation or dialogue. Often it feels like, in my head, I am really arguing with that person('s spirit) already. It has the benefit that with each mock argument I have with that person's spiritual self, I get better, sharper, quicker. My arguments become more thought out, I might realize where I have actually been at fault myself and/or might just resolve some of the conflicting energies beforehand. It is a bit like my own little, private debate class. As a kid I was always fascinated by people who could argue quickly, sharply and come up with twists and turns – outside the box – but to the point and logical. Obviously with age comes more experience, but I do believe that this anticipating of difficult situations and arguments has helped me a lot to develop similar skills.

Another example why one might want to use past experience and think about future events would be when e.g. drinking. It stands to reason that inebriated you are often happier than sober and with it more worry-free and in the 'here and now'. But based on these happy feelings alone you might be tempted to just keep drinking. If then remembering that blinding headache, depression and so on after the last big night out, thinking of such a likely future, you might be more cautious, enjoy your drinks a little slower, have a few soft drinks in between and feel better for it later. Not all happy here and now feelings are necessarily divine; they might be manic or carry the risk of wanton impulses and urges.

Being attuned to Ultimate Good as much as possible, I have little choice but to be relatively present most of the time. There is just too much energy coming through, keeping me awake and present to simply wander off (too far) with my thoughts. It is great to be attuned to Ultimate Good, and I am happy that I am, but it can be hard work! I am more aware of the confusions around me too. I am more aware of suffering I experience or which happens around me. The suffering does not always just vanish because I am present in the here and now and attuned. If healing is sent into these felt sufferings, they eventually vanish, which I experience more presently as well, and which can be a beautiful experience. Sometimes such resolve of negative energies takes seconds or minutes, but many a problem can take hours, days or more. It is still funny though to look at my past romantic notion that being strongly attuned and in the 'here and now' would be the solution to all ails, and where I would find instant bliss and happiness. There are, I am sure, places on Earth where the energies are 'cleaner' and more harmonious and where being in the here and now is going to be more blissful and quite effortless too. Maybe if I find some such places, I'll move there someday.

I guess what I am trying to say is that I think it is okay to wander into past or future; I just think that the intention behind this should be constructive i.e. feeding the growths of happiness not suffering. In my experience 'just' becoming aware of the present is not always going to solve one's problems. Some LLEs might leave because they get bored or annoyed that one does not fall for their traps anymore, by shifting one's attention away from them or ignoring them. When something really heavy attacks though – mindfully watching butterflies is not really going to dissolve much. In my experience one then needs outside (Ultimate Good) help etc.

Furthermore books and movies on the subject are often oversimplified, giving the impression that you are just a single thought away from 'being present'; but I find it can be a multitude of thoughts and emotions, all active at the same time, which try to draw me out of the present. I think my consciousness has improved over the years. On a good day I might notice more things than years ago; on a bad day I might be worse off than before I started on my spiritual tour. To actually fully experience every detail, every input which our senses could provide us with, at any given time, would result in total information overload.

Last but not least some here and now as well as healing and meditation teachers say that it is imperative to be in the here and now to develop spiritually, give healing etc. They say one has to e.g. be able to concentrate on an image perfectly for extended periods of time. Now I find it boring to just meditate on a single spiritual image and my mind would probably wander. I used to feel guilty if I could not stick to a mantra or drifted off during other spiritual work – I have found though that when push comes to shove, during any healing work, when my strong concentration might be necessary, I will get the energy (and motivation) to be very present. With the occasional client it takes me 1+ hours to get to a more focused state with my mind; I reckon though that I am actually getting their 'hard-time-to-concentrate energies' and that they are not my own. Usually as the massage progresses it gets better and the next client will be fine again etc. Furthermore once I am attuned and 'linked-into' the Ultimate Good energy flow, it does not seem too essential whether I stay with it or think about my grocery shopping list; the energy flows, with or without my input… And then there are obviously days when I am just off and all over the place. With some such confusing energies it just needs a little push to get back to reality, with others I have learned that fighting them takes too much energy; I will actually need all my energy to just stay half decently afloat. I try to not go under and pray that Ultimate Good takes care of the confusing energies – and they usually do!

Another bemusing aspect of the esoteric market is the ever-repeating invention of the wheel. I keep seeing advertisements for the latest, best, strongest healing energies, all 'newly' discovered. You could keep on going to seminars, where you will be taught the same thing over and over, just under different names. I always find it funny how descriptions of such seminars all sound the same too. Some 'better' healer has just discovered the holy grail of healing energies. Compared to 'conventional' healing energies his/her energies are so much stronger, purer and it's a bit like washing powder commercials that keep on promising even whiter laundry! If I enter 'attunements' on eBay right now (2013), there are over 500 results, including Ashta Lakshmi Reiki Attunement; Sacred Geometry Reiki Attunement; New Celtic Christians Reiki Attunement; Divine Light Reiki Attunement; Solar Light Reiki Attunement; Excalibur Reiki Attunement; The Herkimer Diamond Ray of Attunement; DNA Healing Reiki Attunement Course; Atlantic Light Temple Energy Reiki Attunement; Golden Ray Reiki Attunement; Full Spectrum Healing Reiki Attunement… all from as little as £1.50. It is a real supermarket of attunements. Maybe they help some people gain more confidence in their healing/channeling abilities…

Besides conventional Usui Reiki, I got Dragon Reiki and Aura Cleansing Reiki attunements. I did feel something when receiving them, but I cannot say that I felt that much more powerful and/or capable as a result. I did start to consider ultimate good, spiritual, healing dragons as potential helpers, after receiving my Dragon Reiki attunement, but just reading about them would have had the same effect. I do not advertise any other healing modalities other than Spiritual Healing and Reiki either. If I found a healer's Web site, who advertised a multitude of different Reiki attunements, I would question their focus or clarity. I dread to think what non-spiritual people would think seeing the same; might they judge such a healer as a total nutcase?

Perhaps people keep on going to seminars or getting more and more different healing energy attunements because some healings just take a long time to come into effect. Some might not have the patience, conscience or energy to 'ride out' their healing processes and go on looking for the next 'quick fix'. If someone promises stronger and more swiftly working energies, it is tempting to try them. I am fairly certain that there is also a natural evolution many Lightworkers go through themselves, allowing them to channel ever stronger and more capable energies. I cannot say that I never fall for such promises, but generally I have decided to stick with 'just' Ultimate Good. I am confident that Ultimate Good will always provide me with the suitable (strength) energies I need for all my healing needs.

Should humanity progress spiritually, perhaps stronger and stronger energies will become available to us – but I doubt that Ultimate Good would insist on me having to go to seminars to learn about them. Imagine having a client on your healing couch with some severe illness like cancer. Now you have worked with healing energies and practiced as a healer for years already and there is an energy upgrade available, which could really help the client, and which could sensibly be channeled by you and tolerated by the client. Which Ultimate Good helper is going to say, "Sorry you will need to go to that seminar on Grand Master New Age Healing. Sorry, Mr. Client, you will just have to die, the healer you chose is not attuned yet to Grand Master New Age Healing!"

Ultimately most of these seminars and attunements still put all the onus of guilt for illness on the sufferer and healer. If a healing does not happen, it is because the client has too much negative energy in their body and/or the healer is just not strong enough. If you find a strong enough healer, can you heal in an instant? Maybe I am a weak healer? In my experience I can channel energies that can pack quite a punch; I rather choose to believe that the greatest factor in someone's healing from a serious condition is the extent of its LLE backup and the amount of resistance that will be triggered by a healing. Some healing processes simply take their time!

I get cautious if healers impose what I call 'frivolous rules' on their followers or clients, like just wearing white, not eating red meat and no sex for at least one week before a treatment and 40 days after. I talked to someone who had been to a healer, asking such of his disciples. The only reason he could give me was that supposedly by not having sex for 40 days every time one is tempted during this time one is reminded of the healer and the healing and hence re-enforces it. I do not consider sex as unhealthy though (reasonable protection should obviously be adhered to); I rather think it is very healing if between consenting adults and performed to mutually please one another. It will usually create more happiness and happiness is great for healing processes.

I'd say that such 40-days-no-sex rules are so hard to adhere to that many probably do not. If they do not adhere to the rule though, if these clients do not heal completely, the healer can claim – that it is no wonder the healing did not work, as you broke my such and such rule. Besides the likely fact that non-adherent patients might get tormented by feelings of guilt; as they think they might have broken a divine instruction, they might start to believe that they just damned themselves to not heal properly. (Sure, there are zen-ists who might believe that ejaculating leads to loss of Chi, weakening the immune system, so 'no sex' might be a wise enough rule for them (male patients that is). It is a matter of opinion or personal physiology. I do not notice any loss of energy when I ejaculate. On the contrary, really good sex feels far more invigorating than draining. Supposedly men lose zinc when ejaculating and zinc is important for a healthy immune system; but here too, if you are worried you might not get enough zinc in your diet, why not just take a zinc supplement.)

Just because something works for a 'guru' does not mean it will work for everyone else. I had plenty of 'crazy' ideas in the past – but I do not propagate them if they seem to contradict basic creational concepts. For example I went through a phase where I followed an intuition saying that confirming my fears would dissolve them. During Peter's time he claimed that by looking at 'bad' decisions made in past lives, one was actively engaging with one's shortcomings and therefore Creation would forgive you for them. For example – I did not really like cold showers, so I might ask Spirit why and get the answer, "It is your fear of cold water, because you drowned in a past life!" If I then confirmed that fear by affirming it, "I am afraid of cold water, I am afraid of cold water, I am afraid of cold water," the fear/aversion would suddenly dissipate.

However, this goes against anything I believed then and believe today. I am aiming to 'overcome' all my fears and weaknesses, and rediscover/reestablish my divine all-loving, wise and fearless self. Any fear is a temporary illusion. By confirming it, I would confirm my illusory shadow-self and not my true divine eternal Light. I believe that by affirming my true divine, fearless self and committing all fears to healing light I will heal. Though some LLEs try to manipulate me into wandering down a path that does not make any sense, and which initially seems to offer me the quicker results, in the long run that path will likely be a dead end. And if I tell others about these paths, I might end up being ridiculed for them! (By the way, ironically, jumping into the cold sea, on holiday, has never been a problem for me – so all that 'cold shower aversion' and drowning theory does not really make any sense anyway!)

Other 'curiosities' I have encountered included one 'intuitive' healer who claimed to slap his clients. Supposedly just following his gut whether that lead him to lay-on-hands, pet or hit a client. Well, I doubt that slapping is the right thing to do; you would be lucky to escape an assault charge. I have had heartbroken clients, where I had visions of pulling out their heart (perhaps they just wanted to be rid of the apparent source of their pain), but I would obviously never follow that 'intuition'! I think that above 'intuitive' healer was picking up on self-punishment or self-mutilation energies of his clients, and following them through. Healers are supposed to personify the divine though, show their clients that divine love is unconditional and not about punishment, but about forgiveness and healing. Another healer claimed to communicate with souls inside her clients. One example was an overweight woman, who supposedly had the souls of a bunch of children inside her. They starved in a previous life and were therefore keeping their 'host' eating in this one! I cannot guarantee that this diagnosis was wrong, but think it unlikely. Another human soul would be too big or strong to fit in another person (without major personality disorders associated with it). The healer supposedly pulled tens if not hundreds of departed souls from her clients…

I personally love crystals; my house is full with them. I like crystals because I can hold them, touch them – and they last. I love all my Ultimate Good Helpers; I think I can feel them at times, but I cannot hold or touch them. Crystals, with their physical bodies, are comforting to me. I also feel there is something to them having been taken from the ground, polished or beautified and carried into the world. We bring them into the world to admire, love, and use them. I also love to read about crystals and what they can do for spiritual development and healing processes. It sounds like they are little pieces of magic solidified, and I do believe they are! But I have found that descriptions of crystals and their healing properties often sound too optimistic. Like, *this crystal will help you overcome shyness and make you feel confident and courageous.*

Many are called 'high vibration' crystals; labeled as extremely powerful and so on. In my experience these 'high vibration' crystals can be very nice, but work best if I feel good anyway. Most of these crystals are quite small too (well, the ones I can afford) so not much to grasp. If I am under heavier attack though I tend to grab one of my workhorse crystals: a nice chunky, relatively inexpensive Hematite or just a clear quartz wand or pebble. Holding such crystals while sleeping I do not have to worry about dropping them either – they are inexpensive and do not chip so easily!

With the amazing descriptions of their healing properties, I initially assumed that if I carry crystals with me or have them around me, they would help within days, maybe a week or two at the most, to achieve the advertised goals. Nowadays I think that weeks, months or years are more realistic. I feel an immediate strengthening, attuning and calmness if I hold some crystal when meditating. But trying to change character traits or rediscover psychic abilities (as promised by many crystal sellers) seems to take far longer. That does not devalue my crystals. They are like little solidified prayers to me and until the prayer has been fulfilled they can help/will help to channel whatever healing or protection frequency I need, even if it takes a lifetime. I think that it should also be mentioned that, to truly feel the effect of a crystal (and often that is mostly that they help me focus and to stay awake during meditation), I prefer to hold them in a hand, meditate with them. I am certain they help me too if I am not in meditation and focus on them specifically – but out of meditation and without holding them, their help is much less palpable to me.

I feel 'at home' in my house and more protected than elsewhere, and I am sure that all the crystals contribute to that. I could well imagine that the number of crystals a person needs might depend on how much healing resistance they encounter. Someone just working on themselves might require less support than someone who also heals others. I must have about 150kg of crystals lying about, plus I have huge etheric crystal structures on the house, in the walls and I still would not mind purchasing more, but I have run out of space to put them.

I have read about many ways to clean and attune crystals. Most commonly one is supposed to rinse them under cold water or bathe them in saltwater. When I started to buy crystals I still followed that advice. I soon reached my limits though. Besides realizing too late that some crystal did not do well with water – I ruined a selenite wand in saltwater – washing them all regularly soon became far too time-consuming. (You can also have crystals cleansed and recharged by sunshine or moonlight, but I have no proper windowsills or outside space.) So just as I have a standing order with Ultimate Good for regular healings, cleansings, protections and recharges for myself and my bodies, I pray for the same for all my crystals and other beings in my house.

Whenever I purchase a new crystal I talk to it, "Hi there! Thank you for coming to me. I hope you are going to be happy being in my life. You might have noticed already that I have a standing order with Ultimate Good for regular healings, cleansings, protections and recharges for all my crystals and all other helping and supporting beings – including yourself. So you do not have to get your own, but you are welcome to. I only work with Ultimate Good and hopefully so will you! There are loads of other crystals in my house, so hopefully you will have a great time. (Make new friends? Have a party?) I hope you can help me too – me, my bodies, my life – heal, cleanse, protect and recharge them. I have read that you are especially good for (mention specific gift), but am grateful for anything else beneficial you might be able to do. If you help, please only help in conjunction with, in, through Ultimate Good. If you do help, try to not overexert yourself. You do not have to help me, I cannot force you; but you are not allowed to harm me, nor my family, friends, clients, colleagues! Thank you, thank you, thank you. Amen!"

Whenever I have extra time or energy reserves, or feel it good to do so, I meditate, channel for my house and all beings in it. That is pretty much it though! And I do not feel my crystals are storing negative energies. I could be ignorant and lazy, to which I challenge that if one believes that a crystal needs human help to cleanse itself, to be washed or the like, does that not potentially belittle their self-awareness and competence? Who says that crystals in the earth do not pick up negative energies and do not have their own ways of cleaning themselves? They might be buried too deep to be washed by water, sun or moonlight; they might be further away from any water, sun or moonlight than in any human dwelling. They would be in the Earth, but in the end the Earth just consists of more stones and crystals… I think that any cleansing is fundamentally about crystal TLC. As long as a crystal can feel like it is appreciated, loved, respected, it will be more inclined to help and channel good energy.

Last but not least, I got one crystal healer to tell me a method she uses, which is more practical than washing or carrying all crystals outside. Supposedly crystals like thunderstorms, and as one can get thunderstorm soundtracks on CD, she just plays those to her crystals once in a while. I would add that gongs, singing bowls and bells are supposed to work as well, played live or on CD. As well as all other room cleansing methods, such as smudging and incense.

There is one last thing I would like to mention – Healer Associations. I have personal experience with 'The Healing Trust' and have knowledge of a few others, which seem level-headed, not too eccentric/outlandish; which is good, especially if trying to build bonds with the medical community. Internationally there still seem to be vast differences in how spiritual healing is approached though. Some spiritual healing organizations require psychic abilities of a healer to become a member. I.e. healers have to accurately spiritually diagnose a patient's ills (and sources of ill). I am glad The Healing Trust asks its members specifically not to diagnose their clients in that way nor to predetermine an exact treatment plan. For most ailments doctors could not do this with 100% accuracy rate either! Most healers' clients will come with ailments across the spectrum from 'just' stress to severe illnesses, and (again) a healer's diagnostic tools are often more subjective than laboratory blood work commissioned by a doctor for example. I can understand that patients, often paying privately for alternative and complementary therapies, would love to have an exact prognosis; how many sessions they will need to achieve a certain healing result. But it could be an unrealistic expectation at this time. This dilemma does not get any less tricky considering that a client might not feel anything much at all for the first few sessions with a healer, just standing there, holding a hand on or over their body and then 'cash in'. Luckily (in the UK at least) there are 'Healing Centers', where clients can just walk in, receive a healing and are only asked for a donation. You can always do your own meditations too, which should make you more sensitive with time and help discern if a healer is a decent channel or not.

I have only been working in this field for a few years. Perhaps in another five years (or ten) I will be an ace at diagnosing (spiritually) and predicting how many sessions it will take to cure a client of a certain ailment or achieve a certain healing goal. I do not expect that the strength of my healings (the amount of healing energies I can channel) will change too much though. And the ability to accurately diagnose does not mean that a healer's work/healing success will be better either.

Generally I always recommend asking for Ultimate Good (or whatever you call Divinity) protection and support when embarking on spiritual ventures however 'holy' the writer/facilitator/guru is supposed to be. Check facts and rules given by said 'teacher'. My golden rule is to ask myself whether something is likely to make me more free and happy in the long term (without harming others in the process) or not? Especially if considering eternity – if I had this body (or such) forever, would a rule make me happier, keep me happy, or be like a stone around my neck? I also ask how likely it is that divine, utterly loving, happy and wise beings might really care about a specific 'rule' or 'tradition' – does it really matter to them if I dress in e.g. a certain color or style? Or what time of day I meditate?

Chapter 20

The Healing Journey

Chronic Fatigue Syndrome (CFS) plagued me for over a decade up to 2010, taking hold first while I was still in Germany. I was tired all the time; my very bones were pleading for rest. I ached. I fantasized about sleeping for a week or a month – and would have preferred that to any luxury holiday. Even when I slept for over 12 hours, there was no real sense of relief. I would still wake up shattered and in pain. My sleep was restless; I dreamed more, i.e. my sleep seemed less of a rest and more of a nightmarish undertaking. On top of that I suffered from night sweats. I felt as if I had the flu six days a week, with my joints and muscles calling out for respite. I had frequent sore throats, recurrent earaches and I was prone to infections. It was hard to tell where a CFS ache stopped and a potential proper viral cold ache started. I am still not all sure if the accompanying depression was just a result of feeling bad constantly or if it was another symptom.

It was hard to stay positive and hopeful – especially regarding a complete healing of all my symptoms. And the longer the symptoms persisted, the harder it got to keep a positive outlook. Feeling like crap comes with all its own challenges. After realizing that all suffering is pre-chosen and handing over past, present and future suffering to Ultimate Good for deletion – I had expected plain sailing for the rest of my human life. I did not expect misery such as CFS to kick in. Had I loaded too much onto my plate? I had undertaken some big changes: moving countries and embarking on finding a whole new career path. There are other people though that move abroad and change careers, many with even fewer funds than me, maybe looking after a whole family, yet they don't get sick. Some of these people might not even have any beliefs in a Higher Power and 'go it alone'.

I was confident (well, in dark hours it was more just hopeful) that I had all the Ultimate Good Help one can imagine. I had read stories about angels miraculously arranging 'coincidences', how it should be no problem whatsoever to find a job, emergency funds and unless one was stuck in some engrained chronic illness already, before finding Ultimate Good's help and starting to pray (in which case it might take some time to completely heal), one could expect good solid health and all the energy and stamina to go about leading a happy and fulfilled life. Lacking that generally left three possible explanations: the ill must either come from the inside, outside or both! If the cause was inside me, than there would still be some energies inside my body which caused me to feel unwell and which kept on attracting difficulties into my life. That meant I still had some more cleansing and healing to do. How long could it take though to free myself from all negativities inside? My body was not that big! Was there anything I could do to support the healing process physically? Were they energetic (was I possessed) or was there physical damage, like that from a virus? Or there was the thought I might be schizophrenic, bipolar or psychotic. From what I had read schizophrenia often set in, in male patients, at around 25 years of age and is frequently triggered by some outside stressors. Well I had been in the cult around that age, which could have been seen as a triggering traumatic event.

As for the 'outside' theory, something or someone must have been attacking me. For years I had strong tendencies to think it was Peter, but there were other candidates to be considered. Was I cursed? I was continuously praying for perfect spiritual protection. How could these energies get through these protec-tions? Was I doing something wrong, causing the Divine to forsake me? In the 10+ years plenty of potential scenarios went through my head. At times I tended to sway more towards trying to find and heal the ill inside me, at other times I favored the theory of being attacked from the outside. Sometimes I tried to fight at both fronts at once. I had no absolute proof either way. I still don't, but for me now there are strong indications that most of my ills came from the outside.

I tried to remain as objective as possible, plus my efforts were always constrained by the amount of energy, time and funds available. Often I only had the strength to fight on one front. Even if it meant going and fighting through the same thought processes again and again. If I dwelled on the inside theory for long, a diagnosis of mental disease often seemed inevitable. Not a nice stigma to carry around, plus I feared if I gave into it and went for medical help, doctors would try to convince me that all the extrasensory sensations/experiences I had were pathological, even the positive ones. I knew some were, but I was not willing to denounce all Spirit.

If I dwelled on the 'outside' source ideas too long, I feared for those around me. If I was energetically attacked what would stop my family, friends or colleagues suffering the same? Most family members or friends I opened up to recommended I stop thinking about my troubles; that it was all in my head. I tried. But being in my body was like living in an old, badly insulated apartment, with a rock band for neighbors. Even if I found earplugs, every-thing would still vibrate – it was impossible not think about my ill health. I hoped that it would be sorted one day – whether I thought about it and added to the healing with meditation or not. But I found it nigh impossible to remain patient and do 'nothing'. If meditating would shorten my illness by just days, it was worth it – each would be one less day of hell. Even just finding some answers about 'why' and 'what was going on' might help alleviate some of the suffering.

Most of my energy was spent on getting to work, working and then whatever food shopping, cooking and laundry was necessary. I did consider that I might just have enormous drama-queen and self-pity programs running. I prayed to have them healed away or be infused with spiritual sedatives to subdue them. I meticulously monitored my emotions for indications of self-pity, so that I would not dwell on them but instead commit them to healing there and then. But I didn't really fit the drama-queen bill – on the contrary, fearing such traits I potentially sought less help than I could have received. Perhaps I should have set up camp in my GP's waiting room and refused to leave until something was organized, and I was more thoroughly investigated…

Most of the time, I felt rather isolated. At the time I was generally so blocked that it was near impossible to 'feel' any Ultimate Good help either. Whenever I did feel any healing going on, it just seemed to scratch the surface. I could feel some energies shifting outside the boundaries of my physical body, but not really inside, at the core of things. With all the ideas going through my head, I was never too sure if they might be just fake healings too. With time and in conjunction with my studies as a 'trained' healer, I made more healer friends and received more healings from others. But even when receiving spiritual healing, I often felt worse afterwards. Some of them knew about my suspicions that Peter, potentially with the power of his group to fuel him, was still attacking me. None of them refused to give me healing though. Like me, most were careful about making definitive spiritual diagnoses of my troubles, but they did not make me feel like a paranoid psycho either.

In time I came up with the following potential candidates as to my physical issues, some easier to exclude (through e.g. blood work) than others: food sensitivities/allergies; IBS; some kind of chronic viral, bacterial or fungal infection; Diabetes; Hypothyroidism; Depression; Schizophrenia; Psychosis; Bipolar Disorder; Paranoid delusions; electro-smog; ME (Myalgic Encephalopathy) and/or CFS (Chronic Fatigue Syndrome). From all my research ME/CFS symptoms are the best match for my experiences. I have never been officially diagnosed, but since CFS is more of an exclusion diagnosis, i.e. doctors check if you have lymphoma, thyroid problems, diabetes, infections (which I did not – according to my general blood work I was quite healthy), and if all comes back negative one is left with the diagnosis of CFS.

It's not a very thrilling diagnosis. As far as I am aware there are no real lab tests yet that 100% verify it. Since many symptoms such as fatigue and body aches don't necessarily leave any obvious physical signs or change one's blood parameters, it is easy for people to think one is just burning the candle at both ends, or simply lazy. The diagnosis also came with a dire prognosis – a complete recovery to pre-CFS energy levels seems rare. Some people might suffer for years, if not their whole lives. I seem to remember that the prognosis of a full recovery was virtually 0%; today there seems to be more optimism. Western medicine seems to just about acknowledge that CFS is an actual disease, not just all made up by oversensitive, creative patients' minds.

There is not much promising research out yet, I have found, which really pins down CFS's causes and which might lead to reliable treatments. The whole topic is rife with speculation, especially from alternative, naturopathic perspectives, and many an afternoon or evening browsing the subject on the Internet really gave me a headache. One cause that often crops up is 'post viral fatigue', i.e. cell damage caused by a previous viral infection, especially from EBV (Epstein-Barr Virus – cause of Mononucleosis), which is seen as a precursor to CFS.

I had had mononucleosis (also known as the Kissing Disease), but that was about a year before 'finding' Peter. From what I read online there are people who develop CFS after mono years after. The problem with this, in my opinion, is that we, as humans, have so many different factors influencing our lives. Once there is a scary theory out in the world, such as mono can lead to CFS, most who have CFS and had mono will connect the two, even if there are years spanning the two events. It disregards all the other people who have had mono and did not develop CFS, and it disregards the countless other influencing factors.

In the two years between my mono and CFS onset I was a member of a cult, had money worries and other stresses, had colds or flus, had sexual relations with different guys etc. It's a dilemma well known to medics and statisticians that just because one finds a statistical correlation between two events, it does not necessarily mean they are related. Humans usually don't live under laboratory conditions; there are just so many variables. I call this the 'cream cheese' phenomenon. I like cream cheese and I am sure that I had my share of cream cheese between having mono and getting CFS symptoms, yet would one really seek the cause of chronic illness in cream cheese? So many people seem to eat it and not have debilitating effects from it at all. But perhaps the combination of having mono and being a cream cheese lover could be the triggering cause? But would anyone ever include consumption of cream cheese in a CFS patients' questionnaire or interview? For me (and probably many other chronically ill patients out there) it is maintaining hope, staying positive, keeping an open mind and exploring therapies (if not too outlandish), while staying grounded and avoiding profiteering quacks.

Being spiritually minded, I live with the assumption that my thoughts have some creational force. And although CFS is the diagnosis I use when telling someone about my recent, past medical history, as it best describes most of my past symptoms, I do not accept science's dire prognosis as being my fate. I give CFS as little power over me as possible. I would also think that science sees CFS as an illness originating from within a patient's body, whereas today, if I have a tired day, the most likely explanation I have for it is outside LLE-healing resistances, mostly related to my client work. I could imagine living on some tropical island, with only a few (relatively happy and enlightened) people around me; I might always feel perfectly alright, but I might not know till I try!

Generally everything can be healed – it is primarily a question of time. I try not to limit the workings of spirit as to imagining precisely how this will happen. I am very stubborn that way – it will be healed. I do not think spirit would have left me here in this body; there is no use in spending the rest of my days suffering needlessly, especially as I don't believe in working off old karma. I have fallen flat on my face plenty of times, but believing that all will be well has helped me to get up again. I also believe my attitude will make it most uncomfortable for LLEs residing in me or passing through me. I believe that once we resign to a negative fate, like suffering from an 'incurable' disease, we might well open the floodgates to it.

In my search for healing, Western medicine was initially rather a disappointment. I had believed some 'alternative' propaganda, seeing doctors and the pharmaceutical realm as nothing but greedy sociopaths maintaining ill-health. The worst were those who tested on animals and so forth. But surely my London GP would not know about that? I certainly didn't tell him! I was somewhat defensive when the only diagnosis he ever came up with was 'depression'; he never even mentioned CFS. I tried to avoid being labeled as a psychosomatic hypochondriac or as a psychiatric patient. During my psychiatric course at medical school, I remember our lecturer telling us about a case where a woman had been hiking in the Alps. Suddenly she had an experience of extrasensory perception. She saw colors around the trees and flowers. Everything seemed more vivid, as if vibrating. The woman did not have any spiritual or esoteric knowledge, and thought she'd better go and check with her doctor. Her GP must have referred her to see a psychiatrist. She was diagnosed as delusional, medicated and hospitalized for a while.

I respect that a psychiatrist has the choice to be an atheist. Even as an atheist some might not disregard phenomena such as telepathy or telekinesis (there is plenty of compelling scientific literature supporting their existence). They may keep an open mind. For me the risk of being transferred to an atheist and close-minded psychiatrist was too scary though. Getting a stigmatizing diagnosis such as schizophrenia or paranoid psychosis, being committed or put on heavy antipsychotics was a risk I felt was not worth taking. I might be unfair in my judgment, but considering that some companies in the UK make you fill in a medical form, when interviewing, made me suspicious. Telling them I'd be off for a few days, for a bit of treatment in a mental health hospital – could that be good for any career? I couldn't financially afford to lose my job.

Perhaps there was also the desire of fitting in with the 'normal' people, leading a 'normal' life again after the cult. I had lost most my friends during my 'Peter' episode. I was in a new city trying to build a new circle of friends. Imagine, "Hi, my name is Alex and I'm schizophrenic, nice to meet you." But mainly I never believed I was crazy! I am aware this belief could be interpreted (by a psychiatrist) as resistance and seen as a sign of psychosis. As long as I did not lose all control and become a serious danger to myself or others, why should I? I meditated on it several times too and asked to exorcise any energy that might cause any mental disturbances. (Years later I chatted with a friend of the family who is a psychiatrist and who alleviated my fears of mental illness. He is not a believer as such, but did allow for me sensitively experiencing other people's emotions/energies. He thought that either way it would be wrong to not at least allow for such theories. Our chat only lasted about 20 minutes though, so I still might not have an outside all clear, clean bill of (mental) health yet.)

I tried my best to combat all the negative energies I experienced too, whatever level they were on, be it physical, emotional, mental or spiritual. I kept calm and remained an objective spectator – a feat I was successful in to varying degrees. With particularly strong attacks – like paranoid delusions – they did at times almost take over my mind, yet I still managed to go to work and function. I would be wary of accepting any new thoughts (especially the scary ones), however strong and convincing, as set in stone. By continuing to meditate and remain open for Ultimate Good healings and cleansings, any paranoid delusions would usually, sooner or later, come crumbling down. Either by losing strength or me being inspired by reasoning that unraveled their 'logic'.

Most of my 'paranoid delusions' were about spiritual concepts, e.g. are the Christian heavens, angels and so forth Ultimate Good or not? A psychiatrist would struggle to give me a definitive answer. But if I was considered 'crazy', thinking about spiritual concepts or communicating with Spirit, wouldn't we have to lock up priests and devout believers in mental hospitals too? I saw a program where a priest took five of his flock to spend a week in silence in a monastery. The week was spent in contemplation and meditation. By the end of it all five participants reported hearing voices/communicating with the Divine. I feared most psychiatrists would not really have a clue what I was contemplating. Plus I had already spent countless hours 'looking' at energies bothering me, going into them, analyzing them. I did not feel I was all that bad at it, and I could not really imagine that a therapist would be more creative and insightful than me, in conjunction with Ultimate Good.

I did not really feel that my first GP helped much at all. Perhaps he did not take me seriously? I had learned not to let out my frustrations on others. Even through my darkest years, friends and colleagues probably saw me friendly and smiling – I saw no use pulling everyone else down with me. Perhaps a friendly, smiling patient, saying he feels terrible, is taken less seriously? Usually my GP asked me what I wanted to do. I suggested various blood work and candida testing. He consented, but everything appeared fine.

So my GP asked what else I would suggest, making it quite

clear that in his opinion all my symptoms could be explained by depression and that my only option was antidepressants and psychotherapy. So any other diagnosis I would have to come up with myself. I was slightly annoyed; I felt guilty enough arriving late to work because of a doctor's appointment again. I knew from my medical studies that there are usually alternative diagnoses to be considered with just about every symptom. I felt he really did not make much of an effort (and he was a medical teaching professor as well). When watching programs like *House* I could get really jealous of his patient care, never excluding possible rare diagnoses.

I tried to monitor my eating to see if my IBS played up after any special foods. It seemed that eating olive oil, fish and tomatoes had adverse effects. I tried to keep my diet olive oil, tomato and fish free. It wasn't easy, but I made it through 4–5 weeks. It was virtually impossible to find any nice ready meals for lunch during work which did not have any tomato in them. Sure, I could have pre-prepared my own lunch – just that any extra effort to cook and pack lunches took away time I could stay in bed longer or rest when getting home. I got a referral for food allergy testing and six months later that appointment came through, by which time I was totally over the whole allergy thing, having reintroduced olive oil, fish and tomatoes months before (they are after all supposed to be super foods as well).

Still my GP kept pushing antidepressants and therapy. After a few months and running out of ideas of my own, I agreed. I did not like the label of being depressed. I was very frustrated and at times low, because I wanted to live a full life, but was continuously stopped in my tracks feeling fluey 24/7. I felt down, but did not consider myself depressed; neither was I suicidal. Sure, I frequently asked Ultimate Good if they were sure they knew what they were doing. And that if this was what my life was going to be like, it was not worth living! But I did not consider leaving my body through my own physical assistance. I trusted that Ultimate Good would have used the chance to get me out the times I had actually tried before. I figured that if I was still here it meant that there were plenty of fabulous things to come. I just had to sit it out, and hopefully it would not take too long. It did not mean, however, that I would be jumping up and down for joy as long as this part of the journey was still so rough. My physical condition aside, I had little to complain about. Professionally things were going alright. I had no reason to be depressed, except for my ill health. Surely depression would be triggered by unhappiness with other life factors, that depression itself would then make me unwell physically. But it seemed the reverse.

Telling my GP that I am positive and considered myself strong got me the reply, "A lot of depressed people consider themselves strong." Maybe the antidepressants would help by blocking whatever energies were pulling me down? What if my GP was right? It's good to hope. I acceded. I gave it my best shot – I did not want anybody to tell me that I had blocked the antidepressants from working by refusing to believe in any helping potential they may have. I started to take Prozac. They are cheap but apparently can take months to kick in. I took them for six months, but no change. Perhaps I should have tried a different antidepressant? I was given the impression that any antidepressant would have to be 'trialed' for another six months before changing prescriptions though. When I had taken Prozac I had felt more tied to the diagnosis of depression, which I resented. I felt less free to consider other diagnostic options and treatments too. I could be suffering for a much longer time by trying an approach that did not really make too much sense to me in the first place, nor was I given any guarantee that we would definitely find an antidepressant to relieve me of my symptoms. I was also wary that the antidepressants might make me dependent or have some other side effects. I decided not to try any others.

My GP wished me luck with any 'alternative' options that I

might try. He still insisted it was depression. He said if I had any 'new', very bad symptoms I could come and see him again. He did not want to potentially miss anything like cancer. I did not expect that to be the case. Funnily enough after two years in his care I had to suggest he at least give me a physical examination, like palpating my gut, to check for lumps or such. I had learned in my medical studies that physical examination is the first thing one does in patient anamnesis – and I displayed all those IBS (Irritable Bowel Syndrome) symptoms. Luckily (or annoyingly) there were no lumps though.

I decided to try to look for alternative help. Traditional Chinese Medicine (TCM) has been around for thousands of years. TCM practitioners are aware of Chi and healing intent, perhaps I could find more suitable help there. There was a shop near my work. I figured a medical tradition that goes back thousands of years will have survived so long for a reason. I did as much as I could afford; unfortunately the NHS is limited when it comes to alternative therapies, so I had to pay privately. I liked that the Chinese doctor did spend more time with me. She even touched me – pulse diagnostic and tongue diagnostic. I could not afford all the acupuncture and massage she recommended, so I went for the individually prescribed and combined herbal infusions alternative. Every two weeks or so I'd go for a checkup and pick up more prepared herb mixes. Considering the time the practitioners dedicate, the cost of the herbs, shop rent, the amount these TCM shops charged seemed reasonable. Still, it was about a third of my disposable monthly income – so plenty enough for me. I had to cook the herbs and let them simmer for about 30 minutes. The brews tasted and smelled disgusting. My flat mates loathed me cooking them in our shared open plan kitchen/living room; for about six months they really stank up the place. I did not experience an improvement (if anything I felt worse), so I quit. The Chinese doctor claimed the 'slow' response was due to the severity of my symptoms. Apparently I'd have to keep drinking the teas much longer and accompany that with daily acupuncture sessions. There was no way I could afford that though, unless I slept under a bridge or stopped eating. I tried regular Chinese acupuncture and massage a few years later, this time without the teas. I was a little better off and thought it deserved a try. I went for a few months but again without any real improvement.

And I wasn't keen on the fact that most TCM therapists I met also implied that theirs was the only one, viable therapy. Any mention of me taking Western herbs and vitamins or practicing healing meditations was usually answered with a polite smile and a little rolling of eyes. It is hard to put my finger on it, maybe the TCM therapists were just empathic, but often I left a consultation feeling rather sorry for myself. Maybe I was ungrateful about their empathy and commiseration, but I usually felt there was no use in 'pulling' me down in such manner. I knew there was something wrong with me, else I would not feel so bad, but I wasn't dying! Also I had made it clear that I had no more money to spend, yet still they insisted (with every visit) that if I added this and that to my routine with them it would help even more! I do not claim that TCM is useless, but I have put it in the draw of 'more masochistic' therapies. The herbs tasted and smelled awful, the acupuncture was alright, definitely relaxing, but the massage and cupping were often very rough.

My sister kept telling me I should try homeopathy, so I decided to give it a try. I have great respect for good homeopaths. They dedicate a lot of time to patient interviews (obviously some think that this alone creates a placebo healing effect). They collate a lot of patient data during their interviews and then have the very hard task of sorting and prioritizing that data. Then they have to match the received information with the most suitable remedy. To find the right remedy homeopaths have to evaluate which, out of several symptoms fitting remedies, fits best and furthermore decide on a suitable dosage (again having a lot of different dosages to choose from). There are so many variables to consider, it is mind-boggling.

I found a nice therapist. His fee was slightly less than what I had paid for my TCM consultation and herb packages. Ideally I only had to see him every 4–6 weeks too. Plus he was there for me via e-mail, in case I required some advice between sessions. There was no charge for this! Homeopathic remedies are relatively inexpensive too. I saw him for about 18 months. During this time I did pretty much get rid of my IBS symptoms, but I would not definitely say it must have been because of the homeopathic treatments I received. I did take some herbal remedies too – mostly recommended by him, plus I did plenty of spiritual work – prayer, meditation etc.

My homeopath seemed capable, but he did not work according to some essential(?) rules. For example most times my homeopath prescribed a remedy straight away, at the end of each session. This was more practical for me too, as I could purchase the remedy straight away from him or the homeopathic pharmacy in the same building. I was disconcerted though as I had learned that it 'should' take a homeopath hours or days to decide upon the perfect remedy. Considering all the variables I had learned that most homeopaths will research remedies in the Materia Medica (encyclopedia of homeopathic medicines) before prescribing! But maybe my homeopath was just that experienced or had a perfect memory?

Besides having had some basic introduction to homeopathy during my medical studies, I now read a few books on homeopathy too. If anything they made me more paranoid. I wasn't sure how my chances for a complete healing success were stacking up anymore. I figured my symptoms were pretty chronic, but, according to one book, supposedly chronic illnesses (especially with mental factors) have a relatively low chance of being successfully treated. Also I read that there is a theory in homeopathy which states that to achieve perfect health one has to run through all the illnesses one has ever had, in reverse order. That includes all childhood illnesses – and I had been sick many times as a kid. And what happens if this reverse order is screwed up by contracting something 'new' during therapy? What about the bit of carbon monoxide poisoning I had around that time because my landlord had not done proper maintenance on the chimney, and the boiler vented through the fireplace in my room? Also was homeopathy suitable if as I expected (at least some of) my symptoms were caused by spiritual, psychic attacks? I mean would an ingested remedy actual treat an attacking outside force? (Obviously the same consideration had plagued me with antidepressants and TCM too.) Well, perhaps the remedies could heal potentially destroyed or harmed energetic protections of mine. I still feared, or hoped, that my ills might just all be from inside me too. Homeopathy furthermore believes some 'symptoms' to be pathological which I do not necessarily see as such, like hearing voices. I agree this could be termed pathological if I heard the wrong kind of voice in my head; if it were from divine source though – surely that should not be 'healed' away as well?

My biggest problem was that I never felt any better after taking a remedy. The entire 18 months was like one big healing crisis – just without the effect of feeling better afterwards. I'd take a remedy, feel even more 'crap' for 2–3 weeks and then slightly better, but not really any better than before taking the remedy. At which point it was time to see my homeopath again for the next prescription. I was frequently concerned about how my homeopath might prioritize my symptoms too. I had a hard enough time to say which was the graver and more essential problem: my extreme fatigue and exhaustion, the whole-body fluey aches, the nightmares, the low mood or perhaps the at times severe stomach cramps? Considering that you have to tell your homeopath all the symptoms you experience be they physical, emotional, mental or spiritual – I spent a lot of my free time analyzing myself.

My symptoms would change all the time, and when talking to him I was uncertain if certain symptoms were still there, or not. I read about the remedies I had been prescribed and about 'proving' a remedy. Proving is the process with which the symptoms of a remedy are gathered. Healthy individuals take a remedy and then note down any changes in their well-being. If several testers report the same symptoms, they become the drug picture according to which they are prescribed. I noticed that at times I 'displayed' remedy picture symptoms, which I had not had before the prescription. Was I so sensitive that I was starting to prove the remedies I took? Was the healing crisis I experienced actually a proving of remedies? I had enough dealing with my own symptoms, thank you.

My homeopath asked me to not read about the drug pictures anymore. Perhaps he was right – it did not do me much good. My problem, perhaps out of desperation, was not being able to sit back and wait to see what was happening. I wanted to be an active part of my therapy. After all I was the individual in the world I trusted most. I couldn't just hand over all control to a therapist – I had tried that with Peter for a while and look how that turned out. It was hard to just 'relax' into a therapy, especially if it seemed to make me feel worse a lot of the time.

There were other things that niggled me about homeopaths – like their aversion to coffee. Coffee and peppermint can annul a remedy's healing properties. I needed one or two big espressos a day, otherwise I would fall asleep in the office! I tried not to 'fear' the coffee, but in my mind if a remedy did not seem to do much, it might be because I had had a cup. You can obviously just take a remedy again, but you might be dealing with a slow start of a remedy's workings (you have to give each remedy a 'fair' chance of getting to work for at least 2–3 weeks), and the more you take a remedy, the greater a chance of proving it...

In homeopathy you have the option to heal negative

symptoms received from taking a substance, e.g. chemotherapy, by taking a homeopathic preparation of the same substance. My therapist never seemed too fond of this theory, maybe because one does not require a homeopathy degree to apply that part of the teachings? I did try taking homeopathic nutmeg at one point, just in case my 'self-induced nutmeg poisoning' had left any damage, but it did not do much. I was getting really tired of all the 'what ifs' with homeopathy. But I had one last hope. I made my own remedy. Since I had started feeling worse and worse since seeing Peter, I figured that most likely he had attached some LLEs to me that I still had to get rid of. Even if I was schizo-phrenic (i.e. pre-Peter damage) or had ME, these were energies inside my body that, if removed, should enable me to heal completely. The divine self that I am was/is perfectly healthy and sane – anything deviating from this are just clouds around the sun inside.

So what if I made a remedy from my current body? Any negativities therein should be included and I would not heal away the actual healthy me! I took a drop of blood, some saliva and some sperm of mine and mixed them all up. I kept the mix with me for several hours to add any negative purely energetic energies inside my bodies and then made a remedy of this mix by diluting it 1/100 and percussing the mix 40 times each – 250 times. You need to concentrate. I lost track a few times and had to start over. I was confident this was the way to go; I might have stumbled upon the holy grail of homeopathy! But… it didn't affect much. I received one more remedy from my therapist after this. He had purposely just marked it as remedy X, so I could not look it up. It gave me the most horrendous mouth ulcers, so painful and debilitating that I could hardly eat or speak. This really pissed me off! A healing crisis (if unavoidable) is supposed to exacerbate symptoms one has had before only! Well I had never had mouth ulcers in my life. I asked my mum too, but she could not remember me having any as a child either. That was it, homeopathy was filed away as a masochistic way of healing too!

I don't want to create an anti-homeopathy movement. Homeopaths and their patients have enough problems already with skeptics that claim remedies are just diluted water and, if at all, work on a placebo level only. I don't believe that, and there seems to be some scientific proof from the biophysics camp that it is not just water too. But don't take my word for it, make your own enquiries. I mainly refer back to the book *The Field* by Lynne McTaggart. It just didn't work for me very well. (But as mentioned before too, ME sufferers supposedly often react adversely to alternative healing therapies.) I actually encountered homeopathy two times more over the years since. A few years later I thought I'd help out a friend, who was studying to become a homeopath, with her case studies. I actually took a remedy again too, but again ended up with severe mouth ulcers within a couple of hours.

Then a year later, during my Hawaiian massage course, my teacher used her own massage oil on me, demonstrating. When I got up, she said, "Is the oil not wonderful, it has all these great homeopathic remedies in it too!" Lo and behold within a few hours my mouth was a sea of sores again. Now there is such a thing as the no-cebo effect (a negative placebo effect), but somehow I feel that my spiritual protections would probably fend most of those off – and I do not usually get strong side effects if I take allopathic medications either. Some alternative remedies have given me vegetative side effects, such as having to pee a lot, wooziness, nausea or loose bowels, but nothing as dramatic as these mouth ulcers. If homeopathy would really just be water or sugar pills, I'd say my reactions were quite remarkable…

In the years to follow I mostly concentrated on spiritual healing and spiritual tools to heal myself. At least with Ultimate Good energies helping me, I did not have to worry about my Ultimate Good Helpers getting the dose wrong. I just had to suss out why the healing took so long. I also experienced a fear of electromagnetic radiation. During times of feeling especially unwell and working in an open plan office, surrounded by PCs, printers and air-condition units, it did make me anxious. Playing into this fear was the fact that I seemed to feel worse during work hours than after work and on weekends. However, it did not explain all the fluctuations in my well-being. If electro-smog had been the cause of my troubles I presume my symptoms should have increased over each working day, worsening as the week progressed. During busy times in the accounting year, I would sometimes go into the office on the weekend. In my near vicinity there were just as many PCs running as usual, but I would feel remarkably calmer, more peaceful and happier when working on a weekend.

Over the years I acquired a peace lily and several crystals – mainly amethyst, which are all meant to neutralize and protect against electro-smog, and which I strategically placed all over my work desk. I bought a little 'high-tech' pendant to protect me against electro-smog, but none of these measures really made any significant difference to my health and well-being. The notion of blaming all my ills on electromagnetic radiation was tempting, especially if you could protect yourself with pendants, plants and crystals. The chance of it being the cause of all my troubles was becoming less logical though. Should I not have felt better than most humans who don't even pray and ask for spiritual healing and protections? Regardless of my desk boasting said peace lily and several crystals I was still the most 'poorly' person in my team.

I believe we don't just have an immune system for our physical body, but there is in-built, self-healing on all energetic levels. Even if we were to receive little holes in our aura from electro-smog, who says that our bodies cannot repair those easily? Similar to UV rays. We need the Sun to synthesize vitamin D3, but UV radiation can also damage our DNA. Our cells have the tools to fix UV damage to a certain extent. Considering the benefits of electricity: warmth in winter, refrigeration, lighting, I wouldn't want be without it. Was my body just too weakened to fix electro-smog damage? Why? I don't deny that the whole 'Peter/cult' experience and consequent year had been traumatic. I had eaten healthily, invested a lot of time into healing any spiritual wounds and tried my best to completely forgive myself for the experience. Even when sick, I believe our bodies retain basic healing abilities. One does not get automatic skin cancer by just going out into the Sun a few times, even if suffering from other severe illnesses. I was neither willing to spread potential paranoia of electro-smog amongst my peers, nor did I have the holidays or funds to move to some Buddhist monastery somewhere – beyond electricity.

Even if I did go on an 'electricity free' retreat, would I feel better for having been able to rest in a more peaceful environment or because I was electro-smog free? If the latter would possibly be true, I might just open the door to a lifetime of fear being around anything electrical… My goal was to heal myself and live a 'normal' life – not make it more difficult and eccentric. Having the benefit of several more years of observing myself, my health took some time to very slowly improve after leaving my office job. I would have expected it to improve much faster after leaving the office and 'just' having to deal with the one PC at home had I suffered from electro-smog damage.

I still tried everything which promised any kind of healing support. There was an American product – Liquid Oxygen drops. I knew we breathe in liters of air every minute and that generally our blood is oxygenated about 95–98% anyway – so how a 10ml bottle of oxygenated water, taken drops at a time, could improve anything puzzled me a bit. There were just so many positive testimonials on the company's Web site though – would they just make them all up? All I seemed to get from taking them was diarrhea! I also drank liters of self-made colloidal silver; supposedly it kills pretty much all bacteria and viruses. Maybe some of my symptoms were due to some bug – the flu-like symptoms did feel the same as when I had viral infections in the past. There were no marked improvements here either. I might actually have wrecked what little healthy gut flora I had left with it. I admit to falling for the colloidal silver marketing. It is widely propagated as 'the' natural kill-all antibiotic (+ antiviral), but upon further inspection the study this claim is based on is in vitro. That does not necessarily translate to what happens inside a human body – toilet cleaner kills bacteria and viruses too, but I would not drink it. Whenever I did get what seemed to be a proper bacterial infection I never got any healing effects from it that equaled taking medical antibiotics either. Later I read that some people's skin can turn irreversibly blue-green after ingesting colloidal silver – a risk too far for me, being vain and all.

Then there was Hulda Clark's 'Zapper'. According to Hulda pathogenic microbes can be killed with electromagnetic frequencies. One is supposed to hold copper electrodes in one's hands, which are connected to a battery-powered frequency generator. Her site does try to sell one countless other naturopathic products as well, all supposed to be essential, but the Zapper does promise total virus, parasite and bacteria kill, so why spend hundreds more on her other products if one wants to kill some bug? I zapped away for hours on end – for a good few weeks. But no amelioration, and the herpes and the plantar warts I had did not disappear either.

I learned that even though some products are marketed as naturopathic/alternative remedies, one cannot assume that they are anything but a ploy to get money from sick people. Many probably so sick, they are desperate and will give anything a try. I beware of products that claim to be panaceas – the long-lost cure-all that doctors and the pharmaceutical industry do not want the public to know about, because they'd all be bankrupt tomorrow if everybody started taking them today! And if a Web site makes you read through a zillion supposed positive, raving feedbacks, then click through three more links before even quoting the price (which will probably be a one-day-special), be assured it is all just hot air! If I still think the actual product might potentially help, I'll just go on eBay and usually find it for a fraction of the cost!

On my self-healing quest I learned too that some alternative marketing was filled with at least as much, often more, defamation and hate towards Western medicine as that which skeptical, non-believing doctors can hold against alternative or complementary therapies. It shamed me; weren't complementary therapists supposed to be more unconditionally loving, wise and forgiving than most doctors, who might never even have heard about an aura or a chakra? And at least doctors will probably just tell you that you are wasting your money trying alternative therapies, whereas alternative therapists will scare you into believing that all medical treatments are going to kill you. A common stratagem of the alternatives is to discredit a medical therapy before raving about their own. You get told how many people get damaged or killed by a medical therapy and how perfect theirs is. As a reader or listener, that usually creates the (probable) illusion that their alternative therapy will work in 100% of cases. I doubt that though; many such advertised herbs, vitamins and the like did not help me. Comparatively doctors are more honest by usually not hiding that a medication is successful in x% of cases only.

I also read that fatigue and grumpiness in the morning can be because one 'binges' on sweets in the evening. It creates a sugar rush, an insulin peak and then one crashes thereafter and wakes up the next morning with a sugar hangover. I was not too sure what to make of that one. Sweets were one of the last few things I did still enjoy during my CFS years. Plus it felt like I needed the energy and possibly the analgesic sugar properties. Having some sweets in the evening in front of the TV helped me relax. They made me feel a bit more normal, a bit more like I had normal amounts of energy and fewer aches. Furthermore, I believed there is a reason why one says one wishes for a 'sweet' life. I believe that life is about happiness and enjoyment. Taking all the 'sweetness' out of it (literally) did not feel right.

Still I knew that the above sounds a bit like an alcoholic's rationalization for drinking, *I just want to forget my worries*. I did not think I overdosed on sweets; if anything I needed to gain weight, not lose it! Nor was I escaping my problems; I did confront them regularly in meditation and so on. But fear and desperation are hard to resist. I figured that even if the whole sugar thing was a delusion, if I cut out sugar and felt good for it, my body and soul could need the respite from feeling sick all the time. So I did give up on sweets. It must have been about 4–6 weeks. I only allowed myself some fresh and the occasional bit of dried fruit for any sweetness, but made sure that I did not start to 'just replace' refined sugars with natural sugars. But, perhaps fortuitously, I did not feel any better so I added sugars back to my diet.

I also question sugar's addictive theory for the fact that when I go on a summer holiday, spending at least a few hours in the Sun every day, I have no desire for my nightly sweetie intake. I might have a fresh fruit smoothie, but I'll happily pass on dessert at night. I'll crave more fresh vegetables and salad too. The same applies to caffeine; some health gurus will tell you it is highly addictive and guarantee that if you drink a lot of coffee, you'll need more (and more) to stay awake and will end up grumpy and with a bad headache when trying to cut back. The other week I had a guest staying and I felt under attack from her associated LLEs. I was as exhausted as I used to feel when suffering with CFS. It took at least one more triple espresso and two energy drinks in the afternoon/evening to get anything done. As soon as she left, my extra coffee and energy drink need went. No headache or grumpiness to speak of either. All that said, when initially trying to give up smoking I displayed most of the classic withdrawal symptoms. The LLEs associated with some addictions can be strong, so if you are an 'ex-something-holic' it is still safer not to partake in whatever substance or behavior which made you dependent. But if one does pray to be delivered of the complete addiction program, including the whole easy relapse 'shebang', it might very well disappear too. The above are my experiences; I cannot guarantee that they are transferable! And I might be lucky that my brain does not get as easily addicted as other people's.

Regarding addiction in general – there is a very interesting study which shows that happy rats actually do not want heroin. The authors postulate that drug addiction in rats is mainly triggered by their 'unhappy' living conditions, as most rat studies will have them living in small wire cages. When one places rats in a 'rat park', an artificial, but species-appropriate environment and gives them a choice of either sugar-laced morphine solution or plain tap water, happy rats will choose significantly less drug water (which impedes their social life) than normal water. Considerably less than control caged rats. See:

Alexander, BK; Beyerstein, BL; Hadaway, PF; and Coambs, RB. "Effects of early and later colony housing on oral ingestion of morphine in rats," Pharmacology Biochemistry and Behavior, Vol. 15, issue 4, 571–576, 1981

In the last years I have come to be more at peace with Western medicine. Sure some doctors probably practice because they like the money and the prestige that comes with their profession, but of all the doctors I have met the vast majority strive to do their best for their patients, and they invest a lot of sweat and tears in their education and training too. Some years after my first go with antidepressants I gave them another try. I had been made redundant from my accountancy job and was trying to establish a spiritual healing practice. My very first endeavor was to rest though.

I took six weeks out. I mainly just slept and meditated, with a bit of eating and TV thrown in. I had dreamt of being able to do this for years; now with a bit of severance money in my pocket, I could indulge it. Sadly it made little difference. The only hours of the day I was half-awake and alert, and did not feel too crummy, were in the evening. A friend told me of his success with a particular brand of antidepressants – more expensive than Prozac. My new GP was much more sympathetic and did not fuss over prescribing them. Almost straight away they gave me a boost of energy. Beforehand I needed about three hours of meditation after breakfast to feel half-decent; now I just got on with my day. The effect did not last very long, a few weeks maybe; after that my energy levels dropped somewhat again. But still taking the pills was a comforting crutch to hold onto for the next four years. Another impressive feat was taking 'Varenciline' – a stop-smoking drug. I had managed to stop smoking for a few months before, without any help, but relapsed after it did not seem to make much of a difference to my well-being. This was much more comfortable. I took Varenciline and after 2–3 weeks my appetite for cigarettes just stopped. I pretty much forgot to smoke. I discontinued them somewhat earlier then recommended, as they are reported to have psychotic and depressing side effects – I did not want to push it.

Last but not least, I am gay and have friends who are HIV+. Two of them are quite spiritual too. They eat healthier than me (being full vegetarians), and do some spiritual work too. They tried some natural remedies initially, after having been diagnosed, but funnily their CD4 dropped and their viral load rose much faster than with other HIV+ friends, who are generally much unhealthier in their lifestyles, taking regular recreational drugs etc. Still all of them, once starting on Highly Active Antiretroviral Therapy (HAART), had their viral load drop to undetectable (i.e. the virus load drops so far that it is not measurable anymore and they become virtually infection free). I rarely hear anyone still having side effects from their HAART therapy, and if they do usually a change in medication fixes that. They seem to have a normal life expectancy again! Considering that HIV is one of the first viruses that can actually be treated (remember there still is no treatment for the common cold), I find the recent rapid development of these drugs is nigh on miraculous! Some years ago I might have 'condemned' anyone giving in to Western medicine and using pharmaceuticals to help themselves. I would have told them to meditate instead, become vegetarian, go on a juice fast, drink a few liters of colloidal silver and so on. In the case of HIV, had they followed my advice it might very well have been a death sentence!

I am sure that some people might still say that my two friends, mentioned above, probably just did not meditate enough. They could have beaten HIV had they alkalized their body PH more. Maybe. But I suspect that, giving it any chance whatsoever, they might have had to meditate 12 hours a day and not eat anything except for freshly squeezed juices etc. – for years. Who has the time for that, or the money? And what would the quality of life be under such a regime? If one watches documentaries about the early years of AIDS, scores of people dying and the love and dedication which went into helping the victims, the demonstrations and so on, one can just about imagine the incredible amounts of love and prayer that went into helping the sick and trying to find a cure! To then turn around and say that modern HAART is of the devil seems narrow-minded!

In 2009 I even underwent sessions with a psychotherapist, a psychologist and a psychoanalyst. I was self-employed and less worried about my 'mental health' image – and I had also read about cults, brainwashing and the damage they may cause. The books had been written by psychotherapists and psychologists. Perhaps there was some understanding about spiritual matters in their community after all? The books were American though, so when trying to find support for post-cult recovery for UK citizens I could only find one psychotherapist who advertised being specialized in the subject.

Fortunately he was in London, so I met up with him and we had an extensive chat. Regarding any potential psychological damage I might have received from my cult experience: he was positive and judged that I seemed to have dealt with all my issues sufficiently rationally. He figured that I did not really need him for more sessions. It was just a question of not giving in to any lingering episodes of emotional fear or guilt whenever they came up – but I should be able to cope with those by myself.

I mentioned that his personal story and attitude helped me overcome my fear that Peter might still attack me, and be strong enough to get through. For anyone reading this, who has recently gotten into a 'fight' with some questionable guru or the like, I would like to mention though that I am pretty confident that some gurus (/gurus' energies) do attack. After a lecture from a 'Shaman' a few years back, where I had my doubts (and criticized openly in front of the seminar group), I had debilitating mouth ulcers thereafter. This time they also affected my throat, esophagus and trachea. I ended up having to take a week off work. I also once treated a client who was seeing a renowned South American healer. From what I heard and read, I doubt that this healer is all that 'holy'. His whole setup smacks of 'cultism' and dependency. The client had, from what I felt, two huge wounds in his light body, as if two of his chakras had been ripped out. Something I had never encountered to such an extent before. These were big wounds, regardless of the client being very spiritual. It could have been caused by his high-powered job, but I suspected it was related to the healer. I told him so (I knew him privately too, so was comfortable sharing my intuition); funnily enough the next day I developed bad mouth ulcers again and lost a few days of work. (NB. Since the initial homeopathy mouth ulcer attack I only had severe cases when taking homeopathic remedies again or 2–4 times when having run-ins with gurus or the like.)

I believe that with strong, charismatic, manipulative gurus the main driving force lies in powerful life limiting energies pulling the strings in the background. If one looks closely, the gurus are not much more than over-inflated balloons. That is why they pop so easily, get so enraged when you dare to question them publicly. They have little backbone and true self-confidence, even if they have the life force of their devoted followers at their disposal. If one has been a member of a destructive, manipulative cult and leaves, i.e. affronts the guru and the energy behind them, one might very well get attacked and feel those attacks. It might take a while to sort this out, and one might have very uncomfortable physical, emotional, mental and/or spiritual ill effects thereafter. I do believe though that if you ask for as many and far-reaching Ultimate Good healings and protections as necessary, possible, available and sensible – the problem will be sorted. It might take a few weeks, even months, but I doubt it will take years. You might also have to make sure you cleanse out any other negative energies the cult-facilitating-LLEs might have placed inside your being, as long as you were still totally open and trusting towards the guru, and which might attempt to trigger desperation or make you return to the cult.

So why don't cults collapse after you have left and asked for perfect healings? Strictly speaking it is not your responsibility to free all remaining cult devotees – just because you have seen the true face of the guru. (Family are excluded, you can fight for them!) Everybody else, who is an adult, can be told your truths and realizations, but it is their decision as to how to react. You can obviously pray for them, ask that they get the strength and find the wisdom to get out. You could even try an intervention, give them a book about cult psychology. I would not recommend interventions that try to use manipulative techniques – you wouldn't be much better than the cult. Don't get me wrong, if the guru did anything criminal against you, rape or other abuse, do pursue them legally. Ultimate Good will help dismantle your personal cult-ghost-train, but if that does not automatically collapse the other cult followers' ghost trains too, the cult will go on for a while yet. Even if background cult-enabling-LLEs are removed, others might take their place...

The psychotherapist I had found myself, but I was referred to the psychoanalyst by my GP. I only sat through one session with him. I know he had been informed, by my GP, that I had been in a cult, so he should have deducted that I had been subject to brainwashing and manipulation. Yet he still chose manipulative techniques to attempt to force me to open up to him. He scarcely greeted me, just a nonchalant, "Hi" – no smile or handshake. Then he told me to sit down and said something along the lines of *We have 45 minutes... Go.* There was no building up of rapport, no general outline or introduction to psychoanalysis or our session together. I did not expect ten minutes of polite small talk, but his whole demeanor seemed very cold. I could be wrong, but I would expect a therapist, who is potentially going to be my therapist for the foreseeable future, to somehow signal that he is a human being, capable of empathy, especially considering that psychoanalysis can be very intrusive and could easily be abused by a therapist. Knowing my history of cult membership, he should have known that if I had learned my lesson (through the cult) I would not just trust any human outright (and possibly get myself brainwashed again). He would have to 'earn' my trust.

He just sat there and stared at me. I asked him what he would like to know, where he would like me to start... He did not reply. Apparently he figured that his continued silence would be a way for me to lose control and just burst out with all my issues. The next 30 minutes we just stared at each other. If he thought he could manipulate me into trusting my innermost being to someone whose greeting was that frigid, I figured two can play that game. Perhaps I could teach him some common politeness? His conclusion was that I was not strong enough for regular weekly or biweekly psychoanalysis; my conclusion was I really did not feel comfortable with his energy and I'd rather do my own thing. Even if he was not planning to manipulate me, it felt like more sessions would most likely be a waste of my time and energy.

I managed three sessions with the psychologist my GP referred me to next. We figured that I might benefit from CBT (Cognitive Behavioral Therapy). I learned that according to psychological understanding, thoughts, emotions and actions are linked. In other words if I change my thinking, i.e. make it more positive, I should be able to improve my mood and motivation for outside activities. Same if I do some activities, like finally cleaning those windows, that should positively influence my thoughts and emotions too. It was interesting to see that psychology is discovering what religion has told us for millennia. Think positive and it will change your life. This is where spiritually minded people believe, in addition to the above, that the right form of thinking will not only have an effect on one's emotions and deeds, but potentially even attract more positive things into one's life – The Law of Attraction. I don't know why it took me three sessions to realize that what I was asked to do by the psychologist I had already been doing for the last 13+ years. It was a mix of trying not to offend and waiting to see if I might be told something I did not know already. Furthermore the CBT therapist treated me as a total novice with regards to self-awareness. I strongly feel that she projected this incompetence expectation onto me, and I fell for it. It was interesting to learn though that spiritual teachings and Western psychology overlap so much – they just use different termi-nologies.

In retrospect, another reason why I decided to discontinue my CBT sessions was that since I had been checking most of my thoughts and emotions already for the last 13 years, I felt I was being told that, because my mood was still low at times, my best option was to just change my low moods through more outside work – go on clean those windows! However, I didn't clean those windows because I was lazy or indulged in self-pity, but rather because I intuitively felt that resting and meditating instead would be more effective! If I did not have the strength or motivation to get outside chores done, I would meditate! And meditation is a form of activity too, a very powerful one at that. With the healing and energy gained from my meditations, I managed to keep working and paying my bills – that was more important than cleaning windows! I still agree that overcoming the weaker self and doing outside tasks can improve one's mood and thinking – there often will be a sense of self-satisfaction for outside things accomplished and some LLEs, having tried to incapacitate one, might leave, as they understand that their attempts are futile. Still I find today that for me whether I meditate or do some chore, when I'm blocked by dis-motivation or depression energies depends on the strength of their attack. Weaker or medium strength LLEs can be 'ignored', but powerful ones I rather meet in meditation, time permitting.

I did learn one more thing from my psychoanalysis and psychology sessions – to try my best not to give into assumptions with my massage and healing clients. I am e.g. tempted at times to tell my clients off if their muscles feel like they don't get any regular exercise, or they do not seem to stretch sufficiently. I have learned though that it is better to ask first if they do exercise or stretch regularly. If they actually do, and I would just accuse them of not doing enough, that would hardly be good motivation. For example, there was one client who had hardly any muscle mass at all. My first instinct was to have a go at him, but instead I asked if he did take any exercise. It turned out that he has hit the gym 2–3 times a week (with a personal trainer) for the last two years! Admittedly he'd gone 40+ years beforehand doing very little. Still, I am pretty confident that had I just opened with, *You really need some exercise*, it could have been quite de-motivating for him and embarrassing for me.

I trawled the Internet for anything else that promised restoring my happiness and energy levels to normal. I tried many vitamins, minerals, herbs and so on. Two especially made a palpable difference. The first being strong probiotics. I make my own kefir (a fermented milk drink). I had read that CFS sufferers might experience many of their symptoms because they have too many negative bacteria in their gut. The negative bacteria have grown in numbers because they have not been hemmed in sufficiently – either due to stress, trauma or antibiotic use. In turn these negative bacteria release toxins into the bloodstream, which weaken and irritate nerves and the immune system. (The article actually stemmed from a Belgium Professor of Medicine!) The suggested therapy was powerful antibiotics, to try to eliminate the bad bacteria. But I figured I'd rather try to just push the negative little critters out (if actually there) with high powered probiotics. Since drinking kefir regularly the fluey, achy feelings and frequent throat aches have pretty much gone. It took my second recommendation, vitamin D3 supplementation, to get the number of infections down, which had kept me off work regularly.

In the beginning vitamin D3 even managed to up my energy levels nicely too, but it appears that whatever energies managed to make me weak and ill managed to recover some lost ground and some of the initial energy gains were leveled out again. Still, not getting sick all the time is a vast improvement, and with more of a steady ability to work comes more financial stability (and less financial worries) too. Furthermore I am pretty confident that vitamin D3 has helped me quit smoking and stay off cigarettes, as well as get off antidepressants. There are several different guidelines about recommended vitamin D3 dosage. Going higher should be discussed with your doctor (you could ask to get your serum levels checked) and/or be at your own risk!

And there are some other supplements which I think are worth mentioning like CoQ10 (supposedly good for one's energy levels, anti-ageing and keeps gums happy); vitamin C (the time release kind); multivitamins; zinc; (odorless) garlic pills (a natural anticoagulant, antibiotic and antiviral – not reliable, however, I have had bacterial infections regardless of regular consumption); milk thistle (a strong herbal antioxidant for the liver; spiritually the liver is supposed to be responsible for digesting emotions – I figure it's a good organ to support); sea buckthorn oil (Genghis Khan is said to have fed sea buckthorn to his warriors for faster wound healing); vitamin B3 (good for schizophrenics, CFS, general health and rejuvenation as it widens the capillaries, so flushes out plenty of toxins! I take it at night); maca (power food of the Incas); Lysine (helps keep HSV at bay); and folic acid (vitamin B9 – good for mucous membrane health; since taking it I have not had any mouth ulcers). I purposely don't include any dosages with the above, because I would not want any readers to go out and buy the same supplements (and dosage) just because I take them. Please read about the products yourself to see if you think they could help you.

Other supplements I have taken have not proved so beneficial, or had uncomfortable side effects, and include: evening primrose oil; resveratrol (had to pee like mad); black seed oil (no palpable effect); tongkat ali and yohimbine (could make me too hyper and diuretic as well as had laxative side effects) – there was a concern too, because tongkat ali's and yohimbine's sources are supposedly quite finite and their continued widespread use currently not sustainable.

I had this phase where I bought all my supplements in the

organic shop, but these days I use eBay or the Internet. It may be that some are more easily absorbed by the human gut if plant derived and in liquid form, but the organic versions are often 4–5 times as expensive as the non-organic supplements. I did start off with an organic liquid multivitamin and mineral mix. It was delicious, but expensive. After taking it for a few months and not really feeling much better, I figured a cheaper tablet version may help to counter the stress of forking out £30 for a month's supply of just one of all my supplements. Any other successes on the road of my continuous and steady endeavors back to pre-Peter energy levels, and perhaps even beyond, I attribute to spiritual healing and spiritual insights rediscovered. I have touched on quite a few already, so now I would like to share with you some of those I have not had a chance to talk about…

My healing journey was not just for physical well-being, but just as important was my emotional/spiritual wellness. I always tried to hold onto my belief that every ailment is spiritual and that it should therefore yield to spiritual healing. Even if we can attribute an infection to physical bacteria – in its essence those bacteria are spiritual beings. Matter is just a thicker form of spiritual energy. Harmful bacteria are just LLEs with a physical body. Our bodies are a conglomerate of spiritual energies working and influencing each other and which vibrate at different frequencies. I do try to stay grounded and remember that physical energy is often harder to shift and manipulate than finer frequency energies – so if it is more effortless to take antibiotics for something, I will. I can then concentrate on dealing with the finer energies, which potentially enabled the bacteria to settle in the first place.

Feeling pretty miserable for about a decade obviously made it hard to keep desperation and paranoia away. I always tried to keep a cool and grounded head on my shoulders, but it was not always easy. Today I can still have tired and depressed days, sometimes worse; but I do not consider myself a CFS sufferer anymore as I am usually pretty sure that I am dealing with outside healing resistances. Even if I get attacked by energies, which might be successful in keeping me more tired and down for up to a week or so, it is remarkable how quickly you can recover when such attacks dissipate. Just feeling good and right again for a few hours will enable me to 'forgive' any attack and 'remember' that it must have been inevitable and beneficial for my long-term happiness. And I do get a bit of a feeling of rebirth every time I come out of an LLE swamp. I have mentioned several guilt traps, fears and so on that I have fallen for during my spiritual journey; there are a few more I'd like to mention now though.

During my dark years only my mind, divine intuition and continuous observation helped me. Some fears took longer to debunk than others. One of the most common fears I experienced was the question of whether I was doing too much or too little of something – especially spiritual work. I tried to be in the zone, i.e. connected to Ultimate Good constantly, not because I was greedy, but because I constantly felt attacked and unwell. Sure enough there were frequent energetic attacks, in the form of guilt, telling me that I was greedy because I did not believe that Ultimate Good only needed say ten minutes per day to provide me with enough healings, energy recharges etc. If I were to believe strongly enough, ten minutes would be more than enough to heal anything! I used to fear that if I meditated and felt better, I should show gratitude rather than a desire to feel even better. I might feel less achy or just be lethargic after a two-hour meditation; was it really greedy to then want to feel perfectly healthy and happy? And whenever I had one of those rare days where I actually could feel a little that I loved and enjoyed life, I'd be attacked by thoughts of, *Okay, so now you have felt good for a few hours, that should be enough, you might as well die now.*

Fearing I was doing too much did not stop fears of not-doing-enough plaguing me, even at the same time. I felt guilty if I fell asleep when sitting or lying down to meditate; when not meditating on something else or for someone else; for not meditating differently; for not exercising more; eating more fruit or drinking more water or when I lacked the energy to study. I have learned that it is true that you can only do as much as you can at any given time. There is no use fretting about how much it is much more sensible to just pray and ask to always 'perform' – think, feel, act – to your optimum, while being fully supported in your undertakings by Ultimate Good. You then just do whatever you have the time and energy for.

Coming back to the hologram theory, that everything is in everything, this too plagued me for some time. Mishaps were easier to excuse now, as their energetic effect would spread out across the Universe; on the downside this theory can create fears that one has to heal the Universe to heal oneself completely. I feel that that would be too strenuous an undertaking, so I doubt that it is so! We might be connected to everything, being part of All-That-Is, but I strongly feel that there are mechanisms that enable us to disengage/keep disengaged from other beings' suffering. The further away and the more unrelated, the more mechanisms. There is no use if we get depressed because light years away a comet crashes into a moon…

Some people would try to convince me that you cannot heal yourself. The common analogy given is that when falling into a swamp, you cannot pull yourself out by the hair. In other words you will always require another person to give you healing. Some apply even more stringent rules, that for effective healings you require a healer of the opposite sex. Not sure where these claims are coming from. I remember hearing them in connection with psychoanalysis as well – that one will not be able to judge and/or view oneself objectively, that you need the outside profes-sional psychoanalyst to untangle, understand and heal your psyche. I had a hard enough time trusting anyone. Nor did I have the money to pay for all the hours of healing I gave to myself every week. I tried some healers, but felt no better. The whole thing did not make much sense to me. True, to have the advice and help of someone more experienced is usually helpful – but I reject that it is impossible to analyze or heal yourself by yourself. In the end I know myself best! And I can look at many more facts and memories inside my brain than I would ever be able to verbalize to someone else in the same amount of time. Besides with a psychotherapist or analyst one might not be free of mutual projections, i.e. if a psychotherapist had certain expectations of me they might twist my thought processes to deliver their self-fulfilling prophecies.

As to why some healers believe that they cannot heal themselves is beyond me now, but I cannot deny that there were some dark hours where I feared it might be so. I recalled, however, that when performing healing work we are never really 'alone' anyway; there are always Ultimate Good energies and beings that will guide or assist. I also feel that in spirit gender is irrelevant, but even if a butch, macho healer required softer feminine energies to heal himself, Ultimate Good will just send more feminine energies or the like. Still, should you feel as if there is some blockage preventing you from giving healing to yourself effectively, just pray for its removal and send healing into it.

I had other theories as to the origin of my dis-ease. I really did not know how 'auras' operate. What happens to the aura in tight confined spaces, like the London Underground? If my aura extended, say one meter beyond my physical bodies (and in healing courses, when other healers tried to feel my aura, it was supposedly five meters wide), would it then not 'fuse' with other people's auras when I got close to them? So even if I cleaned/healed my aura when I meditated, could I be getting everybody else's confused energies when travelling on the Tube? Or almost worse, if my un-wellness was intrinsic might people around me get some of mine too?

I disengaged this paranoia by changing my understanding of my aura. I thought to understand that my auric bodies were perhaps not 'solid' but just a shine – e.g. the emotional, yellow solar plexus chakra energy shines 50 centimeters beyond my physical body, and the spiritual, purple crown chakra energy one meter beyond my physical body. The actual shining light bulb would be where the main chakras meet inside my physical body and somewhat beyond. Now if everybody just shines, if the veneers intermingle, there is no risk of infecting each other. My understanding of my aura has since further evolved. After some time I once again believed that my aura bodies are solid, but that they would be quite malleable and that they can squeeze tight or expand to full size, depending on how much room is available and thus could avoid 'cross-contamination'.

Currently I work on the assumption that my aura does not extend beyond my physical body, again. I believe so, as supposedly everything has an aura, including animals, objects etc. It is easier to understand when imagining ourselves swimming. If water has an aura too extending beyond its physical extend, it would potentially penetrate our aura and vice versa. What about the air surrounding us? We are always surrounded by other matter (with their auras), so unless our auras would fuse (making it very hard to build up effective energetic protections), our auras would always be 'squeezed' to the size of our physical bodies anyway.

Then there were the reincarnation theories. I could have been a villain in my past life and still be connected to all the beings I hurt, and/or was I a holy man and people still prayed to me and sent me their suffering? The first option could have been possible, but I had thought about it years ago and had prayed for complete forgiveness, deprogramming and disconnection, so it was unlikely I would still get any ill effects from it. The second option was pretty improbable too. I would hope that, even if true, all such prayers would have been 'forwarded' to Ultimate

Good helpers to deal with in my absence – I doubt that any being can hear and answer millions of prayers anyway. For example if I pray to Archangel Michael – I see it more as 'Team Archangel Michael'. There are probably millions of Archangel Michaels, all different individuals, but wearing a similar uniform. Had the holy man theory had any merit, I should have felt much better after asking that prayers sent to my ex-life persona be forwarded to Ultimate Good helpers. I did not feel better though. I would not have minded a reprieve, but then again no improvement was comforting. Else one might have argued that Ultimate Good had made a mistake by allowing prayers (directed to an Ultimate Good Saint) to end up with a reincarnated being that does not have the capacity to answer them.

Similarly other healers have suggested that I take on my clients' suffering out of commiseration. This might sound noble at first; many a Hollywood movie glorifies self-sacrifice, but I find that this should only happen if the help can be provided as effortlessly as possible and does not 'damage' the helper. It 'feels' understandable that a mother, for example, would want to take an illness from her child – take on its suffering, but if a nurse or doctor did the same for all their patients it would quickly become unbearable. I have been even more callous in this regard since understanding that suffering is pre-chosen. I love to help, but if I get hurt because I help then I suffer, even though I do not want to suffer anymore. One obviously has to also look at long-term implications. A mother not helping her child, in every possible way known to her, might find life not worth living if anything really bad happened to her child. As for me, I may have a greater capacity for bearing suffering because I can stay more detached from it and have Ultimate Good support. Experiencing some of my clients' suffering is just part of my job. Still, I reject that I consciously invite my clients' suffering in by commiserating with them. I do ask for as many protections as necessary, available and sensible between me and my clients – and all associated energies.

I do not go looking for suffering unnecessarily, because of some deep-seated guilt or the like. I also 'pass on' to Ultimate Good any negative client energies which might end up inside me. It did take some years to understand, and be confident in that understanding, that I am not a masochist (seeking suffering) when I do end up with other people's LLEs, but rather a soldier in a battle, ending up in a cross fire.

Looking back, even though I could have done without most of the suffering I endured, it has made me more confident in my beliefs and better master my fears. Even during quite terrifying encounters, when it e.g. felt like there was a true devil in the room with me, my first thought is to ensure that I am in the Ultimate Good zone and that I affirm as much Ultimate Good help as available and sensible. Staying in the 'zone' at such times helps me to stay (more) calm and focused; I can just get on with breathing and being a channel for Ultimate Good light. That still does not make it a pleasurable experience, but it helps me not to panic.

I am reminded of a guy I saw on TV who trained himself to not react to cold water. Where others would freeze to death within minutes, he can swim for half an hour. His theory was that the 'fear' reaction to cold water kills so quickly, not the cold water itself. He also thinks anyone can learn his skill. Just thinking about it now, that seems a far tougher task than learning to fight Life Limiting Energies. And after all, combating such negativities might just be of more use in life than mastering the threat of falling into ice-cold water...

Afterword

The Ultimate Weapon

I finish by giving you a wonderful tool. The following prayer sums up everything we should ask for, to make our lives as loving, happy, effortless and free from suffering as possible. It can be said aloud or introspectively to be heard by True Ultimate Good forces. This prayer just has to be said once. It serves as a 'standing order' – the ultimate, all-encompassing request/plea. You are more than welcome to give thanks, whenever you remember, for Ultimate Good's continuous help and support. In times of crisis though, I don't want to just stand by so I might repeat this or other prayers again. Feel free to adjust prayers to the needs at hand. For example if I was looking for a job, I'd thank Ultimate Good for their perfect help in finding the perfect job. When I feel I should write a book, I ask for specific help with that. Nothing is too big or small to ask help for – especially if you want to be free of the suffering it causes.

Dear Ultimate Good, my wonderful Healers, Helpers, Guides, Cleansers and Protectors, I would like to ask and thank you for all of the following:

For your assistance (/continued assistance) in perfectly helping me, my bodies and my life to heal, cleanse, be protected and recharged. Perfect help, wherever, whenever and whatever, as minute, or far-reaching and complex as necessary, possible, available and sensible – albeit in the past, present and/or future.

Thank you that your help is as strong, speedy and safe as applicable, necessary, possible, available and sensible at any given time. Thank you that all healings are as pain free and effortless as possible, available and sensible – if ever possible that there are no negative, uncomfortable side effects or healing crises before, during or after any healing. I give you carte blanche with regard to how much, how, where, when and how frequently you help – and please ignore any restrictions I might still hold in my mind and subconscious which restrict the amount or type of help I wish for, expect or believe possible. Thank you that you help me live and work with and in the Light and that should I go astray, you always lead me back to it. Thank you for helping me to completely forgive myself for any suffering chosen – past, present or future. Thank you for being understanding, for bearing with me at all times – ignoring any doubts and fears I might have, receive or give into. My sincerest apologies should I ever misjudge you and blame you for misfortune I might encounter, which are none of your fault.

Thank you for helping me become ever more unconditionally loving, my actual divine self. Thank you for your help that my life becomes ever more effortless, joyful, and successful. Thank you for your strong and perfect protections – that you protect me and those dear to me against negativity from the inside and outside and the outside against us and negativities associated with us – as applicable, necessary, possible, available and sensible. Please protect yourselves as necessary and don't overexert yourselves on my behalf.

Thank you for always removing all negativities coming out of me, through me or which are set free through my healing work anywhere else, as safely as necessary, possible, available and sensible. Please take them away for rehabilitation, safekeeping or for whatever else you see fit. Thank you for continuously helping to diminish the overall, long-term suffering bottom line for myself, my bodies and my life, and that due to all healings associated with my life, no other being suffers an increase in its overall, long-term suffering bottom line. Thank you, Thank you, Thank you. Amen.

I thank you for reading this book and hope it has brought more clarity to you and your life and that in turn it will be more loving, happy, colorful and effortless. I have had great fun writing this book, and am a bit sad it is finished now, but I look forward to new adventures. Perhaps I will move back to the continent, maybe even finish my medical studies. Live long and prosper!

Acknowledgements

My dearest thanks to all the physical as well as spiritual beings which have helped me with this book. Who have inspired me and given me strength and patience.

Special thanks to my family. I am grateful for late night telephone calls and an always sympathetic ear.

Last but not least thank you, Kate Osborne, my editor at Solarus Ltd. Thank you for sharing my vision for this work and all your dedicated work, help, patience and advice. It has helped greatly to round this book and make it a better read.

And whoever invented spell-check, thank you.

About the Author

Alexander King was born and raised in Germany, starting his spiritual quest from scratch as there hadn't been any 'healing' or psychic leanings in his family. He came across the topic of 'Spiritual Healing' while studying medicine. It ignited the 'spiritual' spark within that set him along his journey to eventually become a healer. Initially, looking for a spiritual teacher, Alexander slid head first into a cult. It was a baptism of fire, where his budding spiritual sensitivities and his analytical, scientifically-trained brain engaged in battle with the cult's subtle brainwashing techniques and manipulative teachings. To his credit Alexander saw through the charade 'exposing' the mystical guru for the rather less grandiose cult leader he really was, and freed himself of their stranglehold.

But his trials were not over. Soon after he fell ill with Chronic Fatigue Syndrome for years. However, Alexander's tenacity and stubborn mindset enabled him to fight through this and all his trials without giving up on his beliefs. Preferring to triumph through adversity, he used these challenges to become stronger and to help him understand the dynamics of 'energy' and the causes of suffering on this planet. He stresses though that he received a great deal of spiritual help to persevere.

Alexander now works as a healer and masseur, endeavoring to help people discover the powerful assistance and great love that can be found in Spirit, without creating false, often transient, unrealistic hopes. His cult experience has taught him that it is best to analyze and test spiritual teachings for yourself. In this his first book, *Tours and Cures of a LightSoldier: Surviving the Path to Enlightenment*, he not only shares his fascinating life story, but applies analytical and constructive criticism to an esoteric market (that still lacks strong, honest self-regulatory mechanisms), in order to make enlightenment as transparent and transformative as it was meant to be.

Sources & Glossary

The following sources are listed in order of appearance:

The Power of Your Subconscious Mind Joseph Murphy

Unfinished Symphonies: Voices from the Beyond Rosemary Brown

Bringers of the Dawn Barbara Marciniak

Urban Shaman Serge Kahili King

Hands of Light Barbara Brennan

The Sermon on the Mount Emmet Fox

Take Back Your Life: Recovering from Cults and Abusive Relationships Janja Lalich & Madeleine Tobias

Recovery from Cults: Help for Victims of Psychological and Spiritual Abuse Michael D. Langone

Combatting Cult Mind Control Steven Hassan

The Field Lynne McTaggart

The Secret Life of Plants Peter Tompkins & Christopher Bird

On Life After Death Dr. Elisabeth Kübler-Ross

Dan-Tien: Your Secret Energy Center Christopher Markert

The following is a glossary of terms deemed most relevant:

Aura Our energetic bodies make up our aura. Most Lightworkers seem to believe/feel/see that there are seven main aura bodies, each fed by a front and back chakra, where energies flow in and out. Different aura bodies are responsible for different qualities of our being, be they material, emotional, mental or spiritual. All aura bodies together make up our body or being. Usually it is taught that each aura body has a different color and that most aura bodies extend beyond our physical bodies. It remains to be discussed if what can be psychically perceived as going beyond the physical body are indeed aura bodies or more of an energetic shine…

Aura Body One of seven layers that make up our aura.

Backlash The effect that a Lightworker might experience after having given healing or having sent healing into something. It is most likely due to LLEs not happy and trying to resist the healing processes or 'wanting out' and attempting to use the Lightworker's being for this. It can affect all levels – physical, emotional, mental or spiritual and can come in different strengths.

Body Dysmorphic Disorder (BDD) This is a mental condition where the sufferer is preoccupied with his/her body image and can develop severe, potentially debilitating concerns about minor or imagined perceived flaws of their physical body. BDD often co-occurs with depression, anxiety, social withdrawal, and social isolation.

Chakra Derived from the Sanskrit word wheel but better translated as light vortex. Chakras are energy centers that feed our aura bodies and where pure energy can enter and exit an aura body. They are often depicted as funnels of energy.

Chi/Ki Energy force in Chinese culture and often used as a synonym for Life Force, Prana or healing energy in spiritual/esoteric circles. It can be likened to air, food and drink required to sustain our physical bodies, as sustenance for our light bodies or the soul.

Chronic Fatigue Syndrome (CFS) A condition where persistent fatigue and exhaustion disaffects everyday living and does not go away after rest and sleep, often accompanied by recurring infections, throat aches, muscle and joint aches, IBS, depression and sleeping problems.

Collective Subconscious The collected thoughts, emotions and beliefs making up a nation's culture and trends (or that of a religious group, family, profession etc.). Being part of a collective subconscious we help sustain or shape it without individual thoughts, emotions or beliefs but are in turn influenced by it. The collective subconscious energies in turn feed back and influence our thoughts, emotions, beliefs and ultimately actions.

Collective Subconscious Life Limiting Energies (LLEs) LLEs fed by more than one individual and making up and to varying degrees controlling and protecting collective subconscious structures.

Collective Unconscious See 'Collective Subconscious'

Cult Initially a cult was a group of people worshipping a deity, but nowadays it often has derogatory connotations, where a cult or sect is usually an organization/group of people (religious, political, psychoanalytical, family or other) where one or a few individuals impose their beliefs onto the rest of the group. These gurus, leaders etc. often use manipulative methods and/or coercion. With time the disciples become brainwashed, dependent and have a harder and harder time to free themselves from the control of the leader(s).

Energy Body See 'Aura Body'

Healing Mode The state of a Lightworker being attuned to higher energies, linked in and in the flow. Healing energies can flow through the healer's being for the benefit of the recipient.

Higher Self Understood as our true self, the individualized divine that we are. It is pure and has all the divine abilities, such as divine all-love, wisdom, all-understanding, all-knowing and is connected to 'All-That-Is'. As Lightworkers we strive to be in touch with our higher selves whenever possible and overcome potentially less pure parts of our being such as our lower (emotional or animalistic) self and ego.

Highly Active Antiretroviral Therapy (HAART) Medication prescribed to suppress HIV replication.

Homeopathy Healing modality after Hahnemann, who discovered that ingesting certain substances can create symptoms similar to certain diseases, e.g. quinine poisoning creates symptoms such as in Malaria. But when administering quinine to a Malaria sufferer it can cure – *similia similibus curantur* (similar heals similar). Hahnemann found that this effect seemed to persist, and even improve, if diluting substances repeatedly. Skeptics argue that many homeopathic remedies theoretically do not contain a single atom of the original substance anymore and that healings therefore cannot be anything but placebo.

Huna Hawaiian shamanic tradition. Huna sees all beings (animate and inanimate) as alive and conscious – and as such one can communicate with all beings (on a spiritual level).

Karma Stems from the Indian religions and is the law of cause and effect. According to Karma the energies we put out through thoughts, emotions, beliefs and deeds eventually come back to us, i.e. if we do good, good will come to us – if we do bad, similarly bad things will happen to us. Supposedly Karma can be carried across lives, so bad things happening to us now (even if we are a good person in this life) could have been caused by ourselves in previous lives. Karma does not necessarily try to punish us, but just tries to teach us what our actions onto others feel like. Bad Karma might be dissolved through acts of forgiveness. Once we realize that everything we experience on this planet is pre-chosen Karma teachings lose (some of) their value, even more so if we realize that between lives we are more enlightened and would forgive accumulated Karma.

Life Enhancing Energies (LEEs) Thoughts, emotions and beliefs which enrich our lives and make them happier and more loving – such as happiness, empathy, love, joy, respect, tolerance etc; energies which affirm our divine self and being and which sustain or increase our well-being.

Life Limiting Energies (LLEs) Thoughts, emotions and beliefs which take away from our life (force) – such as stresses, fears, angers, guilt, sadness, resentment, hate, jealousy, envy etc. Such energies usually limit or diminish our life force and hence well-being.

Lightbody See 'Aura Body'

Lightsoldier A Lightworker who concedes that working for the Light/Divine can be a battle at times, and that cuts and grazes might be unavoidable. See 'Lightworker'

Lightwork Work performed by Lightworkers for the good, such as meditation, prayer, visualization, good deeds etc. Lightwork seeks to create healing for yourself or others.

Lightworker A person working and acting for the Good/Light/Divine and who consciously (or subconsciously) tries to use Lightwork to achieve healing for themselves, their lives or those of others.

LLE Booby Traps Energetic traps created by LLEs. Created to go off when a Lightworker tries to heal something or a particular LLE. Booby traps are designed to dissuade Lightworkers from healing away particular LLEs completely or from healing off similar LLEs. Asking for perfect, divine healing help will usually diffuse booby traps before they are triggered. Also see 'Backlash'

Meditation Mode See 'Healing Mode', but especially pertaining to being in meditation.

Myalgic Encephalopathy (ME) See 'Chronic Fatigue Syndrome'

Ouija Board A board game which usually depicts letters and a 'Yes' and 'No' field. Players place their fingers on a pointer or an overturned glass and ask questions to 'Spirit(s)'. If successful Spirit(s) will help to involuntarily move the players' fingers and steer the pointer towards letters or YES or NO, forming answers. There has always been a perceived risk of 'inviting' in either benevolent or malicious spirits. In movies such as *The Exorcist* the board serves as the entry gate for demons.

Prana See 'Chi'

Prelash See 'Backlash', but affecting the healer/Lightworker before the actual performed healing/spiritual work. In my experience the general intent of the LLEs creating prelash is mostly to try to stop the healer from going through with an actual healing.

Psychic Abilities Also called 'sixth sense' or 'extrasensory perception' are attributes beyond our physical senses and include: Precognition, Remote Viewing, Dowsing, Psychic Diagnosis, Telepathy, Clairaudience, Clairsentience and Clairvoyance.

Psychic Diagnosis Using psychic abilities to diagnose a patient's illness and (physical, emotional, mental or spiritual) sources, roots of their ailment(s).

Regression Therapy The act of looking at supposed past lives. Some see therapeutic value in this, as it is said to help us understand that we are indeed eternal souls. But it could also help to understand current relationships or behaviors or feelings in this life, which might stem from/have been created in previous lives.

Shaman Wisdom Keeper or Holy Person in all aboriginal belief systems, most famously Native Americans, Polynesians and Siberians. Usually understood as a medicine man or woman in a community who tries to help the community, gives healings, officiates at ceremonies (births and deaths) and communes with Nature through spiritual dimensions.

Shamanism What shamans practice.

Spiritual Healer A Spiritual Healer attunes to higher Divine powers, offering his/her body and mind as a conduit to channel healing energies for the recipient's benefit. The healing energies have their own intelligence and know best where to go and what to do, so a Spiritual Healer does their best to step aside and let the healing energies work undisturbed and unimpeded.

Spiritual Healing The healing work undertaken by a spiritual healer given to a recipient.

Subconsciousness Those thoughts, emotions and beliefs of which we are not conscious, but which may influence our conscious thoughts, emotions, beliefs or deeds. Or there are also subconscious processes in the human body, such as our heartbeat or the work of the digestive system, usually outside our conscious control and which are at times attributed to our state of subconsciousness..

Traditional Chinese Medicine (TCM) A broad range of medicine practices sharing common scientific concepts which were invented and developed in ancient China and are based on a medical tradition of more than 9,000 years, including various forms of herbal medicine, acupuncture, massage, exercise, and dietary therapy for treating various diseases, injuries and ailments.

Ultimate Good What I call 'The Divine', and what others may refer to as 'God', 'Creation', 'The Great Mystery'.

Unconsciousness See 'Subconsciousness'

Zero Point Field The quantum state of lowest possible energy or vacuum state. There are no physical particles in a vacuum, but it is not empty and still contains energy, such as electromagnetic waves. This energy is ubiquitous and all permeating. Esoteric theories speculate that such electromagnetic waves could store and transmit sheer endless amounts of information.

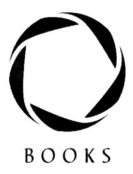

BOOKS

O is a symbol of the world, of oneness and unity; this eye represents knowledge and insight. We publish titles on general spirituality and living a spiritual life. We aim to inform and help you on your own journey in this life.

Visit our website: http://www.o-books.com

Find us on Facebook:
https://www.facebook.com/OBooks

Follow us on Twitter: @obooks